MCAT

Biology
Review Notes

Published by Kaplan Publishing, a division of Kaplan, Inc.
1 Liberty Plaza, 24th Floor
New York, NY 10006

In Partnership with Kaplan's National MCAT Team, 1440 Broadway, 8th Floor New York, NY 10018

Printed in the United States of America

10 9 8 7 6 5 4 3 2 1

ISBN: 978-1-60714-438-0

Kaplan Publishing books are available at special quantity discounts to use for sales promotions, employee premiums, or educational purposes. Please email our Special Sales Department to order or for more information at kaplanpublishing@kaplan.com, or write to Kaplan Publishing, 1 Liberty Plaza, 24th Floor, New York, NY 10006.

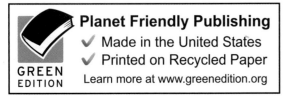

Planet Friendly Publishing
✔ Made in the United States
✔ Printed on Recycled Paper
GREEN EDITION
Learn more at www.greenedition.org

- Manufacturing books in the United States ensures compliance with strict environmental laws and eliminates the need for international freight shipping, a major contributor to global air pollution. Printing on recycled paper helps minimize our consumption of trees, water and fossil fuels.
- Trees Saved: 120 • Air Emissions Eliminated: 12,032 pounds
- Water Saved: 43,648 gallons • Solid Waste Eliminated: 6,466 pounds

Contributors

The Kaplan MCAT Review Notes Series was created by a dedicated team of 45 professionals who worked a combined total of over 11,000 hours.

This text would not exist without the tireless work of Cait Clancy, Henry Conant, Ed Crawford, PhD, Suneetha Desiraju, Marilyn Engle, Christopher Falzone, PhD, Sheryl Gordon, Walter Hartwig, PhD, Jeannie Ho, Jessica Kim, Jeff Koetje, MD, John Linick, Keith Lubeley, Amjed Mustafa, Joanna Myllo, Glen Pearlstein, MD, Dominique Polfliet, Ira Rothstein, PhD, Matthew Wilkinson, and Sze Yan.

Special thanks to: Jesse Barrett, Susan E. Barry, Geri Burgert, Deana Casamento, Robin Garmise, Rita Garthaffner, Chip Hurlburt, Colette Mazunik, Danielle Mazza, Stephanie McCann, Diane McGarvey, Maureen McMahon, Jason Miller, Jason Moss, Maria Nicholas, Walt Niedner, Jeff Olson, Rochelle Rothstein, MD, Lisa Pallatroni, John Polstein, Ron Sharpe, Brian Shorter, Glen Stohr, Martha Torres, Bob Verini, and the countless others who made this project possible.

Using This Book

This book is designed to help you review the science topics covered on the MCAT. It represents one of the content review resources available to you in the Kaplan program.

Additional review is available through the live and on-demand lessons, the library of available practice tests and explanations-on-demand that accompany them, and your flashcards and QuickSheets.

Please understand that content review, no matter how thorough, is not sufficient preparation for the MCAT! The MCAT Biological Sciences and Physical Sciences sections test your reading, reasoning, and problem-solving skills, as well as your science knowledge. Don't assume that simply memorizing the contents of this book will earn you high science scores—it won't. If you want your best shot at great science scores, you must also improve your reading and test-taking skills through the lessons, testing sessions, and the Kaplan and AAMC practice tests in the Training Library. So resist the temptation to reread this book at the expense of taking practice tests! Rather, strike a balance between content review and critical reasoning practice.

At the end of each chapter, you'll find MCAT-style review questions and open-ended questions for study group discussion. These are designed to help you assess your understanding of the chapter you just read.

The last chapter of this book is a special section devoted to what we call the High-Yield Problem Solving Guide. Although not presented exactly in the style of the MCAT, these questions tackle the most frequently tested topics found on the test. For each type of problem, the guide will provide you with a stepwise technique for solving the question and key directional points on how to solve specifically for the MCAT.

Consult the Syllabus in your MCAT Lesson Book for specific reading/practice assignments. Reading the appropriate chapters will greatly enhance your understanding of the lesson material. A glossary and index are included in the back of each review book for easy reference.

This is your book, so write in the margin, highlight the key points—do whatever is necessary to help you get that higher score. It should be your trusty companion as Test Day approaches.

Sincerely,
The Kaplan MCAT Team

About Scientific American

As the world's premier science and technology magazine, and the oldest continuously published magazine in the United States, Scientific American is committed to bringing the most important developments in modern science, medicine, and technology to 3.5 million readers worldwide in an understandable, credible and provocative format.

Founded in 1845 and on the "cutting edge" ever since, Scientific American boasts over 140 Nobel laureate authors including Albert Einstein, Francis Crick, Stanley Prusiner and Richard Axel. Scientific American is a forum where scientific theories and discoveries are explained to a broader audience.

Scientific American published its first foreign edition in 1890, and in 1979, was the first Western magazine published in the People's Republic of China. Today, Scientific American is published in 17 foreign language editions with a total circulation of more than 1 million worldwide. Scientific American is also a leading online destination (www.ScientificAmerican.com), providing the latest science news and exclusive features to more than 2 million unique visitors monthly.

The knowledge that fills our pages has the power to inspire, spark new ideas, paradigms and visions for the future. As science races forward, Scientific American continues to cover the promising strides, inevitable setbacks and challenges, and new medical discoveries as they unfold.

Guide To Margin Notes:

Our Review Notes are designed with ample white space for you to take notes while you work your way through the Kaplan MCAT program. Periodically, you'll come across some of our own comments in the margins. We call these sidebars "margin notes" (pretty clever, right?).

The following is a legend of the five main types of margin notes you'll find in the science Review Notes:

Real World: These notes are designed to illustrate how a concept discussed in the text relates to the practice of medicine and the world at large. Since you are a premed (if not, you're reading the wrong book), we felt that these correlations would both be of interest to you and help solidify your understanding of some key concepts.

Key Concept: These are synopses of the concepts discussed on a page. Typically, we reserved this type of margin note for pages where lots of important and complex information was presented.

Bridge: We use "Bridges" to alert you to the conceptual links that occur between chapters or disciplines.

MCAT Expertise: These are designed to illuminate some of the conceptual patterns that the testmaker tends to focus on when writing MCAT questions.

Mnemonics: Sometimes they rhyme, and sometimes they don't. But we hope that they will all help you recall information quickly on Test Day.

Contents

7 more chapters of Bio

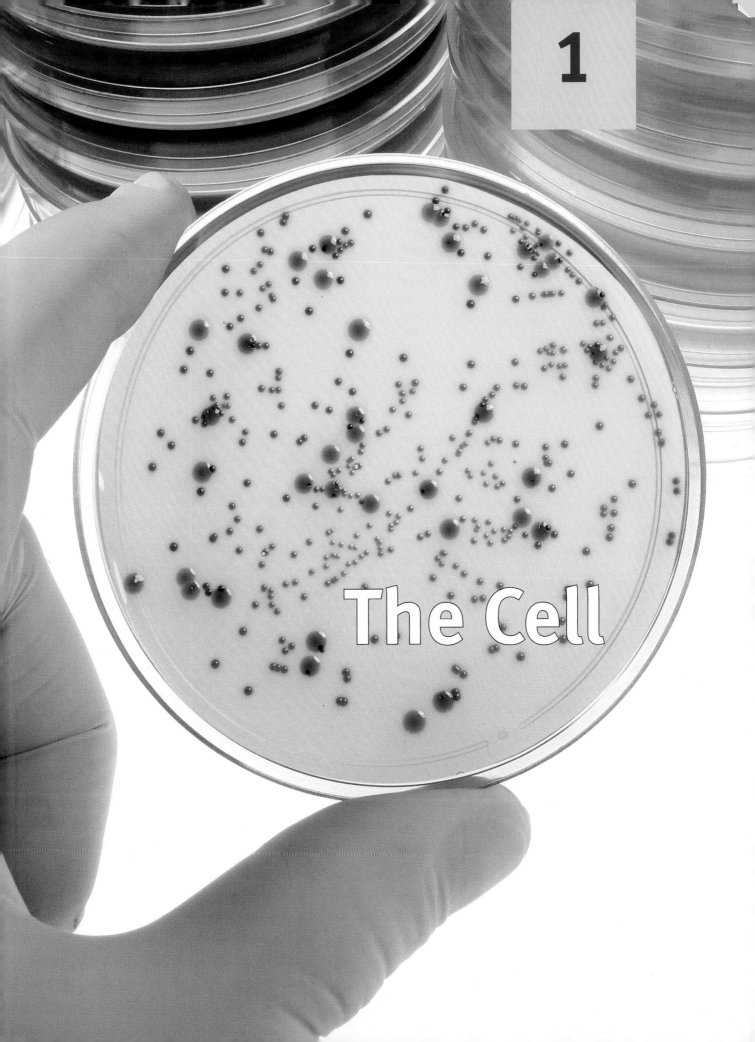

The Cell

I can remember when I was in your shoes. The MCAT loomed large on my proverbial horizon. It was the first test that I can truly say that I was nervous to take before I even cracked a book (and might even have been a little more nervous after I saw how much I needed to learn). Some of you may be a little nervous right now. That's okay! It's perfectly natural to feel some anxiety. But we're here to help you reduce your anxiety and channel your energy into action that will lead to Test Day success. First, take a deep breath (breathing may be the most natural thing we do, yet in a moment of panic, breathing is usually the first thing that goes wrong) and relax. The next few paragraphs won't be tested. Rather, read them with an open and inquisitive mind. They will provide you with a basis to do well not only on the MCAT but also as a physician.

To start, I would like to provide you with a fundamental insight that led me to Test Day and medical school success.

Never be afraid to ask a question.

Sure. It sounds basic enough on the surface of it, but take a second to read it again and really get your synaptic connections firing (I'll wait). Those simple words carry a great deal of meaning. On a surface-level analysis, the MCAT is an exam based on questions: the testmaker isn't afraid to ask you questions, and you shouldn't be afraid to ask questions, either!

To whom exactly should you be directing your questions? Everyone, including yourself. In a very literal sense, a question that you ask now might turn into a correct answer (and another point) on Test Day. The only person you hurt by not asking your questions is yourself.

And beyond the purpose of preparing for the MCAT, you should dig deeper in your thought process and learn to ask difficult questions for which answers are not always clear. I know that you aren't all philosophy majors and some of you may even dread liberal arts, but medicine as a field isn't only about science. It's not enough to know that iron is a critical prosthetic group in hemoglobin and that a deficiency could lead to anemia. Granted, there will be some nights during which you will be responsible for recalling large amounts of information on only a few hours of sleep, but that's just a means to an end, not "the end in and of itself," to crib Kant.

The practice of medicine requires a physician and patient working together to provide ideal treatment for a specific situation. It's not enough for you (the doctor) to just state, "Take two aspirin and call me in the morning," as the old saying goes. How do you arrive at the answers your patients (and you) seek? By asking questions. Believe it or not, many times patients are afraid to question their doctors. It's almost hard to imagine as professionals trained in the art of asking questions! Your patients will come to see you, pay you for your advice, but may be afraid to ask questions such as "why?" (which can be both profoundly simple and profoundly complex). Why this drug? Why this treatment? Why is this happening to me? The way you ask questions will be a model to your patients as you engage them as partners in the greater cause of seeking health and wellness.

To ask—and answer—these questions correctly, ethically, and fully in your future medical practice, you will need to make complete use of your *critical thinking* skills—which snaps you back to the MCAT and the next few months of your life.

The MCAT is designed to test your critical thinking. The testmaker knows that in order for you to be successful physicians tomorrow, you need to learn how to ask questions today. In order to answer the questions your patients ask you, you must ask questions of them. Similarly, to answer the questions the MCAT asks you, you must ask questions of it. But learning to ask the right questions is only the first step in the critical thinking process. You also need to learn to assess the value and applicability of what you already know to what you will learn as you ask the questions and gather information. In your medical practice, you will seek additional information from your patients, colleagues, lab tests, imaging studies, and journal articles. For example, you will be expected to be able to come up with a list of possible reasons for why your patient might have low iron (what's called the "differential diagnosis"), how to test for it, and how best to treat it. On the MCAT, you will gather information from the passages and question stems upon which the test is based and relate this information to what you already know and understand.

Kaplan's Review Notes and Test Day strategies are integral to the development of your critical thinking skills. The information contained in these pages is high-yield and essential for Test Day success. I assure you that we have done our homework in researching the topics that are included on the actual test. The topics included in this book are likely to appear on your MCAT with varying degrees of emphasis. Content areas not tested have been intentionally excluded from our discussions here, so that we do not waste your time and energy. Pay attention not just to our discussion of content, but also to our approach to solving MCAT problems. Learn and practice our methods until they become your methods. Upon the foundation of strong content understanding and time-proven methods, you will build your critical thinking skills. These are the skills that will allow you to reach to the greatest heights of Test Day success.

So I encourage you to question yourself about your own knowledge and goals as we take this journey through biology together. Take caution as you study these notes. Beware of the extreme answer on practice questions. And don't question *everything*; I promise that biology is not a conspiracy theory. It is, after all, based on chemistry, which is based on physics. (And let me assure you now, in spite of how some of you may feel—and quite strongly too—physics itself, is not a conspiracy theory!)

Our first chapter will introduce us to the cell. To get us going, let's look at a fun fact. There are approximately 10 trillion cells in our body (that's 10,000,000,000,000, to be exact) and approximately 100 trillion bacteria living in our gastrointestinal tract. Bacteria outnumber us in our own bodies by a cell ratio of 10:1. This, to say the least, gives new meaning to John Donne's famous saying that "No man is an island unto himself." As we figuratively digest that fact, we ought to begin to think about what we humans have in common with the lowly bacteria living in our gut. Although we are markedly different, we share some fundamental characteristics. The fundamental unit of the human body and of each of those bacteria is the cell. Our goal in this chapter will be to understand the basic structure and organization of the cell so that as we expand our focus to the larger organ systems, we will have a solid foundation for MCAT success.

Cell Theory

Consider that biology has always lagged behind physics and chemistry in terms of fundamental facts. Moreover, the majority of techniques that we now use to study cells required advancements in other fields, especially chemistry and physics. Biology doesn't stand on its own legs. Physics allows us to understand the fundamental laws of interaction in the universe; chemistry builds upon those laws by explaining how reactivity occurs; biology expands the discussion at a meta-level to discuss how organisms interact. It wasn't until the development of microscopes in the 17th century that we were even able to look at our own components "beneath the surface," if you will, of visibility with the naked eye. Over time, and through repeated examination at the microscopic level, we came to recognize fundamental similarities among all living things. As with all good scientific models, we start with a theory. This is one of the MCAT's favorite topics, and we should take careful note of the basic tenets of the Cell Theory. The **Cell Theory** holds true for all organisms, whether they be unicellular or multicellular:

- All living things are composed of cells.
- The cell is the basic functional unit of life.
- Cells arise only from preexisting cells.
- Cells carry genetic information in the form of **DNA**. This genetic material is passed on from parent to daughter cell.

The Cell Theory may seem pretty basic, but complex systems are built from these elementary rules. Consider that our own bodies (very sophisticated machines in their own right) are ultimately a collection of cells all living by these four rules! Pretty incredible and definitely test-worthy.

Methods and Tools ★★☆☆☆

One of the primary obstacles that prevented early scientists from being able to study cells was their size. Ironically, we had lenses allowing us to peer into the depths of space and predict where planets were stationed; yet it wasn't until we turned these lenses inward that we began to understand our own "inner space." Today, our primary techniques for examining the organism at the organ, tissue, cellular, or subcellular levels are **microscopy, autoradiography, and centrifugation**.

MICROSCOPY

Of all the items in the biologist's toolbox, the microscope is not only the one most commonly used, but also the one most commonly tested on the MCAT. Two basic concepts that we should recall from the physics topic of light and optics are **magnification** and **resolution**. We're used to seeing these topics in the Physical Sciences section on MCAT, but as we previously noted, biology and physics are quite intertwined in real life! **Magnification** is the increase in the apparent size of an object; basically, "How much bigger does it look?" Imagine a tiny splinter painfully wedged into a friend's pinky finger. Many of us would search for a magnifying glass, because it enlarges the splinter's image. **Resolution** is the ability to differentiate two closely placed objects. Meaning, once we position our magnifying glass and have a tweezer ready to attack, we're going to want to make sure we pull out only the splinter—and not a layer of our friend's skin!

Compound Light Microscope

This is the most commonly used type of microscope. Similar to telescopes and other systems of lenses that we discuss in physics, a compound light microscope uses two lenses or a system of lenses to magnify the object. The total magnifwication power is the product of the two lenses: the eyepiece (often 10×) and the objective (4×, 10×, 20×, or 100×). In other words, the bacteria we might look at under a microscope may appear 100 times (or more) larger than their actual size. Such organisms are truly microscopic. While the MCAT isn't likely to test us on the specifics of compound microscopy, knowing the basic components can translate into easy points on Test Day when such questions do appear.

1. The **diaphragm** controls the amount of light passing through the specimen, which is important for image contrast. Our cameras have diaphragms for the same reason. Imagine taking a photo with the sun in the background. The image doesn't develop clearly; rather, it appears washed out. The diaphragm can

be adjusted to change the amount of light allowed to pass through the lens. Without a diaphragm, it probably wouldn't show up at all.

2. The **coarse adjustment knob** roughly focuses the image. It does this by moving the stage (platform on which the slide sits) up and down.
3. The **fine adjustment knob** finely focuses the image. Its function is the same as the coarse knob's, but it works over a smaller range of focus.

By and large, compound light microscopes are for nonliving specimens. In order to increase contrast, samples are usually sliced into thin sections, prepared by using various chemical reagents, and then coverslipped. Sounds pretty brutal, huh? Not surprisingly, the organisms usually die sometime during that process. An example of a commonly used dye (which you don't need to memorize for the MCAT, but will once you get to medical school) is hematoxylin, which will show nucleic acids (**DNA** and **RNA**) within the cell by binding to their negatively charged sugar-phosphate backbone moieties.

Phase Contrast Microscope

Although knowledge of the phase contrast microscope isn't commonly tested on the MCAT, we should know it for one major reason: it allows for the visualization of living organisms. Samples are not prepared as described above; rather, the microscope relies on differences in refractive indices among the different subcellular structures. (we said that we'd see some physics!) This system provides a tradeoff: we are able to view the live organism conducting its cellular activities, but we aren't able to increase the contrast of certain structures specifically by using a dye or preparation technique.

Electron Microscope

The most powerful microscope available to the biologist is the **electron microscope**, which allows us to image down to the atomic level. Let's take a step back and consider how this process works. What is the limiting factor in the resolution of the light microscope, or any microscope for that matter? It is the medium that is used to transmit the image. For example, in a light microscope, the resolution of the image is limited by the wavelength of light, which is on the order of nanometers. Images cannot be resolved further as light cannot distinctly transmit the information. An electron microscope uses a beam of electrons; thus, its resolution is at the atomic level on the order of picometers. Electron microscopy has paved the way for major advances in the understanding of subcellular structures: for example, the ability to visualize the interface between the inner and outer mitochondrial membrane. The major drawback is the preparation technique: samples must be sliced very thinly and usually impregnated with heavy metals (often OsO_4) to allow for appropriate contrast. This requires the death of the organism.

MCAT Expertise

Don't overfocus on the physics here; concepts such as refraction are much more likely to be tested in the Physical Sciences section.

Bridge

We'll hear more about the mitochondrial membranes in Chapter 3 as we discuss cellular metabolism.

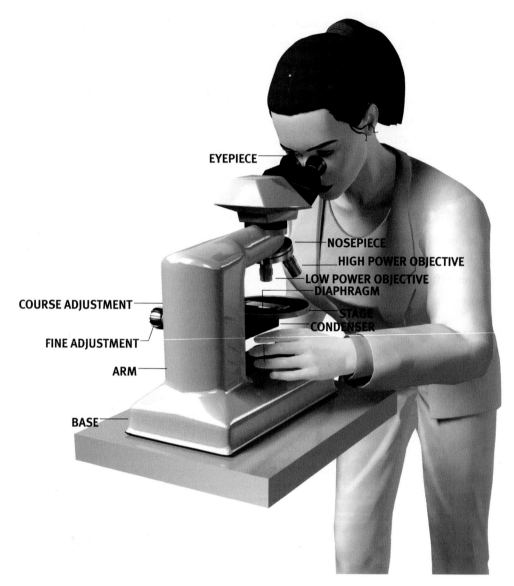

EYEPIECE

NOSEPIECE

HIGH POWER OBJECTIVE

LOW POWER OBJECTIVE

DIAPHRAGM

COURSE ADJUSTMENT

STAGE

CONDENSER

FINE ADJUSTMENT

ARM

BASE

Figure 1.1

AUTORADIOGRAPHY

Another technique that relies on advances in chemistry and physics is autoradiography. Recall that radioactive compounds decay or transform into other compounds or elements through various processes such as alpha or beta decay. We harness this power in various medical technologies including x-rays, radioactive tracing, and nuclear medicine. For example, x-rays are capable of penetrating the body and generating an image. We've all had the routine visit to the dentist, during which images of our teeth are generated and used to identify cavities. We should note that x-rays (and electromagnetic energy in general) can be harmful. This is why it's necessary for us to wear a lead apron during the procedure: The heavy metal absorbs the high-energy rays and limits the exposure of radiation to our vital organs.

On a cellular level, we can use radioactive decay to follow the biochemical processes that occur in the cell. In a basic setup, cells are exposed to an essential compound (glucose, nucleotides, amino acids, etc.) that they need to survive. We manufacture these compounds such that they include radioactive atoms (e.g., tritium, an isotope of hydrogen). The cells are incubated for a given amount of time and then fixed and put onto glass slides for microscopy. Each slide is covered with a piece of photographic film and then kept in the dark to develop for a given amount of time depending on the material used. The appearance of an image on the photographic film shows the distribution of radioactive material within the cell and where the biochemical reactions of interest took place. The developed picture is a way to track processes of interest within the cell.

CENTRIFUGATION

Yet another common biological technique that relies on physical principles is **centrifugation**. Recall that a centrifuge, by spinning at very rapid speeds, is capable of increasing the apparent force on the object in the tubes. The contents of the sample settle toward the bottom of the tube at different rates depending on the shape and density of the particles (measured as the sedimentation coefficient). We discuss the relative strength of the centrifugation in relation to the force of gravity. Thus, a centrifuge that spins at 12,000 g exerts a force on the sample that is 12,000 times greater than the force of gravity. If you think about the last time you were on a roller coaster, you can imagine the same forces in effect. When the roller coaster went through the upside-down loop, why didn't you fall out? Sure, the lap bar helped, but centrifugal force pushed you into your seat. (The centrifugal force is the apparent force equal to and opposite the centripetal force, and is due to the object's inertia.)

Centrifugation is like a mini roller coaster for test tubes. It's a useful technique because it allows cells to be fractionated into their various components based on density. Why would this work? The force will have a greater effect on objects with a greater density (e.g., ribosomes) and pull them to the bottom of the tube while less dense objects (mitochondria and lysosomes) will remain closer to the tube's opening. These can then be carefully removed to study a specific set of subcellular organelles.

Prokaryotes vs. Eukaryotes

The first major biological distinction we can make between living organisms is whether they are **prokaryotes** or **eukaryotes**. We'll discuss viruses later; they are in a class by themselves because they violate multiple tenets of the Cell Theory.

Now, are you ready to learn some Greek? Of course, there is no foreign language section on the MCAT, but a basic understanding of some word roots will give you quick hints on Test Day. The prokaryotic/eukaryotic distinction comes from the lack or presence of a nucleus, respectively. *Karyon* is Greek for *kernel* or *nucleus*. *Pro–* means *before*, and *eu–* means *true*. Thus, prokaryotes existed before nuclei, and eukaryotes have true nuclei.

PROKARYOTES

Understanding prokaryotes won't just help you on the MCAT; they'll be part of your continuing education for the rest of your lives as physicians—because many pathogens are prokaryotic! Prokaryotes are the simplest of all organisms. They include all **bacteria** as well as blue-green algae. Their outer **cell wall** does not enclose any membrane-bound organelles (such as nuclei or endoplasmic reticulum). The genetic material of the organism is contained in a single circular molecule of DNA concentrated in an area of the cell called the **nucleoid** region. We will discuss the reproduction of this genome in Chapter 4. Prokaryotes also have the interesting ability to carry other pieces of genetic information in small, circular pieces of DNA called **plasmids**. These are much smaller than the nuclear genome and often contain only a few genes. However, these genes are quite important. The difference between a bacterial strain that is susceptible to antibiotics and one that isn't may be due to a plasmid in the latter strain that confers resistance to a given antibiotic. These plasmids replicate independently of the nuclear genome, and copies of the plasmids can be transferred from one bacterial cell to another, which helps explain why bacteria are capable of passing resistance to other bacteria. It's a good bet that the bacteria you learn about in medical school will have evolved and changed a great deal by the time you attend your 20-year medical school reunion, thanks to plasmids.

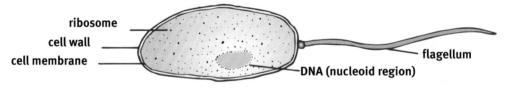

ribosome
cell wall
cell membrane
flagellum
DNA (nucleoid region)

Figure 1.2

Most bacteria exist in one of two shapes. Spherical bacteria, known as cocci, include common pathogens like *Staphylococcus aureus* (see Figure 1.3a). Rod-shaped bacteria, like *Escherichia coli* (see Figure 1.3b), are also known as bacilli.

All bacteria contain a **cell membrane** and **cytoplasm**, and some have **flagella** (see Figure 1.4), which can also be found in eukaryotic cells (like sperm), where they

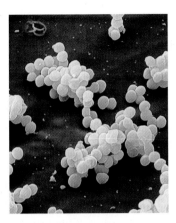

Figure 1.3a

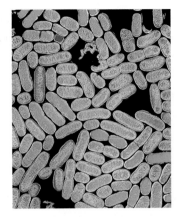

Figure 1.3b

give the cell motility. Since these structures are also found in eukaryotic cells, it is difficult to develop antibiotics that may target them. Instead, drugs tend to attack structures specifically found in bacteria. For instance, if you have ever taken azithromycin for a cold, you took a drug that specifically interfered with bacterial ribosomes, which are smaller than eukaryotic ribosomes. Before we move on, let's stress that not all bacteria are bad. In fact, our existence depends on some of them! We'll learn in a later chapter that bacteria in our large intestine help break down food. Others even produce vitamins for us.

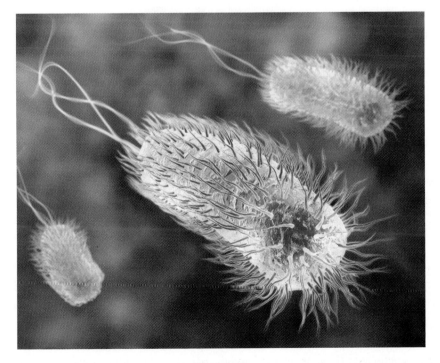

Figure 1.4

EUKARYOTES

Our second, and more testworthy, set of organisms is the eukaryotes. As we discussed above, eukaryotes are made up of cells with true nuclei and membrane-bound organelles. Remember that eukaryotes can be either unicellular or multicellular. We can think of the eukaryotic cell as a city. As we go through each of its structures, we can continue this analogy to help us remember key facts for the MCAT. Each cell has a cell membrane enclosing a semifluid **cytosol** in which the organelles are suspended. The cytosol is like the city air. It allows for the diffusion of molecules throughout the cell. Genetic material is encoded in DNA organized into linear strands known as **chromosomes** and found within the **nucleus**. There are some differences between different types of eukaryotes; for example, plants contain both a cell wall and **chloroplasts**, which are absent from animal cells. Let's discuss the organelles in more detail.

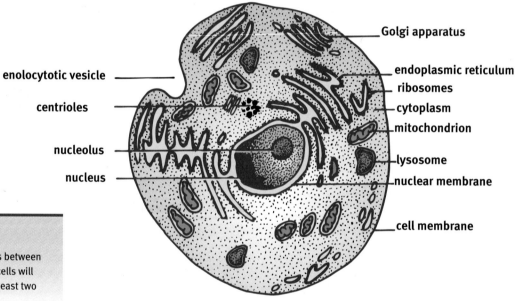

Figure 1.5

Eukaryotic Organelles ★★★★★★

Eukaryotic cells separate their biochemical reactions into distinct membrane-bound organelles, much as cities are divided into different districts and neighborhoods. These organelles are suspended within an aqueous cytosol that contains free proteins, nutrients, and other solutes.

If we continue to think about a eukaryotic cell as a city with distinct sections, we might better remember each of the parts. Every city needs a way to get from point

A to point B, a system of roads and highways. Just as cities have eight-lane highways as well as two-lane roads, so, too, does the cell. The cell has a **cytoskeleton**, which is made up of three types of proteins. From smallest to largest, they are **actin filaments, intermediate filaments**, and **microtubules**. These proteins form structures that allow materials to be moved around inside the cell. The cytoskeleton also provides a framework for anchoring other organelles within the cell.

The major organelles (or city structures) that we need to discuss for the MCAT are the nucleus, ribosomes, endoplasmic reticulum, Golgi apparatus, vesicles, vacuoles, lysosomes, microbodies, mitochondria, chloroplasts, and centrioles.

CELL MEMBRANE

The cell membrane is our city wall. It encloses our cell and selectively chooses who or what to let in and out. Just as a regular wall may be made of bricks, our wall is a **phospholipid bilayer**. The theory that underlies this is known as the **fluid mosaic model**. The phospholipid bilayer is studded with proteins and lipid rafts that can control the movement of solutes in and out of the cell, much as a city gate controls the flow of traffic. These molecules are usually freely mobile within the membrane.

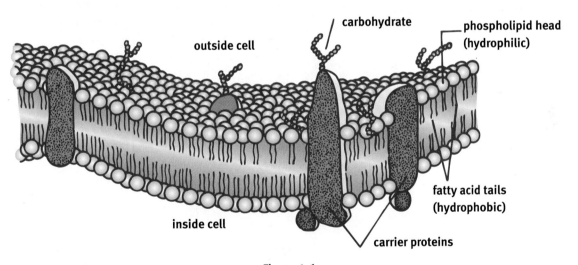

Figure 1.6

These phospholipids have a strongly hydrophobic tail (nonpolar) and a hydrophilic (polar) head. The hydrophilic regions face the interior and exterior of the cell, whereas the hydrophobic tails face each other along the intramembrane space. Cholesterol molecules also are found in the membrane, which help to regulate the fluidity or stiffness of the membrane. Cholesterol sometimes gets a bad reputation, owing to emphasis on its negative health effects, but cholesterol is important; our cells use cholesterol not only to help with membrane fluidity, but also to generate all steroid hormones. Animal cells have the ability to produce cholesterol molecules for inclusion in cell membranes and steroid hormone production. We know, however,

Key Concept

The ability of different molecules to traverse a membrane is critical to cells. The cell must be able to allow nutrients and required compounds in while preventing bacteria, viruses, and harmful compounds from entering. This is a commonly tested MCAT topic.

Key Concept

We will have more to say about receptors as related to the nervous system, digestive system, and endocrine system, just to name a few; they may be tested in many ways including membrane trafficking, isomerism, specificity, and binding kinetics. We can easily see that this is a topic we should keep in mind for MCAT success.

that excessive dietary cholesterol is unhealthy. It has many deleterious health effects such as atherosclerosis. Moderate dietary intake is key.

The proteins we discussed earlier may be visible on one or both sides of the membrane. Moreover, they play a variety of different roles within our cells. **Transport proteins**, which we can liken to border agents that control entry and exit into our city, allow polar molecules and ions to move in and out of the cell, whereas **cell adhesion molecules** (CAMs) are proteins that allow cells to recognize each other and contribute to proper cell differentiation and development.

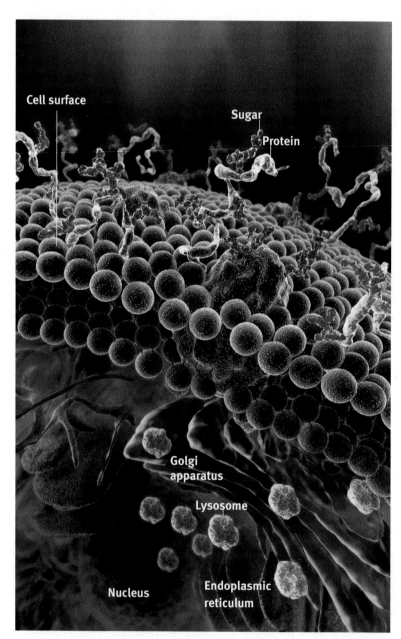

Figure 1.7

Key Concept

We need to appreciate that the more nonpolar a molecule is, the easier time it will have traversing the hydrophobic core of the cell membrane. For example, nonpolar steroid hormones cross the cell membrane and meet up with their receptors inside the cell. By contrast, protein hormones bind to cell membrane receptors and modify cellular activity via an internal secondary messenger (e.g., cyclic AMP).

NUCLEUS

Continuing our voyage through our cellular city, we come to the nucleus, which we can think of as the city hall and the public library. The nucleus is the control center of the cell, and functions much as a cellular city hall. The nucleus is the most commonly tested organelle on the MCAT, so we should focus on its intricacies. Moreover, it contains all of the genetic material necessary for replication of the cell; thus, it is also like the public library in that it serves as a repository for this information. The nucleus is surrounded by the **nuclear membrane** or **envelope**, a double membrane that maintains a nuclear environment separate and distinct from the cytoplasm. Of course, the nucleus cannot be completely isolated from the rest of the cell, so the nuclear membrane is punctured with **nuclear pores** that allow for the selective two-way exchange of material into and out of the nucleus. The genetic material (DNA) is organized into coding regions called **genes**. The linear DNA is wound around organizing proteins known as **histones** and then further wound into linear strands called **chromosomes** (or **chromatids**), just as the books in a library are sorted based on subject and placed on shelves. Finally, there is a subsection of the nucleus known as the **nucleolus**, where the ribosomal RNA (**rRNA**) is synthesized.

RIBOSOMES

Ribosomes are the factories of our city. They are responsible for protein production. Just as a factory takes an order and produces goods so, too, do the ribosomes. They take orders from the nucleus (city hall) and produce goods (proteins) that are necessary for the survival of the cell. Ribosomes come in two varieties: free (traveling tradesmen) and bound (think of large factories that produce specific goods like cars). These central merchants all have the same shipping department, the **endoplasmic reticulum** (ER).

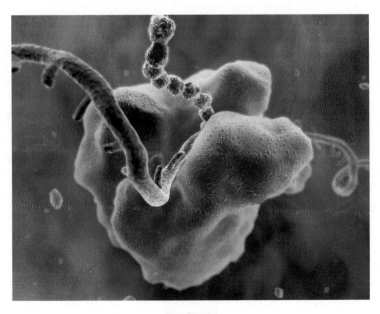

Figure 1.8

ENDOPLASMIC RETICULUM

Just outside the nucleus, the endoplasmic reticulum exists as a series of interconnected membrane-bound organelles. There are two varieties: **smooth** and **rough**. Rough ER's outer surface is ribosome-studded, whereas smooth ER is ribosome-free.

By and large, the ER is responsible for the proper production (via bound ribosomes) and sorting of materials from the cell, especially those destined to be secreted. Think back to our analogy. The ER acts as a giant shipping center, taking the goods that were produced and sending them to the correct location. The smooth ER works toward lipid synthesis and detoxification of drugs and poisons, whereas the rough ER is more directly involved in the production of protein products.

GOLGI APPARATUS

Think about our shipping center. We know that it is going to be busy with getting goods out. Sometimes as the goods get shipped they either reach the wrong destination or have to be repackaged to make sure that they are correctly sorted. Much like this, the Golgi apparatus is the way in which certain products in our cell will be repackaged. The Golgi is a series of membrane-bound sacs; it receives materials from the smooth ER and then repackages them to send to the cell surface. These products are often sent in **secretory vesicles** that release their contents to a cell's exterior in a process known as **exocytosis**. This is analogous to us sending a product

Key Concept

The Golgi apparatus is Packaging Central. It directs materials within the cell.

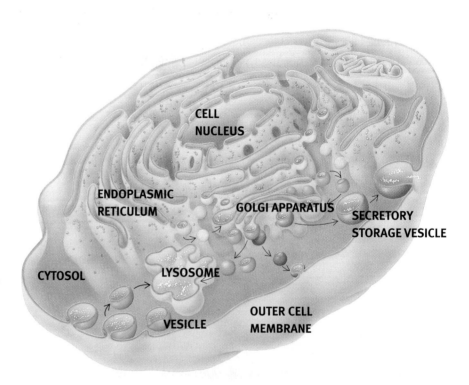

CELL
NUCLEUS

ENDOPLASMIC
RETICULUM

GOLGI APPARATUS

SECRETORY
STORAGE VESICLE

CYTOSOL

LYSOSOME

VESICLE

OUTER CELL
MEMBRANE

Figure 1.9

to a different city, See how much fun our MCAT studying can be when we add in analogies? They may seem silly, but when it counts on Test Day, they will help us remember key facts and achieve a high score.

VESICLES AND VACUOLES

Vesicles and vacuoles are the wrapping we discussed in the previous paragraph. They are used to transport and store materials that are ingested, secreted, processed, or digested by the cell. Vacuoles are larger and more likely to be found in plant cells. Remember that there are many different types of eukaryotes we may be asked about on Test Day. Each of their organelles may be slightly different to fit the needs of that organism.

LYSOSOMES

Lysosomes are the garbage dumps of our cells. They take material brought in by endosomes (specialized vesicles that serve as garbage trucks) and, using hydrolytic enzymes at a lowered pH (5), they break down materials ingested by the cell. Just as we wouldn't want to live by a garbage dump, lysosomes are effectively able to sequester these hydrolytic enzymes from the remainder of the cell, which prevents them from damaging the cell through oxidized intermediates. Lysosomes are also important in the removal of old cellular components and replacement with newer ones, similar to the way buildings may be deconstructed and destroyed during the remodeling process. Finally, lysosomes serve an important purpose in that they can cause the death of the cell in a process known as **autolysis**. By selectively choosing when to release these enzymes, the cell can commit suicide if necessary (e.g., the DNA is damaged). In addition, lysosomes give us recycling properties in that some of the broken-down products can be reused in other cellular processes. You should be familiar with the key organelles (such as the nucleus) whose damage will cause the cell to go through apoptosis. This is great material for an MCAT discrete question.

MITOCHONDRIA

Mitochondria are the powerhouse of the cell or the power plant in our town. What kind of power plant is it? Well, of course, a nuclear one. Remember, we are dealing with eukaryotic cells. The mitochondrion contains two layers: the inner and outer membrane. Just as in a nuclear power plant, the outer membrane is like the walls. It allows in the appropriate materials for respiration primarily based on size. The inner membrane is analogous to the reactor chamber of a nuclear power plant; it contains the molecules and enzymes necessary for the electron transport chain. The inner membrane contains numerous in-foldings known as the **cristae**, which are highly convoluted structures that increase the surface area for the electron transport chain enzymes to sit within. The inner membrane encloses the **mitochondrial matrix**, which contains many other enzymes important in cellular respiration (see Chapter 3). Between the two membranes lies the **intermembrane space**.

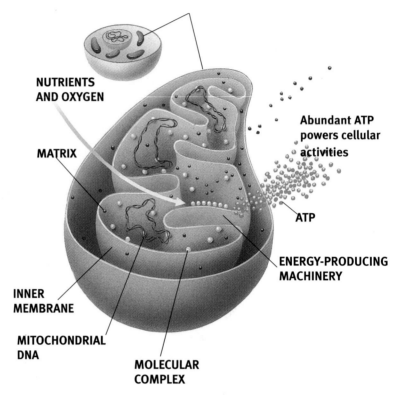

NUTRIENTS AND OXYGEN

MATRIX

Abundant ATP powers cellular activities

ATP

ENERGY-PRODUCING MACHINERY

INNER MEMBRANE

MITOCHONDRIAL DNA

MOLECULAR COMPLEX

Figure 1.10

Real World

Mitochondria can be inherited only from the mother. That means that if a woman has a genetic defect in one of her mitochondrial genes, she will pass it on to *all* of her children; conversely, a man cannot pass it to any of his children.

Mitochondria are different from other parts of the cell in that they are **semiautonomous**. They contain some of their own genes and replicate independently of the nucleus via binary fission. Mitochondria are thought to have evolved from one prokaryotic organism ingesting another in a symbiotic relationship. Just as a nuclear power plant can have a meltdown incident (think Chernobyl), so, too, can the mitochondria. They can release some of the enzymes in the electron transport chain during the process of programmed cell death (**apoptosis**).

MICROBODIES

Microbodies are specialized factories within our cellular city. They catalyze specific types of reactions by sequestering the necessary enzymes and substrates. Two specific microbodies are **peroxisomes** and **glyoxysomes**. Peroxisomes are responsible for the creation of hydrogen peroxide within a cell and are used to break down fats into usable molecules, as well as catalyze detoxification reactions in the liver. Glyoxysomes are important in germinating plants, where they convert fats to usable fuel (sugars) until the plant can make its own energy via photosynthesis. Remember that the MCAT may test you on some of the specific functions of organelles, so you should be filing these away as you study.

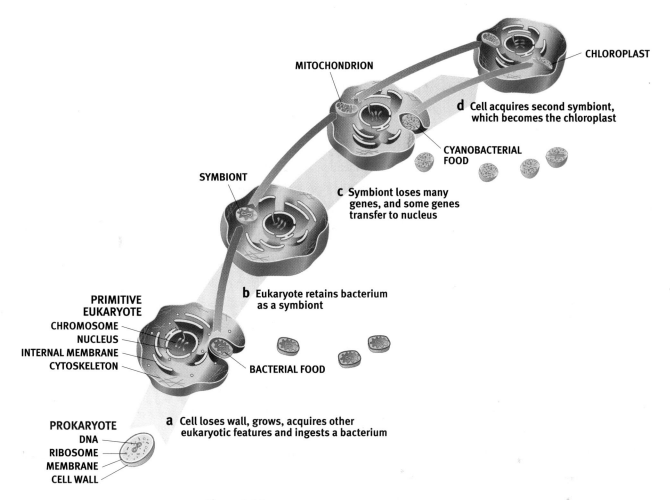

MITOCHONDRION

CHLOROPLAST

d Cell acquires second symbiont, which becomes the chloroplast

CYANOBACTERIAL FOOD

SYMBIONT

c Symbiont loses many genes, and some genes transfer to nucleus

b Eukaryote retains bacterium as a symbiont

PRIMITIVE EUKARYOTE
CHROMOSOME
NUCLEUS
INTERNAL MEMBRANE
CYTOSKELETON

BACTERIAL FOOD

a Cell loses wall, grows, acquires other eukaryotic features and ingests a bacterium

PROKARYOTE
DNA
RIBOSOME
MEMBRANE
CELL WALL

Figure 1.11

CHLOROPLASTS

If the mitochondria are nuclear power plants, the chloroplasts are solar power plants. Chloroplasts are found in our more ecologically concerned organisms (plants and algae). They contain chlorophyll and are responsible for the generation of energy using water, carbon dioxide, and sunlight. They also contain their own DNA and may, like mitochondria, have evolved via symbiosis.

CELL WALL

Sometimes the basic cell membrane (our city wall) isn't enough of a deterrent to foreign organisms. We need to reinforce it with stronger barriers and structural supports. Many eukaryotic cells are surrounded by a cell wall for both defense and increased stability. All plant cells have a cell wall composed of cellulose; fungi have walls made of chitin; animals do not have cell walls.

Key Concept

Not all cells have the same relative distribution of organelles. Form will follow function: cells that require a lot of energy for locomotion (e.g., sperm cells) have lots of mitochondria; cells involved in secretion (e.g., pancreatic islet cells) have lots of Golgi bodies; and cells such as red blood cells, which primarily serve a transport function, have no organelles at all!

CENTRIOLES

Nothing more than a specialized type of microtubule, the centrioles are part of our highway system within the cell. They are important for spindle formation and are not membrane bound. Animal cells have a pair of centrioles that are oriented at right angles to one other. Plant cells do not have centrioles.

CYTOSKELETON

As we previously mentioned, the cytoskeleton is the highway system of our cell and provides a transport system as well as structural strength. There are three components: microfilaments, microtubules, and intermediate filaments.

Microfilaments are made up of solid polymerized rods of **actin**. They are the smallest of our roads. Places of use include muscular contraction, where they interact with **myosin** (more on this in Chapter 6). They are also involved in movement of materials within the cellular membrane and amoeboid movement.

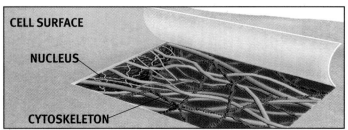

CYTOSKELETON of a cell consists of microfilaments (*bottom left*), microtubules (*bottom center*) and intermediate filaments (*bottom right*), all of which are nanometers wide. The rounded shape near the center in each of these photographs is the cell nucleus. The three components interconnect to create the cytoskeletal lattice, which stretches from the cell surface to the nucleus (*top left*). The molecular structure of each component is shown above the corresponding photograph and is color coded to the top left illustration.

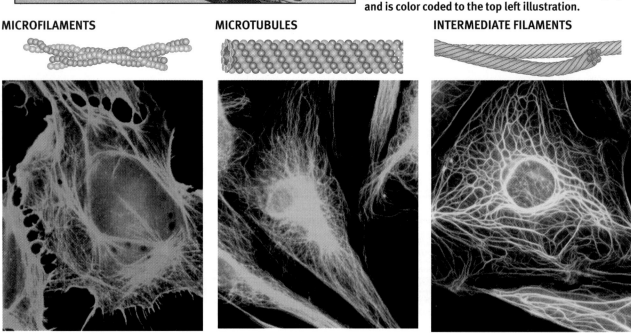

Figure 1.12

Microtubules are hollow, unlike actin. They are polymers of 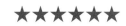 **tubulin** proteins. Microtubules radiate throughout the cell, providing the largest roads (superhighways) for transport as well as structural support. They are involved in chromosomal separation during mitosis and meiosis; they are also the structural basis for **cilia** and flagella, which are structures involved in a variety of processes from trapping foreign matter (see Chapter 8) to providing motility for sperm (see Chapter 4).

Intermediate filaments are a collection of fibers that help maintain the overall integrity of the cytoskeleton.

Movement Across the Cell Membrane ★★★★★★

Because cells spend much of their time and energy setting up membranes to control what passes in and out of the cell, they also need to regulate how substrates are capable of moving across that membrane. This is analogous to the border patrol we mentioned earlier, and we will take a look at these processes in turn. An important point to keep in mind is that all movement is based on concentration gradients, which is an MCAT favorite and will definitely net you points on Test Day. Regardless of what we are moving, the gradient will tell us whether this process will be passive or active.

SIMPLE DIFFUSION

The most basic of all processes, simple diffusion does not require energy; substrates move down their concentration gradient much as a ball would roll down a hill. There is potential energy (see—our MCAT physics is back in action) in a chemical gradient; each of these processes exploits that fact. **Osmosis** is a specific kind of simple diffusion that concerns water; water will move from a region of lower solute concentration to one of higher solute concentration. That is, it will move from a region of higher water concentration down its gradient to a region of lower water concentration. Osmosis is important in several places, notably where the solute itself is impermeable to a membrane. In such a case, water will move until the solute concentrations are equimolar. If the concentration of solutes inside the cell is higher than the surrounding solution, the solution is said to be **hypotonic**; such a solution will cause a cell to swell, sometimes to the point of bursting. The opposite situation is known as a **hypertonic** solution. If the solutions inside and outside are equimolar, they are said to be **isotonic**. A key point here is that **isotonicity** does not prevent movement; rather, it prevents the net movement of particles. They still move; it's just a zero-sum game.

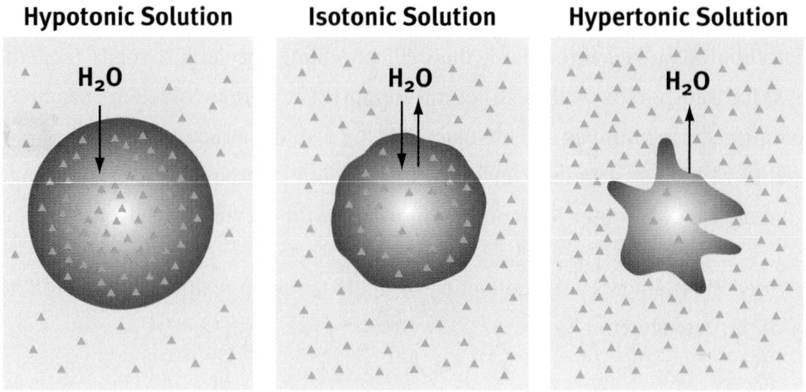

Figure 1.13

MCAT Expertise

Hypertonicity and hypotonicity are commonly tested using an erythrocyte and the Na^+/K^+ ATPase pump, which can control the cell's volume when placed in a stressful environment.

We can liken this process to the movement of people out of a city as it grows. As we have more and more people, some will move down the concentration gradient and out of our city. In real life, this principle can be demonstrated by placing a red blood cell in pure water. Because red blood cells have an osmolarity of 300 mOsm, versus 0 mOsm of pure water, we can determine that water will rush into the cell, causing it to burst.

FACILITATED DIFFUSION

Bridge

Diffusion is the biological version of a ball rolling down a hill—down its potential energy gradient. Active transport is the biological equivalent of pushing a ball up a hill; energy in the form of adenosine triphosphate must be expended, and work is performed.

Facilitated diffusion, also known as passive transport, is simple diffusion for molecules that need a little extra help. For molecules that are impermeable to the membrane (large, polar, and/or charged), the energy barrier (city wall) is too high to cross. Facilitated diffusion allows integral membrane proteins to serve as channels for these substrates to avoid the hydrophobic region of the phospholipid bilayer.

ACTIVE TRANSPORT

Active transport results in the net movement of a solute against its concentrations, just like rolling a ball uphill. Active transport always requires energy. Think about how your cells do this continually; it adds up to quite a Herculean task! This process is used throughout the body, for instance, in the nervous system to maintain the electric potential in neurons, and in the kidneys to conserve useful solutes (e.g., glucose) from the filtrate.

ENDOCYTOSIS AND EXOCYTOSIS

Key Concept

Exocytosis and endocytosis allow the cell to compartmentalize certain functions, creating specific environments favorable to reactions such as digestion.

Endocytosis is the process whereby the cellular membrane invaginates and engulfs material into the cell. The material is kept sequestered from the cytosol by virtue of being in a vesicle, which is important because cells will sometimes ingest toxic substances. **Pinocytosis** is the endocytosis of fluids and small particles, whereas

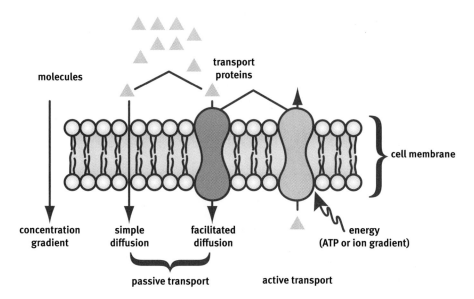

Figure 1.14

phagocytosis is the ingestion of large molecules. Often there will be a receptor to which substrates bind to induce ingestion, much as you might make airplane noises and move the spoon around when you try to make a baby ingest his pureed carrots.

Exocytosis is the reverse process whereby substrates are released from the cell into the outside world. This becomes important in the nervous system and intracellular signaling.

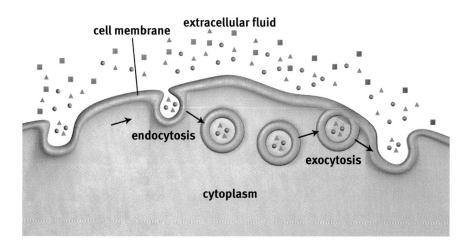

Figure 1.15

Table 1.1

	Simple Diffusion	Osmosis	Facilitated Diffusion	Active Transport
Concentration Gradient	High $\longrightarrow$ Low	High $\longrightarrow$ Low	High $\longrightarrow$ Low	Low $\longrightarrow$ High
Membrane Protein Required	No	No	Yes	Yes
Energy Required	NO—this is a PASSIVE process	NO—this is a PASSIVE process	NO—this is a PASSIVE process	YES—this is a ACTIVE process; requires ATP
Type of Molecule/s Transported	Small nonpolar (O_2, CO_2, etc . . .)	H_2O	Large nonpolar (e.g. glucose)	Polar molecules or ions (e.g. Na^+, Cl^-, K^+, etc . . .)

Tissues

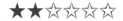

In multicellular organisms, cells may organize into discrete tissues that carry out different functions. To continue our analogy, if cells are like cities, tissues are the states into which they organize themselves. We will be discussing each of the organ systems in turn; several are MCAT favorites, including the circulatory, excretory, and nervous system.

EPITHELIAL TISSUE

These tissues cover the body and line the cavities; they provide a means for protection, invasion, and desiccation. Epithelium is also involved in absorption, secretion, and sensation.

CONNECTIVE TISSUE

Connective tissue supports the body and provides a framework for higher-level interactions. Bone, cartilage, tendons, ligaments, adipose tissue, and blood are all connective tissues.

NERVOUS TISSUE

Neurons are the primary cell in nervous tissue. They make use of electrochemical gradients to allow for cellular signaling and the coordinated control of multiple tissues, organs, and organ systems.

MUSCLE TISSUE

There are three types of muscle tissue: **skeletal, smooth, and cardiac**. Whereas each serves a specific function (which we will discuss in Chapter 6), each exhibits great contractile ability and strength.

Viruses

If we remember back to the beginning of the chapter when we discussed the Cell Theory, we noted that viruses don't fit the definition of a living thing. By definition, viruses are acellular structures composed of nucleic acids surrounded by a protein coat. They may be as small as 20 nm or as large as 300 nm. For reference, prokaryotes are 1–10 μm and eukaryotes are an order of magnitude larger.

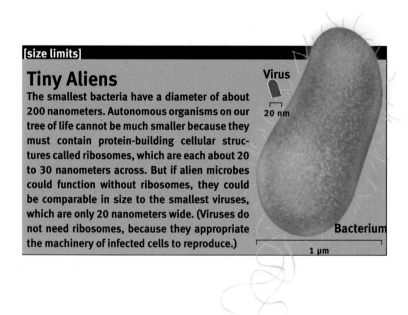

[size limits]

Tiny Aliens

The smallest bacteria have a diameter of about 200 nanometers. Autonomous organisms on our tree of life cannot be much smaller because they must contain protein-building cellular structures called ribosomes, which are each about 20 to 30 nanometers across. But if alien microbes could function without ribosomes, they could be comparable in size to the smallest viruses, which are only 20 nanometers wide. (Viruses do not need ribosomes, because they appropriate the machinery of infected cells to reproduce.)

Virus

20 nm

Bacterium

1 μm

Figure 1.16

The nuclear information may be circular or linear, single or double stranded, and DNA or RNA. The protein coat is known as a **capsid**. Since they cannot reproduce independently, viruses are known as **obligate intracellular parasites**. They must express and replicate their genetic information within a cell because they lack the necessary machinery to do it themselves. After hijacking a cell's machinery, a virus will replicate and turn out new copies of itself known as **virions**, which can be released to infect new cells. **Bacteriophages** are viruses that specifically target bacteria. They do not actually enter bacteria; rather, they simply inject their genetic material, leaving the remaining structures outside the infected cell. Viruses can be likened to spies that hijack our factories and alter orders from the city hall (nucleus) to make their own nefarious products.

Bridge

Consider that viruses evade the immune system differently than bacteria do. Most bacteria never enter a cell, whereas viruses must do so in order to replicate. This has immune system implications that will be discussed later.

Real World

Diseases caused solely by viruses include the common cold, measles, mumps, chicken pox, croup, polio, influenza, hepatitis, and AIDS. It's trickier to use drugs against viruses than against bacteria, because viruses actually live inside host cells and have no organelles of their own (recall that many antibiotics work by targeting specific prokaryotic organelles). To date, the few antiviral medications that exist work by interfering with enzymatic reactions involved in viral replication. More success in combating viruses has been achieved through vaccination. Of the diseases listed above, vaccines currently exist for measles, mumps, chicken pox, polio, influenza, and hepatitis.

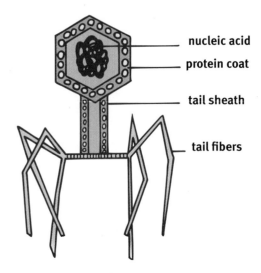

Figure 1.17

Conclusion

Our first chapter introduced the basis of all biology: the Cell Theory. We then introduced some of the techniques used in biology, and it's important for us to know how and when to apply these techniques. This sort of critical thinking is important to doing well on the MCAT. The eukaryotic versus prokaryotic distinction was our next topic of discussion. Eukaryotes will be the primary focus on the MCAT, but a few key facts about prokaryotes will net you a couple of points on Test Day. The subcellular organelles were discussed in detail; learn these well. Finally, we took a quick look at viruses and how they violate parts of the Cell Theory. We will now turn our attention to enzymes, which allow cells to carry out the basic chemical reactions necessary to support life.

CONCEPTS TO REMEMBER

☐ The Cell Theory defines what a cell is. Moreover, it gives us a basis for determining what sorts of organisms fit the biological definition of life.

☐ A variety of tools exist for biologists to study living organisms. Keep in mind that the basis for these techniques is physics and chemistry, and may be tested that way.

☐ Prokaryotes are organisms that lack a nucleus and membrane-bound organelles.

☐ Eukaryotes contain both a nucleus and membrane-bound organelles, although those organelles may differ based on the organism and its ecological niche (e.g., plants have chloroplasts whereas animal cells do not).

☐ Membrane-bound organelles provide a mechanism for eukaryotic organisms to separate biological reactions and functions into discrete compartments. Know the function of each of these compartments.

☐ Passive transport (simple diffusion, facilitated diffusion, and osmosis) transfers solutes down their concentration gradients. No energy input is required. The energy has already been stored in the chemical gradient.

☐ Active transport requires energy and moves solutes against their concentration gradients.

☐ Endocytosis and exocytosis provide a mechanism whereby a cell can either engulf or excrete substrates. Moreover, it provides a way to isolate these compounds from the cytosol.

☐ Cells of similar type will organize together into tissues that can carry out higher-level functions.

☐ Viruses violate several tenets of the Cell Theory and are not considered to be alive.

Practice Questions

1. All of the following are components of the Cell Theory EXCEPT

    A. all living things are composed of cells.
    B. all living things possess mitochondria.
    C. cooperation among cells allows for complex functioning in living things.
    D. all cells arise from preexisting cells.

2. Upon bacteriophage infection, the host cell is directed to synthesize viral protein. A scientist wishing to study the location of this process in the cell might use

    A. centrifugation.
    B. autoradiography.
    C. electrophoresis.
    D. phase contrast microscopy.

3. A student is trying to determine the type of membrane transport occurring in a cell. She finds that the molecule to be transported is very large and polar, and when transported across the membrane, no ATP is used. Which of the following is the most likely mechanism of transport?

    A. Active transport
    B. Simple diffusion
    C. Facilitated diffusion
    D. Exocytosis

4. Which of the following is NOT a type of tissue found in the human body?

    A. Connective tissue
    B. Nervous tissue
    C. Adipose tissue
    D. Cytoplasmic tissue

5. Which of the following types of nucleic acid will never be found in a virus?

    A. Single-stranded DNA
    B. Double-stranded DNA
    C. Single and double-stranded RNA
    D. All of these can be found in a virus.

6. Which of the following activities occurs in the Golgi apparatus?

    A. Synthesis of proteins
    B. Modification and packaging of proteins
    C. Breakdown of lipids and carbohydrates
    D. Photosynthesis

7. Mitochondrial DNA

    A. is circular.
    B. is self-replicating.
    C. is important in the synthesis of mitochondrial ribosomes.
    D. both A and B.

8. Which of the following is NOT a function of the smooth endoplasmic reticulum?

    A. Lipid synthesis
    B. Poison detoxification
    C. Protein synthesis
    D. Transport of proteins

9. What is the main function of the nucleolus?

    A. Ribosomal RNA synthesis
    B. DNA synthesis
    C. Cell division
    D. Chromosome assembly

10. In which of the following organelles is pH the lowest?

    A. Lysosomes
    B. Mitochondria
    C. Rough ER
    D. Chloroplasts

11. Which of the following is NOT a difference that would allow one to distinguish between a prokaryotic and a eukaryotic cell?

    A. Ribosomal subunit weight
    B. Presence or absence of the nucleus
    C. Presence or absence of the cell wall
    D. Membrane-bound vs. no membrane-bound organelles

12. Prokaryotic and eukaryotic animal cells both have

    A. DNA.
    B. ribosomes.
    C. a cell wall.
    D. both A and B.

13. Which of the following is NOT involved in cell movement?

    A. Cilia
    B. Flagella
    C. Actin
    D. Centrioles

Small Group Questions

1. Can glucose freely diffuse through the cell membrane? Why or why not?

2. Explain why mitochondria and chloroplasts possess similar characteristics.

3. Cystic fibrosis is a genetic disease characterized by thick mucus secretions that block air passages in the lungs. This disease results from faulty chloride channels that allow Cl^- and Na^+ to remain in the cells that line the airways. How does this cause the mucus in the airways to become thick?

4. Most biologists consider viruses to be nonliving because they are unable to replicate independently. How might you argue against this position? What characteristics do viruses have that make them lifelike?

Explanations to Practice Questions

1. B

The Cell Theory can be summarized by four main ideas: 1) all living things are composed of cells; 2) the cell is the basic functional unit of life; 3) cells arise only from pre-existing cells; and 4) cells carry genetic information in the form of DNA. From the given choices, all of them are components of the Cell Theory, with the exception of (B). The presence or absence of mitochondria is not a component of the Cell Theory, making (B) the correct answer.

2. B

The best way to identify the location of synthesis of viral proteins is to label amino acids with radioactive isotopes. This technique is used in autoradiography, which utilizes radioactive molecules to trace and identify cell structures and localize biochemical activity. Autoradiography, (B), is therefore the correct answer.

3. C

We are asked to identify the type of transport that would allow a large, polar molecule to cross the membrane without any energy requirement. This scenario describes facilitated diffusion, which uses a transport protein (or channel) to facilitate the movement of large, polar molecules across the nonpolar, hydrophobic membrane. Facilitated diffusion, like simple diffusion, does not require any energy, which explains why no ATP was consumed during this transport process. (C) is therefore the correct answer.

4. D

The four basic types of tissue found in the human body are epithelial (skin), connective (bone, cartilage, tendons, ligaments, adipose tissue and blood), nervous (neurons), and muscle (skeletal, cardiac and smooth). There is no such thing as cytoplasmic tissue, making (D) the correct answer.

5. D

In a virus, the nucleic acid can be either linear or circular, and is found in four varieties: single-stranded DNA, double-stranded DNA, single-stranded RNA and double-stranded RNA. Thus, all types of nucleic acid can be found in a virus, making (D) the correct answer.

6. B

The Golgi apparatus consists of a stack of membrane-enclosed sacs. It receives vesicles and their contents from the smooth ER, modifies them (e.g., glycosylation), repackages them into vesicles and distributes them. Therefore, from the given choices, only (B) matches the function of the Golgi apparatus.

7. D

Mitochondrial DNA, or mDNA, is circular and self-replicating, which allows the mitochondria to be semi-autonomous. Mitochondria are capable of synthesizing some of their own proteins and can replicate via binary fission. However, mitochondria are not entirely independent from the rest of the cell, as many of their components (e.g., ribosomes) are produced in the nucleolus of the cell, along with the other ribosomes. (D) is therefore the correct answer.

8. C

The smooth endoplasmic reticulum is involved in the transport of materials throughout the cell, in lipid synthesis and the detoxification of drugs and poisons. Proteins can cross into the smooth ER, where they are secreted into cytoplasmic vesicles and transported to the Golgi apparatus. Thus, from the given choices, protein synthesis is not a function of the smooth ER, but rather of the ribosomes associated with the rough ER. (C) is therefore the correct answer.

9. A

The nucleolus (not to be confused with the nucleus) is a dense structure in the nucleus where ribosomal RNA (rRNA) is synthesized. Ribosomal RNA is the main component of the ribosomal subunits. (A) is therefore the correct answer.

10. A

A low pH indicates an acidic environment. From the given choices, only lysosomes maintain an acidic environment since they contain hydrolytic enzymes involved in intracellular digestion. These enzymes are maximally effective at a pH of 5 and need to be enclosed within the lysosome–in an environment that is distinct from the neutral pH of the cytosol—to prevent them from digesting the cell itself. When a cell is injured, it can commit suicide by rupturing the lysosomal membrane and releasing hydrolytic enzymes into the cell. (A) is therefore the correct answer.

11. C

The main differences between prokaryotes and eukaryotes are: prokaryotes do not have a nucleus, while eukaryotes do; prokaryotes have ribosomal subunits of 30s and 50s, while eukaryotes have ribosomal subunits of 40s and 60s; and prokaryotes do not have membrane-bound organelles, whereas eukaryotes do. Lastly, it is important to note that while a cell wall is present in most prokaryotes, fungi and plants are the only eukaryotes that have cell walls. Therefore, the presence or absence of a cell wall does not definitively differentiate between prokaryotes and eukaryotes, making (C) the correct answer.

12. D

Among the similarities between prokaryotes and eukaryotes are the presence of DNA and organelles (such as ribosomes). While most prokaryotes have a cell wall, fungi and plants are the only eukaryotes that have cell walls. As such, (D) is the correct answer.

13. D

From the given choices, all of them are involved in cell movement, with the exception of (D). Centrioles are composed of microtubules and direct the separation of chromosomes during cell division. Therefore, they are not involved in cell motility making (D) the correct answer.

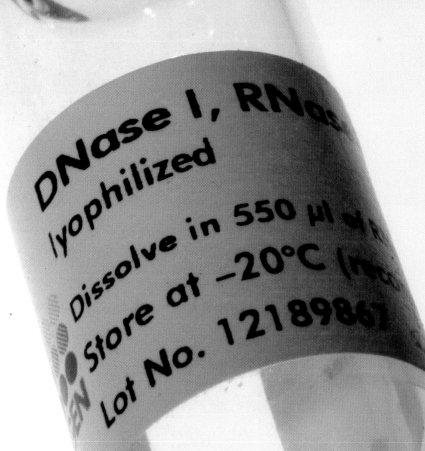

2

Enzymes

Introduction

Tune into the national news on any given night, and you are likely to hear a report on hypertension—what causes it, how we can avoid it, and most urgently, what we can do to treat it. The risk of hypertension, or high blood pressure, is especially high in individuals whose weight and body fat percentage classify them as obese, which means that as the obesity epidemic becomes more widespread, hypertension does as well. Increased sodium intake and pregnancy can also lead to hypertension, but luckily, neither of these risk factors are permanent.

Millions of Americans are told each year to alter their diet, add exercise to their daily regimen, or even take prescription drugs to control their hypertension. Many of these medications fall under a category called ACE inhibitors. ACE, short for angiotensin-converting enzyme, converts a peptide called angiotensin I to angiotensin II. Angio-tensin II goes on to stimulate a hormone that raises blood pressure. Let's back up a little bit. In response to a drop in blood pressure, specialized cells in the kidney, known as juxtaglomerular cells, release an enzyme called renin. Renin converts the dormant precursor angiotensinogen into angiotensin I, which is cleaved by ACE to angiotensin II. Angiotensin II stimulates aldosterone, a steroid hormone that allows the kidney to reabsorb more sodium, and because water generally follows sodium, water re-enters blood as well. The blood's volume increases, thus the hydrostatic pressure against blood vessels also increases. Another name for hydrostatic pressure against blood vessels? Blood pressure. So without ACE, angiotensin II can't stimulate aldosterone, and blood pressure stays low. This is how ACE inhibitors work.

So there are natural enzymes and hormones that actually raise blood pressure? Doesn't that contribute to the problem? Well, it's not supposed to. The human body must always remain in a very delicate stable state known as homeostasis. If that balance is tipped even a little bit, chemical messengers rush to correct it. In other words, when we're dehydrated or injured, we'd be goners without ACE. Enzymes are crucial proteins that dramatically increase the rate of chemical reactions. They're used to regulate homeostatic mechanisms in every organ system, and are regulated by inhibitors themselves, like the ACE inhibitors used to treat hypertension. They're kept safe and ready to go in inactive forms like angiotensinogen and are sent on their way when needed. In this chapter, we'll learn all about how enzymes work and how different conditions influence their activity. We'll also see how enzymes are regulated, which will help us tie concepts together in every organ system we learn for the MCAT.

Thermodynamics and Kinetics ★★★★☆

Recall that thermodynamics relates the relative energy states of a reaction in terms of its products and reactants. An **endothermic** reaction is one that requires energy input, whereas an **exothermic** reaction is one in which energy is given off. Remember that *endo*– means *in* and *exo*– means *out*; so endothermic reactions take energy in to go forward, whereas exothermic reactions release energy out as they go forward. We can look at a reaction diagram to see this demonstrated more clearly.

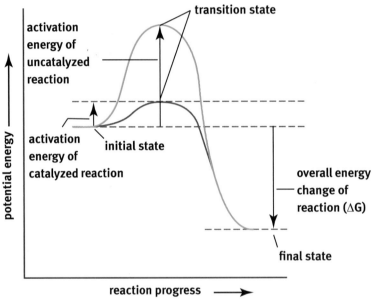

Figure 2.1

The reaction shown here is exothermic. Note that the ΔH for this reaction is negative. A very important characteristic of enzymes is that they do not alter the overall enthalpy change for a reaction, nor do they change the equilibrium of a reaction. Rather, they affect the rate (kinetics) at which a reaction occurs; thus, they can affect how quickly a reaction gets to equilibrium but not the actual equilibrium state itself. As catalysts, recall that enzymes themselves are unchanged by the reaction. What is the functional consequence of this? Far fewer enzymes are required relative to the overall amount of substrate. Think back to general chemistry and recall how catalysts exert their effect. They lower the activation energy; in other words, they make it easier for the substrate to reach the transition state. Imagine having to walk to the other side of a tall hill. The only way to get there is to climb to the top of the hill and then walk down the other side. Wouldn't it be easier if something could bore a tunnel through the center of that hill so you wouldn't have to climb as high? That's exactly what enzymes (and all catalysts) do for chemical reactions.

Most reactions catalyzed by enzymes are technically reversible, although that reversal may be energetically unfavorable and therefore unrealistic.

Enzyme Specificity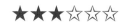

Enzymes are picky; they tend to catalyze a single reaction or class of reactions. For example, urease catalyzes the breakdown of only urea. Chymotrypsin, on the other hand, can cleave peptide bonds around the amino acids phenylalanine, tryptophan, and tyrosine in a variety of polypeptides. Although those amino acids aren't identical, they all contain an aromatic ring, which makes chymotrypsin specific for a class of molecules.

NORMAL ACTIVITY OF ENZYME

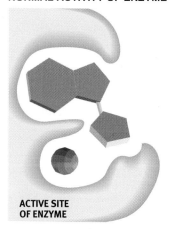

ACTIVE SITE
OF ENZYME

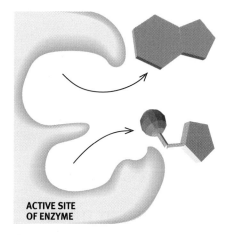

ACTIVE SITE
OF ENZYME

Figure 2.2

Most enzymes end in the prefix *–ase*. The molecule upon which an enzyme acts is known as its **substrate**. Biochemists cleverly named the complex between the enzyme and substrate the **enzyme–substrate complex**. The **active site** is the location within the enzyme where the substrate is held during the chemical reaction. Two competing theories explain how enzymes and substrates interact, but one of those two is generally more accepted than the other.

THE LOCK AND KEY THEORY

This theory is aptly named. It suggests that the enzyme's active site (lock) is already in the appropriate confirmation for the substrate (key) to bind. No alteration of the tertiary or quaternary structure is necessary upon binding of the substrate.

Bridge

Consider that enzymes often break down or create molecules (H_2O_2, OCl^-) that would be damaging to the cell if they were released into the cytoplasm. Think back to the last chapter's discussion on how cells deal with these oxidants and/or reactive oxygen species, which are necessary for certain reactions.

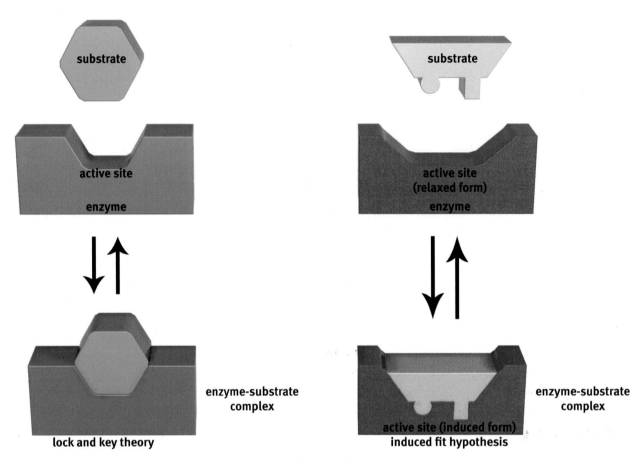

Figure 2.3

THE INDUCED FIT THEORY

The more scientifically accepted theory is the induced fit theory, and it is the one we are more likely to see on Test Day. Imagine this: the enzyme is a foam stress ball and the substrate is a frustrated MCAT student's hand. What's the desired interaction? The student wants to release some stress and relax. As his hand squeezes the ball, both change conformation. The ball is no longer spherical and his hand is no longer flat because they adjust to fit each other well. Ball squeezing takes energy, and therefore, this part of the reaction is endothermic. Once the student lets go of the stress ball, we have our desired product: a relaxed, more confident test taker. Letting go of the stress ball is pretty easy and doesn't require extra energy. This part of the reaction is exothermic. Just like enzymes, foam stress balls return to their original shape once their crunchers (substrates) let go of them.

What would happen if we tried to cure an earache using a stress ball? Well, unfortunately, inner ears don't really have any ability to grab stress balls. Try holding a stress ball up to your ear; it's a good bet that nothing would change shape. Similarly, a substrate of the wrong type will not cause the appropriate conformational shift in the protein, which allows for exposure of the active site. No reaction occurs.

Table 2.1

Enzymes:
1. Lower the activation energy
2. Increase the rate of the reaction
3. Do not alter the equilibrium constant
4. Are not changed or consumed in the reaction (This means that they will appear in both the reactants and products.)
5. Enzymes are pH and temperature sensitive, with optimal activity at specific pH ranges and temperatures
6. Do not affect the overall ΔG of the reaction
7. Are specific for a particular reaction or class of reactions

Cofactors

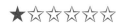

Many enzymes require nonprotein molecules called **cofactors** to be effective. Enzymes without their cofactors are called **apoenzymes**, whereas those containing them are **holoenzymes**. Cofactors are attached in a variety of ways ranging from weak noncovalent interactions to strong ones. These tightly bound factors are known as **prosthetic groups**. Cofactors are a topic that we are likely to see on Test Day, so we should know they are essential.

Two important types of cofactors are small metal ions and small organic groups. The latter organic cofactors are actually called **coenzymes**. If we think back to the introduction of the previous chapter and recall all the bacteria living in our gut, this turns out to be a good thing, because some of these bacteria make biotin, a necessary human cofactor. The vast majority of these coenzymes are vitamins.

Enzyme Kinetics

Enzyme kinetics is a high-yield topic that can score us several points on Test Day. Just as the relief our student derives from squeezing a stress ball depends on a number of factors such as size or shape of the ball, enzyme kinetics are dependent on conditions such as temperature, pH, and concentrations of substrate and/or enzyme.

EFFECTS OF CONCENTRATION

The concentration of the substrate [S] and enzyme [E] greatly affects how quickly a reaction will occur. Let's say that we have 100 stress balls (enzymes) and only 10 frustrated students (substrates) to squeeze them (high enzyme concentration relative to substrate). We will quickly reach equilibrium (students letting go and feeling

Real World

Deficiencies in vitamin cofactors can result in devastating disease. Thiamin is an essential cofactor for several enzymes involved in cellular metabolism and nerve conduction. Thiamin deficiency, often a result of excess alcohol consumption, results in diseases including Wernicke-Korsakoff syndrome. In this disorder, patients suffer from a variety of neurological deficits including delirium, balance problems, and, in severe cases, the inability to form new memories.

Bridge

Vitamins come in two major classes: fat and water soluble. This is important to consider in digestive diseases, where different parts of the gastrointestinal tract may be affected by different disease processes. Loss of different parts of the gastrointestinal tract may result in different vitamin deficiencies.

relaxed) as there are many active sites available. As we slowly add more substrate (students), the rate of the reaction will increase and more people will be happy in the same amount of time because we have plenty of available stress balls for them to squeeze. However, as we add more and more people (approaching 100), we begin to level off and reach a maximal rate of relaxation. There are fewer and fewer available stress balls until all sites are occupied. Unlike before, inviting more students to the room will not change the rate of the reaction. It cannot go any faster once it has reached **saturation**. At this rate, the enzyme is working at **maximum velocity**, denoted by V_{max}. If you don't yet understand this, keep reading and look at the diagram. This concept is essential for Test Day.

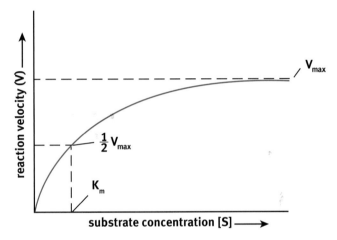

Figure 2.4

The Michaelis-Menten equation proposed in 1913 suggests the following. Enzyme–substrate complexes form at a rate k_1. The ES complex can either dissociate at a rate k_2, or turn into E + P at a rate k_3. Note that in either case, the enzyme is again available.

$$E + S \underset{k_2}{\overset{k_1}{\rightleftharpoons}} ES \overset{k_3}{\Rightarrow} E + P$$

Some important and Test Day–relevant math can be derived from this equation. When the reaction rate is equal to $\frac{1}{2} V_{max}$, K_m = [S] and can be understood to be the point at which half of the enzyme's active sites are full (half the stress balls are in use). When [S] is less than K_m, changes in [S] will greatly affect the reaction rate. In contrast, at high [S] (many students), [S] exceeds K_m and approaches V_{max}.

EFFECTS OF TEMPERATURE

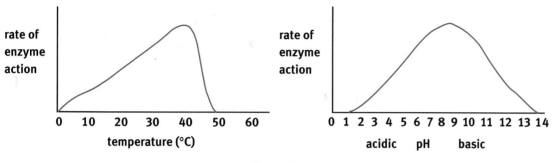

Figure 2.5

Enzyme-catalyzed reactions tend to double in rate for every 10°C increase in temperature until the optimum temperature is reached; for the human body, this is 37°C. After this, activity falls off sharply as the enzyme will denature at higher temperatures. Some enzymes that are overheated may regain their function if cooled. A real-life example of temperature dependence occurs in Siamese cats. Siamese cats are dark on their faces, ears, tails, and feet but white elsewhere. Why? The enzyme responsible for pigmentation, tyrosinase, is mutated in Siamese cats. It is ineffective at body temperature, but at cooler temperatures becomes active. Thus the tail, feet, ears, and face (cooled by air passing through the nose and mouth) have an active form of the enzyme and are dark.

EFFECTS OF pH

Most enzymes also depend on pH in order to function properly. For enzymes that circulate and function in human blood, this optimal pH is 7.4. This means that a pH of 7.3 in human blood is termed acidosis even though it's more basic than chemically neutral 7.0. The MCAT assumes that we know this, so let's commit it to memory now. Where might exceptions to this occur? Both are in our digestive tract. Pepsin, which works in the stomach, has maximal activity around pH 2, whereas pancreatic enzymes, which work in the small intestine, work best around pH 8.5. We will discuss the pH levels in the stomach and intestine in Chapter 7.

Regulation of Enzymatic Activity

Although enzymes are useful, we want to be able to control when they work. This may be accomplished in a variety of ways; two test-worthy ones are **allosteric effects** and **inhibition**.

Key Concept

Consider how the human body uses this. What part of the human body might require enzymes that work at a lower temperature? The answer will appear in Chapter 4.

Bridge

Consider that digestive enzymes chew up fats, proteins, and carbohydrates—the very same compounds of which our body is made. How do these enzymes know to digest your food but not your body? Simply put, they don't! So, we regulate their activity in a coordinated manner using feedback mechanisms and other substances.

ALLOSTERIC EFFECTS

Enzymes that are allosteric have multiple binding sites. The active site is present as well as at least one other site that can regulate the availability of the active site. These are known as **allosteric sites**. **Allosteric enzymes** alternate between an active and an inactive form. The inactive form is incapable of carrying out the enzymatic reaction. Binding in the allosteric site may consist of either **allosteric activators** or **allosteric inhibitors**. Binding of either causes a conformational shift in the protein. The effect is what differs. An activator will result in a shift that makes the active site more available for binding to the substrate. An inhibitor will make it less available. In addition to being able to alter the conformation of the protein, binding of activators or repressors may alter the affinity of the enzyme for its substrate. For example, the binding of one molecule of oxygen to hemoglobin shifts the entire molecule such that there is an increased affinity of the remaining subunits for oxygen.

INHIBITION

The activity of an enzyme may be regulated by one of its products (feedback inhibition) or other molecules that can bind to the enzyme (reversible and irreversible inhibition).

Feedback Inhibition

A large number of biological reactions are regulated through feedback inhibition. Once we have enough of a product, why create more? In feedback inhibition, the product may bind to an enzyme or enzymes that acted earlier in its biosynthetic pathway, thereby making the enzyme unavailable for other substrates to use. This is schematically represented below, as we see product D feeding back to inhibit the first enzyme in the pathway. Let's be sure we have a good handle on this concept before we move on, because it appears often in endocrine pathways (Chapter 12) and is commonly tested on the MCAT.

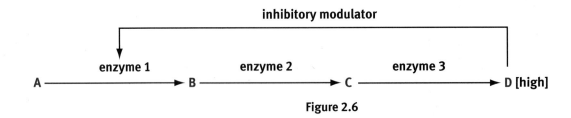

Figure 2.6

Reversible Inhibition

There are three types of reversible inhibition: competitive, noncompetitive, and uncompetitive. Competitive inhibition simply involves occupancy of the active site. Substrates cannot access enzymatic binding sites if there is an inhibitor in the way. Competitive inhibition can be overcome by adding more substrate, so that the substrate-to-inhibitor ratio is higher. If more molecules of substrate are available than molecules of inhibitor, then the enzyme will be more likely to bind substrate than inhibitor (assuming the enzyme has equal affinity for both molecules). What about noncompetitive inhibition? This term describes inhibitor binding to an allosteric site instead of the active site, which induces a change in enzyme conformation. Since the two molecules do not compete for the same spot, inhibition is *noncompetitive* and cannot be overcome by adding more substrate. Once the enzyme's conformation is altered, no amount of extra substrate will be conducive to forming an enzyme–substrate complex.

Irreversible Inhibition

In this type of inhibition, the active site is made permanently unavailable or the enzyme is permanently altered. A real-world example is aspirin. Acetylsalicylic acid (aspirin) irreversibly acetylates cyclooxygenase. The enzyme can no longer make its products (prostaglandins), which are involved in modulating pain and inflammatory responses. To make more prostaglandins, new cyclooxygenase will have to be synthesized through transcription and translation.

Inactive Enzymes ★★★☆☆

Certain enzymes are particularly dangerous if they are not tightly controlled. These include the digestive enzymes (e.g., trypsin), which, if released from the pancreas in an uncontrolled manner, would digest the organ itself. To avoid this danger, these enzymes and others are secreted as inactive **zymogens** (e.g., trypsinogen for trypsin). Zymogens contain a catalytic (active) domain and regulatory domain. The regulatory domain must be either removed or altered to expose the active site. Apoptotic enzymes (caspases) exhibit similar regulation.

Conclusion

Our current study focused on the way in which cells are able to carry out the reactions necessary for life. We began with a thermodynamics and kinetics review in relation to enzymes, which are biological catalysts. We went on to discuss the factors that may affect enzyme activity, including substrate concentration (think Michaelis-Menton kinetics), cofactors, temperature, and pH. All of these are likely to appear on Test Day. Enzymes need to be regulated; we analyzed the basics of inhibition, primarily mediated via negative feedback. Finally we talked about inhibitors of enzymes that may be reversible or irreversible. The difference between competitive and noncompetitive inhibition is a key Test Day concept. Let's move on now to discuss cellular respiration, a series of chemical reactions designed to generate energy for the cell. These reactions depend on the assistance of enzymes.

Key Concept

Reversible Inhibition

Competitive Inhibitor	Noncompetitive Inhibitor
Binds to active site	Binds to site other than active site
Can be overcome by adding more substrate	Cannot be overcome by adding more substrate

Real World

The concept of competitive inhibition has relevance in the clinical setting. For example, methanol (wood alcohol), if ingested, is enzymatically converted to toxic metabolites that can cause blindness and even death. Administration of intravenous ethanol is the treatment of choice for a patient suffering from methanol poisoning. Ethanol works by competing with methanol for the active sites of the enzymes involved.

CONCEPTS TO REMEMBER

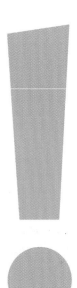

- ☐ Enzymes are biological catalysts that lower the activation energy necessary for biological reactions.

- ☐ Enzymes do not alter the enthalpy change (ΔH) that accompanies the reaction; rather, they change the rate (kinetics) at which equilibrium is reached.

- ☐ Enzymes have an active site that is where the relevant chemistry occurs.

- ☐ Each enzyme catalyzes a single reaction or type of reaction with fairly high specificity.

- ☐ Some enzymes require cofactors to be active. These tend to be either metal cations or small organic molecules.

- ☐ Temperature and pH can both affect the enzyme's activity. Temperature and pH can result in denaturing of the enzyme and loss of activity owing to loss of secondary, tertiary, and, if present, quaternary structure.

- ☐ Feedback inhibition provides a way for an enzyme to slow its activity. If product builds up, the enzyme has completed its task and can stop working so rapidly. Often it is the product that binds to an allosteric site of the enzyme to cause this change.

- ☐ Reversible inhibition can be competitive or noncompetitive. Competitive inhibition may be overcome by increasing the amount of substrate.

- ☐ Irreversible inhibition alters the enzyme in such a way that it is no longer available and never will be. New enzyme molecules must be synthesized from scratch.

- ☐ Some enzymes that could be harmful to the parent organism (e.g., digestive enzymes such as trypsin) are secreted in inactive forms to prevent their unintended activity.

Practice Questions

1. Consider a biochemical reaction A → B, which is catalyzed by A–B dehydrogenase. Which of the following statements is true?

    A. The reaction will proceed until the enzyme concentration decreases.

    B. The reaction will be more favorable at 0°C.

    C. A component of the enzyme is transferred from A to B.

    D. The free energy change (ΔG) of the catalyzed reaction is the same as the uncatalyzed reaction.

2. Consider the following enzyme pathway.

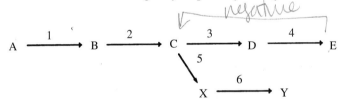

An increase in [E] leads to the inhibition of enzyme 3. All of the following are results of the process EXCEPT

    A. an increase in [B].

    B. an increase in [Y].

    C. decreased activity of enzyme 4.

    D. increased activity of enzyme 6.

3. Which of the following statements about enzyme kinetics is FALSE?

    A. An increase in the substrate concentration (at constant enzyme concentration) leads to proportional increases in the rate of the reaction.

    B. Most enzymes operating in the human body work best at a temperature of 37°C.

    C. An enzyme–substrate complex can either form a product or dissociate back into the enzyme and substrate.

    D. Maximal activity of many human enzymes occurs around pH 7.2.

4. At which pH would pancreatic enzymes work at maximum activity?

    A. 5.3

    B. 6.7

    C. 7.2

    D. 8.5

5. Some enzymes require the presence of a nonprotein molecule to behave catalytically. An enzyme devoid of this molecule is called a(n)

    A. holoenzyme.

    B. apoenzyme.

    C. coenzyme.

    D. zymoenzyme.

6. Which of the following factors determine an enzyme's specificity?

  A. The three-dimensional shape of the active site
  B. The Michaelis constant
  C. The type of cofactor required for the enzyme to be active
  D. The prosthetic group on the enzyme

7. Enzymes increase the rate of a reaction by

  A. decreasing the activation energy.
  B. increasing the overall free energy of the reaction.
  C. both A and B.
  D. none of the above.

8. Bonding between atoms within an enzyme such as trypsin is best described as

  A. peptide.
  B. saccharide.
  C. ionic.
  D. van der Waals.

protein

9. In the equation below, substrate C is an allosteric inhibitor to enzyme 1. Which of the following is another mechanism caused by substrate C?

  A → enzyme 1 → B → enzyme 2 → C

  A. Competitive inhibition
  B. Irreversible inhibition
  C. Feedback enhancement
  D. Negative feedback

10. When lactase hydrolyzes its substrate, lactose, which of the following occurs?

  A. Lactase retains its structure after the reaction.
  B. Lactose retains its structure after the reaction.
  C. Lactase increases the activation energy of the reaction.
  D. Lactose decreases the activation energy of the reaction.

Small Group Questions

1. Why do enzymes function at specific pH and temperature ranges?

2. Describe the kinetic effects of increasing substrate concentration while enzyme concentration remains constant.

3. Explain the significance of K_m in enzyme-catalyzed reactions.

Explanations to Practice Questions

1. D

In an enzyme-catalyzed reaction, the rate of a reaction is increased by a decrease in the activation energy. Furthermore, enzymes are not changed or consumed during the course of the reaction. Also, the overall free-energy change of the reaction, ΔG, remains unchanged in the presence of an enzyme. This implies that (D) is the correct answer.

2. A

Looking at the enzyme pathway, we notice that if enzyme 3 is inhibited, everything that is controlled by it will decrease in concentration and activity. That is, the concentration of D and E will eventually decrease. The activity of enzyme 4 will also decrease because it will be acting on a decreased amount of substrate. In addition, if enzyme 3 is inhibited, more of C will be converted to X through enzyme 5. As such, the concentration of X and Y are expected to increase, as is the activity of enzyme 6. Anything before the enzyme 3 should remain unaffected. Therefore, the concentration of B will remain the same, making (A) the correct answer.

3. A

Most enzymes in the human body operate at maximal activity around a temperature of 37°C and a pH of 7.2, which is the pH of most body fluids. In addition, as characterized by the Michaelis-Menten model, enzymes form an enzyme–substrate complex, which can either dissociate back into the enzyme and substrate or proceed to form a product. So far, we can eliminate (B), (C), and (D), so let's check choice (A). An increase in the substrate concentration, while maintaining a constant enzyme concentration, leads to a proportional increase in the rate of the reaction only initially. However, once most of the active sites are occupied, the reaction rate levels off, regardless of further increases in substrate concentration. At high concentrations of substrate, the reaction rate approaches its maximal velocity, and is no longer changed by further increases in substrate concentration. Therefore, the statement in (A) is not entirely true.

4. D

Pancreatic enzymes work optimally in the alkaline conditions of the small intestine. It is not necessary to know the exact pH at which these enzymes work because the only basic pH is seen in (D).

5. B

An enzyme devoid of its necessary cofactor is called an apoenzyme and is catalytically inactive. (B) is therefore the correct answer.

6. A

An enzyme's specificity is determined by the three-dimensional shape of its active site. Regardless of which theory of enzyme specificity we are discussing (lock and key or induced fit), the active site determines which substrate the enzyme will react with. (A) is therefore the correct answer.

7. A

Enzymes increase the rate of a reaction by decreasing the activation energy. They do not affect the overall free energy, ΔG, of the reaction. (A) is therefore the correct answer.

8. A

(A) is correct because enzymes are proteins. Proteins are composed of amino acids linked together by peptide bonds. The other choices are not bonds that would be found in proteins. (B) is a type of bond found in polysaccharides. (D) may be formed between secondary or tertiary structures but is not as good an option as (A).

9. D

By limiting the activity of enzyme 1, the rest of the pathway is slowed, which is the definition of negative feedback. (A) is incorrect because there is no competition for the active site with allosteric interactions. There is not enough information for (B) to be correct because we aren't told whether the inhibition is reversible. In general, allosteric interactions are temporary. (C) is incorrect because it is the opposite of what occurs when enzyme 1 activity is reduced.

10. A

(A) is the correct answer because, by definition, an enzyme remains unchanged by the reaction that it catalyzes. (B) is incorrect because a substrate is changed by an enzymatic reaction. (C) is not true, as an enzyme would decrease the activation energy. (D) is also incorrect since a substrate does not affect the activation energy.

3

Cellular Metabolism

What do vitamin C, omega-3 fatty acids, papaya enzymes, iron, turmeric, Saint John's wort, calcium, and coenzyme Q_{10} (CoQ_{10}) have in common? They are all found in over-the-counter dietary supplements. Some of them have proven benefits, whereas others seem to provide the most for those who believe in them. CoQ_{10} is of special interest in disorders that seem to decrease its natural levels in the body. According to some, these disorders range from Parkinson's disease to Alzheimer's disease, to cancer. It's most commonly used to ward off cancer or in patients who suffer from heart disease.

So what does CoQ_{10} actually do? It's naturally found in the inner mitochondrial membrane of the cell and helps make adenosine triphosphate (ATP). Decreased levels of CoQ_{10} translate to decreased levels of ATP, and increasing CoQ_{10} does the opposite. Increased levels of ATP drive protein production, muscle contraction, and innumerable other biochemical processes, including those involved in immune function. In addition, as an antioxidant, CoQ_{10} counters the harmful effects of free radicals, which we most often hear about in anti-aging face cream commercials. But free radicals aren't just aesthetic obstacles; rather, they are implicated in a number of disorders including cancer, Parkinson's disease, and Alzheimer's disease (sound familiar?).

The truth is, it's not totally proven that CoQ_{10} is a miracle vitamin. In some cases, it works; in others, it doesn't. For some cancers, it helps; for others, not so much. Part of the problem is that controlled studies in humans either have not been run or have not confirmed the effects of CoQ_{10} on the progress of these disorders. In many cases, CoQ_{10} cannot be advised positively or negatively, and it's really up to the patient to try it, if so desired. It *is* advised, however, that all supplements be reported to the managing physician so that potential ill interactions can be avoided.

In this chapter, we'll observe CoQ_{10}'s antioxidant powers in the electron transport chain. We'll also learn about the other processes that harvest high-energy electrons— namely, glycolysis, pyruvate decarboxylation, and the Krebs cycle. Furthermore, we'll look at how some cells metabolize glucose without an electron transport chain. Finally, we'll analyze the energy potential in noncarbohydrate sources.

Transfer of Energy

THE FLOW OF ENERGY

All energy for living organisms is ultimately derived from the sun. **Autotrophs** are organisms that are capable of using the sun's energy to create organic molecules (e.g., glucose) that can store that energy in their bonds. By and large, plants carry out most of Earth's autotrophic functions, through the anabolic process of **photosynthesis**.

These organisms do not require an exogenous source of organic compounds. **Heterotrophic** organisms, on the other hand, derive their energy by breaking down the organic molecules made by plants, and harnessing the power held in the bonds of the molecules. Thus, as humans, we are catabolic in our energy generation.

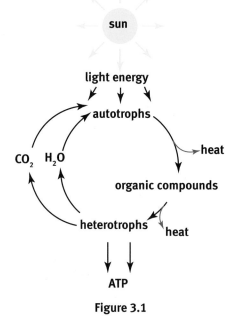

Figure 3.1

Glucose ($C_6H_{12}O_6$) is a central mediator in this process. Like many other six-carbon monosaccharides, it is capable of forming a ring structure known as a pyranose, in either an α or β configuration.

The formation of glucose by autotrophs involves the breaking of C–O bonds in CO_2 and O–H bonds in H_2O. These atoms are then rearranged into glucose while storing energy in the chemical bonds that are being formed. Because the sun's energy powers photosynthetic reactions, it is considered to be an endothermic process.

$$6\ CO_2 + 6\ H_2O + Energy \Rightarrow C_6H_{12}O_6 + 6\ O_2$$

Heterotrophic organisms liberate this energy by breaking these bonds and coupling the energy release to perform useful work. The cellular respiration equation is simply the photosynthesis equation in reverse.

$$C_6H_{12}O_6 + 6\ O_2 \Rightarrow 6\ CO_2 + 6\ H_2O + Energy$$

No machine is perfect, however; some energy must be lost along the way. Our biological systems are no exception; there is energy lost in the form of heat for each of the relevant reactions.

ENERGY CARRIERS

The energy that is released during glucose catabolism must be harnessed to provide any useful value. To do so, our cells use intermediates such as **ATP** and the coenzymes **NAD⁺** and **FAD**. These molecules serve as high-energy electron shuttles between the cytoplasm and mitochondria.

ATP

Adenosine triphosphate is the primary energy currency of the cell. Its rapid formation and degradation allow for energy to be stored and released as needed. Whereas we might equate fat with an IRA or glycogen with a certificate of deposit, ATP is the dollar bill in your wallet. You can use it immediately.

Adenosine triphosphate is generated during glucose catabolism. It consists of the nitrogenous base adenine, the sugar ribose, and three phosphate groups. Can you recall how to tell if the sugar is ribose or deoxyribose? Ribose's 2′ carbon is bound to a hydroxyl group, whereas deoxyribose's 2′ carbon is bound only to a hydrogen. The actual energy is stored in the high-energy phosphate bonds. Let's think back to our chemistry lessons: Why would these bonds be high-energy? Because it is energetically unfavorable to have so many negative charges (such as those found in phosphate groups) in close proximity to one another. To do so requires strong covalent bonding, which, when broken, releases usable energy.

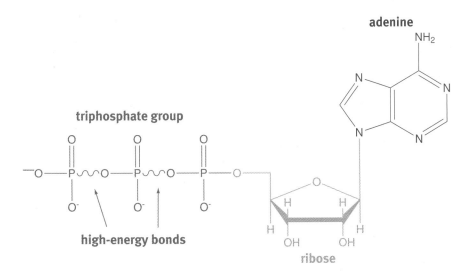

Figure 3.2

Adenosine triphosphate may be broken down into adenosine diphosphate (ADP) and inorganic phosphate (P_i) or adenosine monophosphate (AMP) and pyrophosphate (PP_i). In both cases, the release of energy is approximately 7 kcal/mol.

$$ATP \Rightarrow ADP + P_i + 7 \text{ kcal/mol}$$
$$ATP \Rightarrow AMP + PP_i + 7 \text{ kcal/mol}$$

Processes that require energy, such as muscular contraction or active transport, will be coupled to the energy release from ATP breakdown. Alternatively, glucose catabolism provides the energy necessary to reverse this process and regenerate the high-energy currency.

$$ADP + P_i + 7 \text{ kcal/mol} \Rightarrow ATP$$

NAD⁺ and FAD

Nicotinamide adenine dinucleotide (NAD^+) and flavin adenine dinucleotide (FAD) are coenzymes capable of accepting high-energy electrons during glucose oxidation. These electrons usually come in the form of hydride ions, denoted as $H:^-$. They do not provide energy themselves; rather, they are a means to an end. By passing through the **electron transport chain**, ATP can be generated by using their captured stored energy. It's like returning a shirt that you bought so that you can get the money back (ATP). The unworn shirt is worth a certain amount of money and holds that value until you return it.

Redox reactions are often tested in the chemistry sections, but by no means are they absent from biology. Recall that reduction results in a lowering of oxidation state and oxidation results in an increase in oxidation state. Can we imagine how this will come into play in cellular respiration?

Cellular respiration is just one big series of redox reactions. When NAD^+ and FAD accept hydride ions during glycolysis and the Krebs cycle, they are **reduced** to NADH and $FADH_2$, respectively. The hydride electrons are carried to the electron transport chain on the inner mitochondrial membrane, where they are liberated to produce ATP. That liberation reverses (i.e., **oxidizes**) NADH and $FADH_2$ to their original forms.

oxidized form		reduced form
NAD^+	$\xrightarrow{H:^-}$	NADH
FAD	$\xrightarrow{2H}$	$FADH_2$

Figure 3.3

Bridge

Hydride ions are very strong reducing agents. Two reagents we'll often see are $LiAlH_4$, lithium aluminum hydride, and $NaBH_4$, sodium borohydride.

Key Concept

These redox reactions do not directly produce usable energy. Rather, they transport high-energy electrons to a final electron acceptor (oxygen), which is coupled to ATP generation.

Glucose Catabolism ★★★★★★

At last, we have arrived at meat of this chapter. Heterotrophic cells require glucose as their primary source of fuel. The energy they contain is liberated through two distinct processes: **glycolysis** and **cellular respiration**. As we start examining these processes, recall from earlier chapters that we emphasized the ability of the eukaryote to separate different chemical reactions into different subcellular organelles. We will see that principle in action throughout this chapter.

GLYCOLYSIS

Glycolysis is a series of reactions that break down glucose into two smaller organic molecules. Before we become too worried about the various steps and intermediates, however, let's remember that the MCAT is more interested in our overall understanding of the concepts. We don't need to know a series of reactions. In fact, for our purposes, we can consider all of glycolysis to be one smooth reaction. All we need to know are net inputs and outputs for that "one reaction." We'll guide you through the relevant information in the next few pages.

Glycolytic Pathway

Glycolysis occurs in the cytoplasm, in the presence or absence of oxygen. The pathway is outlined for us in Figure 3.4, but we'll learn just enough to focus on the inputs and outputs. First, let's glance at the products of step 4. **Dihydroxyacetone phosphate** isomerizes into a second molecule of **glyceraldehyde 3-phosphate (PGAL)**. Takeaway? Since we now have twice as many PGALs as glucoses, steps five through nine will all be occurring twice as many times as steps one through four, per molecule of glucose. Starting with organic molecules, let's count our inputs and outputs. Our input is six-carbon glucose, and our output is two molecules of three-carbon **pyruvate**. Next, let's look at our ATP inputs and outputs. Steps 1 and 3 each consume one molecule of ATP. Steps 6 and 9 each produce one ATP and occur twice—a total of four, a net of two. The direct generation of ATP from ADP and P_i is known as **substrate-level phosphorylation**. What about electron carriers? NAD^+ is reduced to NADH twice, so we start with two molecules of NAD^+ and finish with two molecules of NADH.

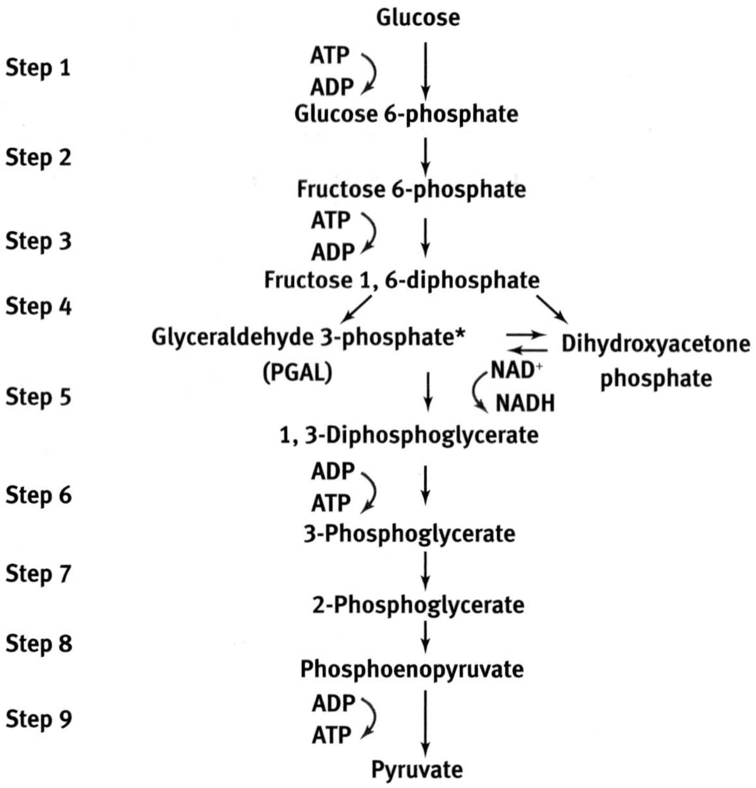
Glucose
Step 1
ATP
ADP
Glucose 6-phosphate
Step 2
Fructose 6-phosphate
Step 3
ATP
ADP
Fructose 1, 6-diphosphate
Step 4
Glyceraldehyde 3-phosphate*
(PGAL)
Dihydroxyacetone phosphate
Step 5
NAD+
NADH
1, 3-Diphosphoglycerate
Step 6
ADP
ATP
3-Phosphoglycerate
Step 7
2-Phosphoglycerate
Step 8
Phosphoenopyruvate
Step 9
ADP
ATP
Pyruvate

***NOTE: Steps 5–9 occur twice per molecule of glucose (see text).**

Figure 3.4

MCAT Expertise

You do not need to memorize the individual reactions of glycolysis for the MCAT. You do need to know the final net inputs and outputs of these reactions. Also know that this reaction is anaerobic. It can occur in the absence of oxygen.

The net reaction for glycolysis is:

$$\text{Glucose} + 2\ \text{ADP} + 2\ P_i + 2\ NAD^+ \Rightarrow 2\ \text{Pyruvate} + 2\ \text{ATP} + 2\ \text{NADH} + 2\ H^+ + 2\ H_2O$$

This process doesn't give us much bang for our buck. Indeed, most of the chemical energy extracted from the sun is still stored in pyruvate's bonds. Pyruvate has two potential fates based on the character of the cell's environment. It's kind of like a choose-your-own-ending novel. In aerobic organisms (those that use oxygen to survive and thrive), pyruvate undergoes further oxidation through the mitochondrial electron transport chain. In anaerobic organisms (those that function without oxygen), pyruvate undergoes an oxygen-free process called fermentation. Some cells are obligate aerobes or anaerobes, meaning that they require that designated environment. Others are facultative and prefer one environment over the other, but can survive in either.

Key Concept

Know the difference between total and net output. Glycolysis has a total energy output of four ATP but a net output of only two ATP, as the other two ATP are required to drive the process.

Fermentation

Take a quick glance back at our glycolysis equation. NAD^+ is a necessary reagent and must be present for glycolysis to occur. At the end of glycolysis, the coenzyme is present only in its reduced form, NADH. One way to regenerate NAD^+ is through oxidation in the electron transport chain, but anaerobic organisms wouldn't participate in that. So, another method is used: fermentation. Fermentation reduces pyruvate to either **ethanol** or **lactic acid**. Recall that redox reactions always occur in pairs. So if we reduce pyruvate, what are we doing to NADH? Oxidizing it back to NAD^+ so that we can recycle it for further rounds of glycolysis.

The term *fermentation* actually refers to all the steps of glycolysis plus the reduction of pyruvate. The postglycolytic reduction does not produce any new ATP, only NAD^+. This means that anaerobic organisms cash out a total of two ATP dollars. Not bad, but the payout could be much larger in the presence of oxygen.

Alcohol Fermentation

This process occurs in yeast and some bacteria; in fact, after acing the MCAT, we might want to celebrate with beverages made through this process! Pyruvate is first decarboxylated to acetaldehyde, which is then reduced by NADH to ethanol, thereby regenerating the NAD^+.

$$\text{Pyruvate (3C)} \Rightarrow CO_2 + \text{Acetaldehyde (2C)}$$
$$\text{Acetaldehyde} + \text{NADH} + H^+ \Rightarrow \text{Ethanol (2C)} + NAD^+$$

Lactic Acid Fermentation

This process occurs in some fungi and bacteria, as well as in our own mammalian muscles when oxygen demand exceeds supply. Basically, many glucose molecules are put through glycolysis, yielding twice as many molecules of pyruvate and NADH. Not all of the pyruvate can be immediately put through cellular respiration, so it builds up. Concurrently, NADH builds up, depleting cells' supply of NAD^+. To keep muscles working, pyruvate is reduced to lactic acid (3C) and NADH is oxidized back to NAD^+. Lactic acid decreases the local pH, which we feel as the burn and fatigue effects of strenuous exercise. Once oxygen supply catches up to demand, the lactic acid may be converted back to pyruvate in a process known as the **Cori cycle**. The amount of oxygen necessary to do this is known as the **oxygen debt**.

$$\text{Pyruvate (3C)} + \text{NADH} + H^+ \Rightarrow \text{Lactic Acid} + NAD^+$$

CELLULAR RESPIRATION

Whereas glycolysis seems to impart little bang for our proverbial buck (glucose), cellular respiration definitely knows how to maximize it. Indeed, it is the most efficient means of glucose catabolism, generating approximately 36 to 38 ATP per

Bridge

The conversion of acetaldehyde to ethanol is a typical reduction reaction of an aldehyde to an alcohol in organic chemistry.

Key Concept

Remember that the prefix *acet–* refers to two-carbon molecules.

molecule of glucose (in other words, a 36- to 38-dollar output for a two-dollar input). Respiration is aptly named; it is an aerobic process using an electron transport chain, with oxygen being the final electron acceptor. We noticed that glycolysis took place in the cytoplasm; we'll see a bit more action in the cytoplasm and then a move over to the mitochondria.

There are three key phases for us to cover: **pyruvate decarboxylation**, the **citric acid cycle**, and the **electron transport chain**. A productive way to keep track of these reactions will be to follow the carbons (again, the inputs and outputs). Recall that glucose has six and our two pyruvates have three each. Thus, we haven't lost any yet… but we will. As we go through the next three processes, note where carbons are split up and how many are lost. Organizing our facts this way helps us organize the intricate details for Test Day success.

Pyruvate Decarboxylation

The first step in aerobic respiration is pyruvate decarboxylation. This step itself does not require oxygen, but it only occurs once the cell commits to aerobic respiration—and that commitment is made only in the presence of oxygen. Pyruvate is transported from the cytoplasm into the mitochondrial matrix, where it is decarboxylated (i.e., loses a CO_2). The remaining acetyl (2C) group is bound to a **coenzyme A** molecule to form **acetyl-CoA**. One NAD^+ is reduced to NADH per pyruvate; in other words, two NAD^+ molecules are reduced per molecule of glucose. Acetyl-CoA is a key intermediate in the utilization of fat, protein, and other carbohydrate energy reserves. Let's keep track of our carbons. We started with six, three in each pyruvate. We are left with two acetyl-CoA molecules that have two carbons each, and release the other two as carbon dioxide molecules.

$$\text{Pyruvate (3C)} + \text{Coenzyme A} + NAD^+ \Rightarrow NADH + H^+ + \text{Acetyl CoA (2C)}$$

Citric Acid Cycle

The citric acid cycle goes by other names: the **Krebs cycle,** after the man who described it, and the **tricarboxylic acid cycle (TCA),** as many of its intermediates are tricarboxylic acids. Regardless of what we call it, the MCAT wants us to know it. The cycle starts with the combination of acetyl-CoA (2C) and oxaloacetate (4C), to generate citrate (6C). Through a series of eight reactions, two CO_2 molecules are released and oxaloacetate is regenerated. As we've mentioned before, we should know the inputs and outputs of the cycle, but the individual steps and intermediates are not particularly test-worthy.

Key Concept

Remember that glucose has six carbons. Two of the original six carbons are lost during pyruvate decarboxylation as CO_2.

Key Concept

Energy checkpoint:

2ATP (from glycolysis)

2NADH (from glycolysis)

2NADH (from decarboxylation of pyruvate)

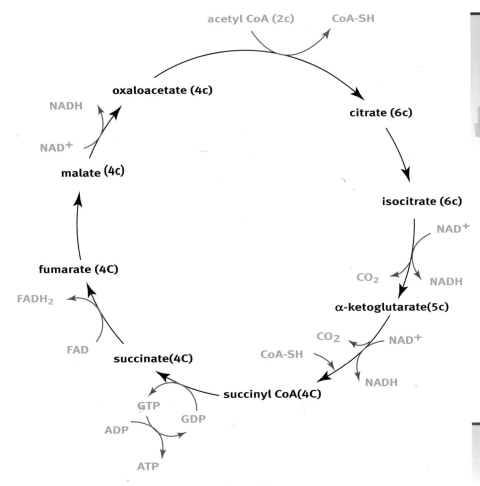

Figure 3.5

MCAT Expertise

We do not need to know the eight intermediates of the TCA cycle. We should know that the major purpose of this cycle is to generate high-energy intermediates that can be used to make ATP. Note that some ATP is generated from GTP directly, through substrate-level phosphorylation.

Key Concept

This ATP is actually made in the form of GTP, which is energetically equivalent.

The citric acid cycle doesn't directly generate much energy. Each turn of the cycle generates one ATP via substrate-level phosphorylation and a GTP intermediate, for a total of two dollars per glucose molecule. Add that to our total from before, and we have four dollars from substrate-level phosphorylation. The value of the citric acid cycle is its ability to generate high-energy electrons that are carried by NADH and $FADH_2$. For each molecule of acetyl-CoA that enters the cycle, three NADH and one $FADH_2$ are produced. Let's summarize our Krebs cycle outputs. We'll multiply all our products by two, to account for the fact that the cycle turns twice per molecule of glucose.

$$2 \times 3 \text{ NADH} \Rightarrow 6 \text{ NADH}$$
$$2 \times 1 \text{ FADH}_2 \Rightarrow 2 \text{ FADH}_2$$
$$2 \times 1 \text{ GTP (ATP)} \Rightarrow 2 \text{ ATP}$$

These coenzymes then transport the electrons to the electron transport chain on the inner mitochondrial membrane, where more ATP is produced via **oxidative**

Key Concept

Energy checkpoint:

2ATP (from glycolysis)

2NADH (from glycolysis)

2NADH (from decarboxylation of pyruvate)

6NADH (TCA cycle)

2FADH$_2$ (TCA cycle)

2ATP (TCA cycle)

phosphorylation. At the end of the citric acid cycle, oxaloacetate is regenerated in anticipation of the next round.

The overall reaction is:

$$2 \text{ Acetyl CoA} + 6 \text{ NAD}^+ + 2 \text{ FAD} + 2 \text{ GDP} + 2 \text{ P}_i + 4 \text{ H}_2\text{O} \Rightarrow$$

$$4 \text{ CO}_2 + 6 \text{ NADH} + 2 \text{ FADH}_2 + 2 \text{ ATP} + 4 \text{ H}^+ + 2\text{CoA}$$

Let's account for carbon inputs and outputs. We had a carbon input of four, two in each acetyl-CoA. Our output is four carbon dioxide molecules (two per turn). No useful organic products are left over.

Electron Transport Chain

Electron Transfer

The phases of glucose catabolism that we have reviewed to this point (glycolysis, pyruvate decarboxylation, and the TCA cycle) have reduced several high-energy electron carriers, but we have not yet been able to use that harnessed energy. In other words, we have a lot of valuable goods but have not yet sold them for cash. The electron transport chain allows us to do so. Oxidative phosphorylation is the process by which electrons from NADH and FADH_2 are passed along an assembly line of carriers that release free energy with each transfer. That free energy is put toward ATP production. Most of these carriers are enzymes known as **cytochromes**. They resemble hemoglobin in that they each contain a central iron atom that can undergo reversible redox reactions as electrons bind and release. Like many other transition metals, iron can be present in more than one oxidation state, which makes it a likely candidate to participate in redox reactions.

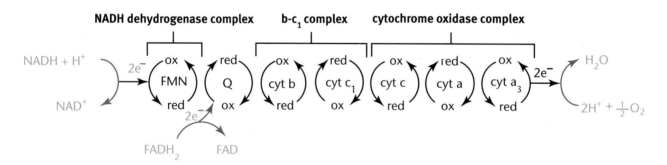

Figure 3.6

These cytochromes are best organized into three major complexes. Take a look at Figure 3.6. The first complex is called **NADH dehydrogenase (complex I)**, next is the **b-c₁ complex (complex III)**, and the last is **cytochrome oxidase (complex IV)**. You'll probably notice that we've left out two things: complex II and carrier Q. Let's get into a bit more detail.

First, NADH gives its electrons directly to **FMN** (**flavin mononucleotide**), which is part of complex I. Those electrons are then passed to **carrier Q** (**ubiquinone**). Carrier Q is a small hydrophobic molecule, not an enzyme (protein) like its neighbors. It's as important as the others, but just isn't named the same way. Carrier Q passes the electrons on to complex III, which donates them to complex IV. Oxygen takes the electrons from **cytochrome a_3**, a protein in complex IV, along with two protons to make water. The energy from each NADH generates three ATP molecules.

The $FADH_2$ molecules each generate only two ATP molecules. Why? Their electrons don't start with complex I. They're actually given directly to **complex II**, **succinate-Q oxidoreductase**. Complex II gives those electrons to carrier Q, and the rest of the pathway is the same as NADH's. Let's visualize complex II directly above carrier Q in the membrane. $FADH_2$'s high-energy electrons travel a shorter distance to get to oxygen, and therefore, less energy is extracted from them.

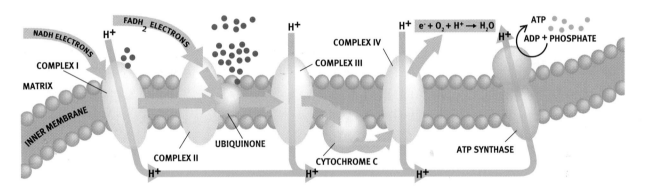

Figure 3.7

$$2 H^+ + 2 e^- + \tfrac{1}{2} O_2 \Rightarrow H_2O$$

When will the electron transport chain not be a viable method of regenerating NAD^+ and FAD? We've already discussed that fermentation occurs concurrently with oxygen debt. In addition, certain poisons can inhibit the system. **Cyanide** blocks the final transfer of electrons to O_2 and **dinitrophenol** (**DNP**) destroys the mitochondrion's ability to generate a useful proton gradient that is necessary for effective ATP generation.

ATP Generation and the Proton Pump

The actual production of energy relies on coupling the energy drops to the phosphorylation of ADP. A **proton gradient** across the inner mitochondrial membrane links the oxidation of NADH and $FADH_2$ to ADP phosphorylation. How is this gradient created? As the reduced carriers give up electrons, free

MCAT Expertise

Our cell compartmentalizes the glycolytic pathway in a location separate from pyruvate decarboxylation, the TCA cycle, and electron transport chain. Knowing the locations where these processes occur is a perennial MCAT favorite.

protons are passed into the mitochondrial matrix where they accumulate. The electron transport chain then pumps these ions out of the matrix into the intermembrane space at each of the major protein complexes. The accumulation of H⁺ in the intermembrane space makes it both positively charged and acidic. In Chapter 1 we learned that such a concentration differential is a form of stored energy. Here, the electrochemical gradient drives H⁺ passively back across the inner mitochondrial membrane into the mitochondrial matrix. This is known as the **proton-motive force**. How does this happen? We should also recall from Chapter 1 that charged species are particularly impermeable to membranes because the energetic barrier is simply too high for a charged species to navigate a large nonpolar region. Instead, we used channels: here, enzyme complexes called **ATP synthases**. As the H⁺ ions pass through these specialized channels back into the matrix, the energy released allows for the phosphorylation of ADP back to ATP. This is the process known as **oxidative phosphorylation**.

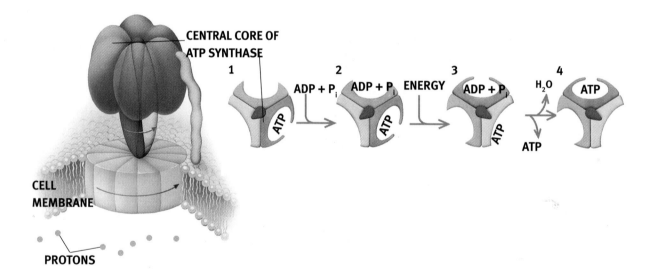

Figure 3.8

REVIEW OF GLUCOSE CATABOLISM

The overall generation of energy in glucose catabolism comes from two sources: substrate-level phosphorylation and oxidative phosphorylation (based on the generation of high-energy intermediates). The total amount of ATP generated depends on these two processes and how much of each occurs. We should be familiar with the relative amount of energy produced by each for Test Day success.

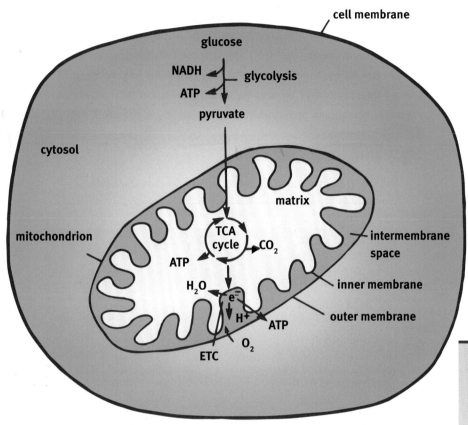

Figure 3.9

Substrate Level Phosphorylation

Degradation of one molecule of glucose will yield a net of four ATP: two net ATP from glycolysis and one ATP per turn of the TCA cycle (it turns twice, once for each acetyl-CoA).

Oxidative Phosphorylation

Follow Table 3.1 as we walk through the steps. First, we will count high-energy intermediates; then we will calculate the total ATP. Pyruvate decarboxylation yields two NADH (one for each pyruvate). Each turn of the TCA cycle gives us three NADH and one $FADH_2$; this means a total of six NADH and two $FADH_2$ because we have two acetyl-CoA molecules that enter the cycle per molecule of glucose. Each NADH can generate three ATP per molecule, except for the two from glycolysis. Those two cannot traverse the inner mitochondrial membrane, and instead give their electrons directly to carrier Q. Thus, they only generate two ATP each. So the total ATP extracted from NADH is four from glycolysis (2×2), six from pyruvate decarboxylation (2×3), and 18 from the TCA cycle (6×3). This leads to a subtotal of 28 ATP from NADH ($4 + 6 + 18$). What about $FADH_2$? There are two total $FADH_2$ molecules generated and at two ATP each, we get a total of four from $FADH_2$. When we add the four ATP generated by substrate-level phosphorylation, we have a grand total of 36. Can you imagine investing two dollars and cashing out 36? These aerobic cells are great financial planners! Prokaryotes are even more successful, they're capable of generating 38 total ATP. Can we figure out why? What is the key difference between prokaryotes and eukaryotes? Nuclei and membrane-bound organelles. Since the NADH molecules from glycolysis don't have a prokaryotic mitochondrial membrane to traverse, they save two ATP (one per NADH).

Table 3.1. Eukaryotic ATP Production per Glucose Molecule

Glycolysis		
2 ATP invested	−2	ATP
4 ATP generated	+4	ATP (substrate)
2 NADH × 2 ATP/NADH	+4	ATP (oxidative)
Pyruvate Decarboxylation		
2 NADH × 3 ATP/NADH	+ 6	ATP (oxidative)
Citric Acid Cycle		
6 NADH × 3 ATP/NADH	+18	ATP (oxidative)
2 $FADH_2$ × 2 ATP/$FADH_2$	+ 4	ATP (oxidative)
2 GTP × 1 ATP/GTP	+ 2	ATP (substrate)
Total	**+36**	**ATP**

Alternate Energy Sources

Certainly there will be times when our glucose stores run low. During those times, we can rely on other sources of energy that will be able to feed into the glycolytic and TCA pathways. These molecules fall into three large categories: carbohydrates, proteins, and fats. We will discuss the ingestion and digestion of these molecules in Chapter 7.

CARBOHYDRATES

Glucose is a monosaccharide. Sugar polymers (carbohydrates) can be broken down during digestion and then stored in the liver for later use in a polysaccharide form known as glycogen. The glycogen will be converted to glucose-6-phosphate, a glycolytic intermediate, when needed.

FATS

Fats are stored in adipose tissue in the form of triglycerides (a.k.a. triacylglycerol). Three long-chain fatty acids are esterified to a glycerol (three-carbon) molecule for long-term storage. Glycerol can be converted to PGAL, which is a glycolytic intermediate; however, the real energy of fats is stored in the fatty acids. Fatty acids will first be activated in the cytoplasm in a process requiring two ATP. They will then be transported to the mitochondrial matrix to undergo sequential rounds of **beta-oxidation**, whereby acetyl-CoA (input for the TCA cycle) will be generated. Each round of oxidation results in creation of one NADH and one $FADH_2$. Triglycerides are usually three fatty acids (16C each) bound to glycerol. Thus, they have 48 total carbons. Because we remove two at a time, we can undergo 24 total rounds of beta-oxidation, generating 24 NADH and 24 $FADH_2$. Close to 100 ATP can be generated by one fat molecule. It is an amazingly efficient form of energy storage. In an average adult human, fat stores are sufficient for one month's worth of energy needs.

PROTEINS

Proteins are polypeptides, which are themselves made up of amino acids. They are used as energy sources only when carbohydrates are insufficient. The removal of the amine moiety from amino acids by **transaminases** results in molecules known as α-keto acids. The vast majority of these acids can be converted into acetyl-CoA or are intermediates of the TCA cycle and can enter into it directly.

Key Concept

The ability of the body to use a variety of energy sources is the basis for several fad diets. Regardless of the intake, however, the same three types of molecules (carbohydrates, proteins, and fats) are used to run the body.

Metabolic Map

The relationship of the three major energy sources is diagrammed below.

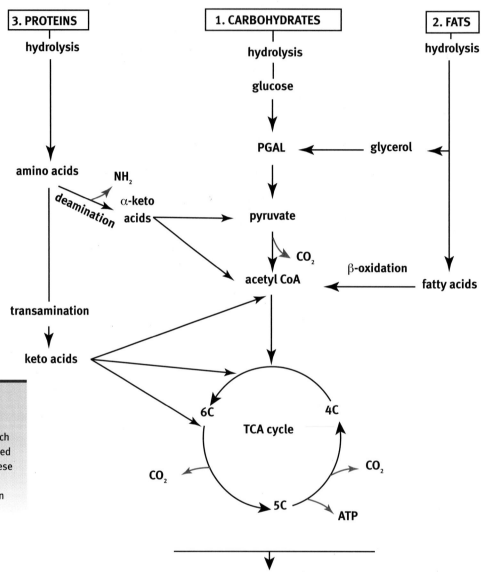

Figure 3.10

Key Concept

Remember to follow the carbons. Glucose is a six-carbon molecule; each of these carbons is eventually removed from the body in the form of CO_2. These carbon dioxide molecules are generated during pyruvate decarboxylation and the TCA cycle.

Conclusion

Cellular metabolism is a complex and intricate topic on heavy rotation on the MCAT playlist. We started by discussing energy generation from a stratospheric view, separating heterotrophs from autotrophs. We then moved on to discuss the basic energy currency of the cell, ATP, likening it to the dollar bill in our wallet. We also took time to examine the high-energy intermediates that may be used to generate ATP. Glucose catabolism made up the meat of this chapter. At a first glance, we discussed catabolism, which provided little net energy for the input; we noted that the vast majority of the energy was still stored in the high-energy bonds of pyruvate. We then went on to examine how this energy could be liberated by going through pyruvate decarboxylation, the TCA cycle, and the electron transport chain. Recall that 18 times as many ATP could be generated from aerobic processes as could be from glycolysis alone. Finally, we noted that because glucose is not our only food intake, there must be metabolic mechanisms to handle other carbohydrates, fats, and proteins. A large amount of detail was presented in this chapter; it's important to identify those points which are critical for MCAT success. As we mentioned several times, it's most important to focus on the inputs and the outputs. Let's move on to reproduction (Chapter 4), where we'll focus on a different eukaryotic organelle: the nucleus.

CONCEPTS TO REMEMBER

- ☐ Organisms may be broadly divided into heterotrophs and autotrophs; the MCAT is primarily concerned with heterotrophs.

- ☐ ATP is the primary energy currency of the cell. NAD^+ and FAD are coenzymes that may be reduced to carry high-energy electrons that can generate ATP.

- ☐ Glycolysis results in the generation of two pyruvate and two net ATP. It can be carried out by all organisms.

- ☐ Eukaryotic organisms separate the different anabolic processes (glycolysis, oxidative phosphorylation, etc.) into different organelles to compartmentalize enzymes and prevent energy loss.

- ☐ Fermentation (ethanol or lactic acid production) provides a means to regenerate NAD^+ in anaerobic organisms or aerobic organisms with oxygen debt.

- ☐ Pyruvate decarboxylation and the TCA cycle generate some ATP but are primarily responsible for capturing high-energy electrons for use in the ETC.

- ☐ Molecular oxygen is the final electron acceptor and results in the formation of water molecules.

- ☐ ATP production depends on the generation of a proton gradient across the inner mitochondrial membrane.

- ☐ The sum total of ATP generated by glucose catabolism is 36 ATP (38 in prokaryotes). The vast majority of this is due to the processes other than glycolysis.

- ☐ The interplay of carbohydrates, proteins, and fats occurs at the level of cellular metabolism; specifically, each of these molecules may be converted into glucose, one of its derivatives, or processing intermediates.

Practice Questions

1. Which of the following INCORRECTLY pairs a metabolic process with its site of occurrence?

   A. Glycolysis - cytosol
   B. Citric acid cycle – mitochondrial membrane
   C. ATP phosphorylation – cytosol and mitochondria
   D. Oxidative phosphorylation of pyruvate - mitochondria

2. Which of the following processes has a net reaction of:

   $2Acetyl\ CoA + 6NAD^+ + 2FAD + 2GDP + 2P_i + 4H_2O \rightarrow 4CO_2 + 6\ NADH + 2FADH_2 + 2GTP + 4H^+ + 2CoA$

   A. Glycolysis   *glucose → 2 pyruvate*
   B. Fermentation   *pyruvate → EtOH + lactic acid*
   C. Tricarboxylic acid cycle
   D. Electron transport chain

3. In glucose degradation O_2
   $C_6H_{12}O_2 + \cancel{H_2O} \rightarrow CO_2 + H_2O + Energy$

   A. oxygen is the final electron acceptor.
   B. oxygen is necessary for ATP synthesis.
   C. water is produced.
   D. Both A and C.

4. Fatty acids enter the catabolic pathway in the form of

   A. glycerol.
   B. adipose tissue.
   C. acetyl CoA.
   D. keto acids.

5. In which of the following reactions is the reactant <u>oxidized</u>?

   A. $FAD \rightarrow FADH_2$
   B. $NAD^+ \rightarrow NADH$
   C. $NADPH \rightarrow NADP^+$
   D. $ADP \rightarrow ATP$

6. Which of the following statements correctly identifies the purpose of <u>fermentation</u>?

   A. To use up excess pyruvate formed as a result of glycolysis
   B. To produce NAD^+ in order to continue glycolysis
   C. To produce NADH in order to continue glycolysis
   D. To prevent further increases in oxygen debt

7. In which part of the cell would you expect to find cytochrome c?

   A. Mitochondrial matrix
   B. Outer mitochondrial membrane
   C. Inner mitochondrial membrane
   D. Cytosol

8. Which of the following is <u>LEAST</u> likely to occur during oxygen debt?

   A. Buildup of lactic acid
   B. Buildup of pyruvate
   C. Decrease in pH
   D. Fatigue

9. Autotrophic organisms, as compared to heterotrophs, convert sunlight into bond energy through photosynthesis. Which of the following best describes the type of process that photosynthesis is?

A. Anabolic — synthesis
B. Catabolic — degradation
C. Glycolytic
D. Fermentation

10. In the course of glycolysis

A. NADH is reduced to NAD^+.
B. NAD^+ is oxidized to NADH.
C. glucose is degraded into two molecules of pyruvate.
D. Both A and B.

11. Which of the following correctly describes the amount of ATP produced from the high energy carrier coenzymes?

A. 1 $FADH_2$ → 1 ATP
B. 1 $FADH_2$ → 3 ATP
C. 1 NADH → 1 ATP
D. 1 NADH → 3 ATP

12. What is the total amount of ATP yielded by the catabolism of one glucose molecule via the Krebs cycle?

A. 6 ATPs
B. 12 ATPs
C. 24 ATPs
D. 36 ATPs

Small Group Questions

1. Oxidation-reduction reactions can involve a variety of molecules. Why are those involving hydrogen and oxygen of such importance in biological systems?

2. If a hole is created in a mitochondrion, can it still perform oxidative respiration? Can mitochondrial fragments perform oxidative respiration?

Explanations to Practice Questions

1. B

In order to answer this question, we have to look at each answer choice in turn. Glycolysis does indeed occur in the cytosol, so we can eliminate (A). The citric acid cycle (also known as the TCA or Krebs cycle) occurs in the mitochondrial matrix, which means that (B) incorrectly pairs the metabolic process with its site. Glancing at (C) and (D), we can confirm that they are true. Therefore, the correct answer is (B).

2. C

It is not necessary to have all the net reactions memorized for each metabolic process. All we need to answer this question correctly is to identify a few key reactants and products. In this case, we start with acetyl CoA and end with CoA. We also notice that in this reaction, NAD^+ and FAD are reduced to NADH and $FADH_2$, and that CO_2 is formed. The only metabolic process in which all of the above reactions would occur is the TCA cycle, also referred to as the Krebs or citric acid cycle. (C) is therefore the correct answer.

3. D

This question is testing our general knowledge of cellular respiration. Notice that all types of cellular respiration (aerobic and anaerobic) start with the degradation of glucose. In aerobic respiration, oxygen is the final electron acceptor, and water is therefore produced at the end of the electron transport chain. While oxygen is needed for aerobic respiration in order to produce 36 molecules of ATP, it is not necessary for ATP synthesis in general; ATP can also be produced via anaerobic processes, even though it will be made in smaller quantities. From the given answers, (D) is the correct response.

4. C

Fat molecules stored in adipose tissue can be hydrolyzed by lipases to fatty acids and glycerol. While glycerol can be converted into PGAL, a glycolytic intermediate, a fatty acid must first be activated in the cytoplasm by cleaving an ATP into cAMP. Once activated, the fatty acid is then taken to the mitochondrion where, through a series of oxidation reactions, it is converted to acetyl CoA. Thus, fatty acids are converted into acetyl CoA, which enters the TCA cycle, making (C) the correct answer.

5. C

In order to answer this question, we must remember that "reduction" is a reduction in charge through the gain of electrons, while oxidation is an increase in charge through the loss of electrons. In the case of the energy storing molecules of cellular respiration, the high potential electrons generally come from hydride ions (H^-). Since the question is asking us to determine in which reaction the reactant gets oxidized, our task is to select the equation in which the reactant loses one hydride ion. From the given choices, the only one that matches our prediction is (C). Another way to look at it is to notice that $NADP^+$ has a +1 charge, which represents an increase from the zero charge that NADPH has, suggesting that the reactant was oxidized to yield the product.

6. B

Fermentation (either alcohol fermentation or lactic acid fermentation) occurs during anaerobic conditions. In order to insure that cells have a minimum amount of energy (in the form of ATP), even during periods of oxygen deprivation, fermentation works to make sure that glycolysis continues its course. As a result of glycolysis (an anaerobic process), 2 molecules of ATP are formed. While this is a modest amount of energy, it is sufficient to maintain some metabolic processes for a limited amount of time. During this process, NAD$^+$ is reduced to NADH. In order for glycolysis to continue, however, the cells have to oxidize NADH so as to form NAD$^+$. Without NAD$^+$, glycolysis would stop and the cells would quickly run out of energy. The purpose of fermentation therefore is to produce the NAD$^+$ necessary for glycolysis by oxidizing NADH. (B) matches with our prediction and is thus the correct answer.

7. C

While you are not expected to know every last detail of cellular respiration, you should recognize the word cytochrome as being part of the cytochrome oxidase complex, which participates in the last part of the electron transport chain. Our task then becomes identifying where in the cell the ETC takes place. (C), the inner mitochondrial membrane, correctly identifies the location of the electron transport chain and is thus the correct answer.

8. B

Oxygen debt refers to the amount of oxygen that would be needed to convert the lactic acid formed through fermentation back to pyruvate. In a way, it is a measure of how far behind on oxygen the cell is. During anaerobic conditions, when the cell is deprived of oxygen, lactic acid fermentation occurs, which results in an increase in the amount of lactic acid, and consequently a decrease in the pH of the cytoplasm. This, paired with the limited amount of energy (ATP) that the cell can produce in anaerobic conditions (through glycolysis) also leads to fatigue. Thus, the least likely to occur during oxygen debt is a buildup of pyruvate. Pyruvate is used up in lactic acid fermentation in order to produce the NAD$^+$ required to maintain glycolysis. (B) is therefore the correct answer.

9. A

Autotrophic organisms (e.g., green plants) convert sunlight into bond energy that is stored in organic compounds (mainly glucose). This is achieved through the anabolic process of photosynthesis, during which carbon dioxide, water, and energy from the sun are processed to produce glucose and oxygen. Since photosynthesis is an energy-requiring process involving the biosynthesis of complex organic compounds from simpler molecules, we refer to it as anabolic. (A) is therefore the correct answer.

10. C

During glycolysis, one molecule of glucose is degraded to form two molecules of pyruvate. In this process, NAD$^+$ is reduced to form NADH, and 2 molecules of ATP are formed in the net reaction. The only choice that correctly describes glycolysis is (C).

11. D

During oxidative phosphorylation, energy is harvested from the carrier coenzymes FADH$_2$ and NADH in order to form ATP. As such, one molecule of FADH$_2$ will be oxidized to produce two molecules of ATP. Similarly, one molecule of NADH will be oxidized to produce either 2 or 3 molecules of ATP (depending on where the NADH was generated) in the electron transport chain. The only answer that correctly illustrates the amount of ATP generated from one of the high energy carrier coenzymes is (D).

12. C

You are asked to use the information provided to calculate the amount of ATP produced per glucose molecule. First, calculate the total amount of ATP produced per acetyl CoA molecule: 3×3(from NADH) + 2(FADH$_2$) + 1(GTP) = 12. Next, since each glucose molecule produces 2 Acetyl CoA molecules, multiply the answer by 2: $2 \times 12 = 24$. The final number is therefore 24, making (C) the correct answer.

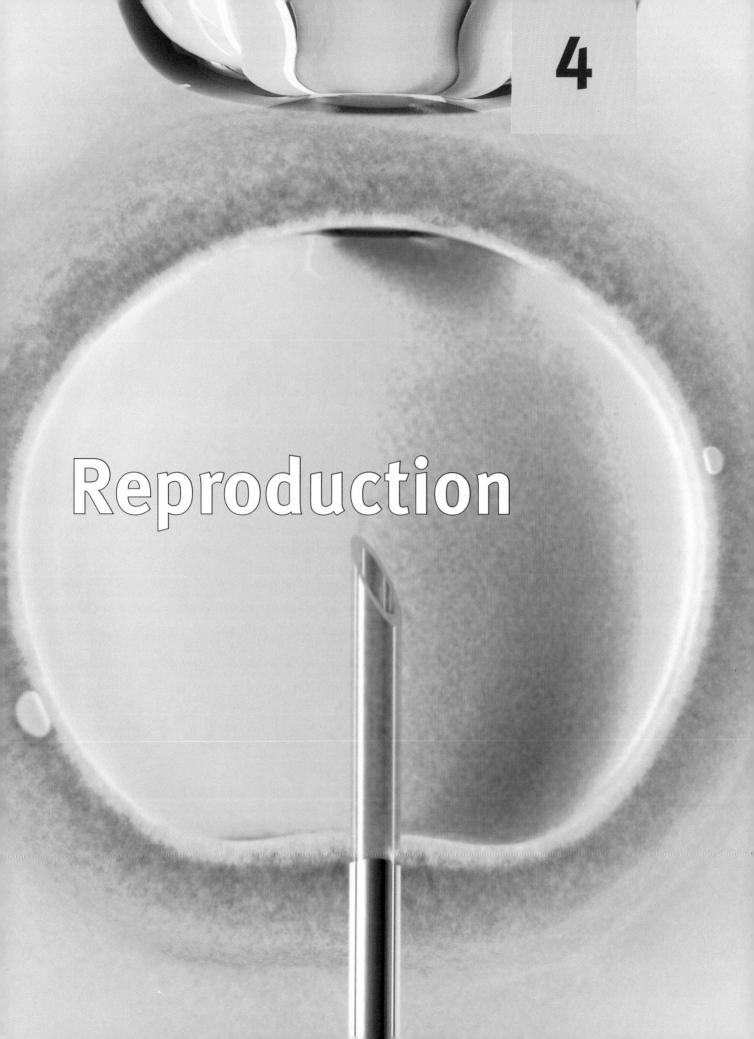

Reproduction

4

All mammals share certain characteristics: milk-producing mammary glands, three bones in the middle ear and one in the lower jaw, fur or hair, heterodont dentition (different kinds of teeth), and both sebaceous (oil-producing) and sudoriferous (sweat) glands. Those all make sense, right? We can all identify with those traits. What about the presence of a placenta during embryonic development? Sure, that's characteristic of eutherians such as humans and bats and whales. But there are two groups of mammals that birth their young a bit differently: prototherians and metatherians.

We've probably all seen illustrations of friendly-looking koalas and kangaroos, our metatherian (marsupial) friends from Australia that appear to carry their young in their pockets. A typical metatherian fetus (joey) undergoes some development in his mother's uterus, then climbs his way out of the birth canal and into her marsupium, or pouch. The pouch protects her nipples so that her joey can have full, safe access to her nourishing milk until he is ready to survive on his own.

What about prototherians? As the word's root should indicate, prototherians are probably more primitive than metatherians and eutherians. And in fact, they share more characteristics with ancestral reptiles (who evolved over 100 million years earlier) than do the other two younger groups of mammals. Reptiles encase their developing embryos within hard-shelled amniotic eggs, and lay them to be hatched. This method of development is referred to as *oviparity*. Prototherians (monotremes), though more advanced than reptiles, are also oviparous. They hold on to their eggs longer than reptiles, but do eventually lay them for hatching. More evidence? Also like reptiles, monotremes reproduce, urinate, and defecate all through the same orifice: the cloaca. In addition, their legs are on the sides of their bodies (think lizard) rather than underneath them (think dog).

Hard to imagine a mammal laying eggs, huh? Keep in mind that in order to be classified as mammals, the two living monotreme species (platypus and echidna) had to share only those specific characteristics that we already discussed with kangaroos, eared seals, and your pet cat. It might seem a little strange that something as essential as reproduction could be so different in other mammals, but the truth is, there are a wide variety of reproductive mechanisms in nature. Many organisms reproduce without a sexual partner. Others are versatile and can reproduce sexually or asexually, depending on environmental conditions. In this chapter, we'll examine some different methods of reproduction and discuss the advantages and disadvantages of each. We'll also get into the fine details of sexual reproduction, at both the cellular and tissue levels.

Cell Division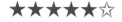

In the simplest sense, organisms must find a way to create more of the cells they are composed of. Babies certainly don't have as many cells as we do as adults. Where do

Key Concept

It's hard to believe but true—all the nucleated cells of our body, regardless of their structure and function, have exactly the same chromosomes. The only exceptions are the sex cells, which have only half as many chromosomes as somatic cells. Thus, different cell types have distinct structures and functions not because their DNA is different, but because the *expression* of what's coded in the DNA is unique to that cell type. We will discuss this in much greater detail in Chapter 5.

those extra cells come from? Cell division is the process whereby a cell replicates its DNA, doubles its organelles and cytoplasm, and then splits into two daughter cells. These cells will be identical in that they have the same genetic complement (much as identical twins have the same DNA). This is a key MCAT point to which we will return later. Cell division results in different fates for prokaryotes and eukaryotes. For prokaryotes (which are all unicellular), cell division provides a mechanism of reproduction. The same goes for unicellular eukaryotes, but for multicellular eukaryotes, cell division also replaces cells that are ready to retire.

First, let's talk about prokaryotes. These organisms divide via **binary fission**, a type of asexual reproduction (more on this shortly). Because prokaryotes have no organelles, the single DNA molecule attaches itself to the cell membrane and duplicates itself while the cell itself grows in size. The cell membrane then invaginates, or pinches inward, to create two identical daughter cells.

Eukaryotic cell division is a bit more complex. That's not a bad thing for us, because it simply means more possible points on Test Day. Since there are multiple chromosomes per cell, organisms must properly segregate these chromosomes during duplication. Moreover, we must also make new cytoplasm and organelles. Eukaryotic **autosomal** cells contain the **diploid (2n)** number of chromosomes. **Haploid,** or germ cells contain the *n* number of chromosomes. For humans, these numbers are 46 and 23, respectively; we inherit 23 of these chromosomes from each parent. Eukaryotic autosomal cells reproduce by a process known as the cell cycle.

THE CELL CYCLE

The cell cycle is a perennial MCAT favorite so let's get those synaptic connections firing as we work our way through its phases: G_1, S, G_2, and M. Mitosis is the stage in which the cells actually divide. The other three phases are collectively known as interphase.

Interphase

This is the longest part of the cell cycle. Cells that divide may spend as much as 90% of their time in this phase. On the other hand, cells that enter terminal differentiation (e.g., muscle and nerve cells) spend all of their time in an offshoot of G_1 called G_0.

G_1 Stage (Presynthetic Gap)

During this phase, cells will create organelles for energy and protein production (mitochondria, ribosomes, and endoplasmic reticulum) while also doubling in size. In addition, the passage into S (synthesis) phase is governed by a **restriction point**. Certain criteria must be met for the cell to pass the restriction point and enter the synthesis phase. Think of it this way: Would we want to go to

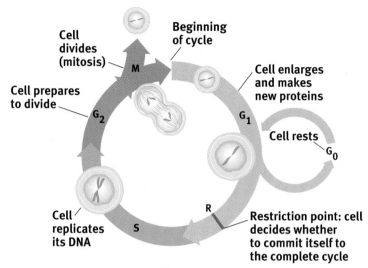

Figure 4.1

the Olympics without a proper trainer and a nutritious diet? Similarly, the cell makes sure all the necessary equipment is available and ready for S phase.

S Stage (Synthesis)

During this phase, we replicate, or synthesize, the genetic material in the cell so that each daughter cell will have identical copies. After replication, each chromosome consists of two identical **chromatids** that are bound together at a specialized region known as the **centromere**. Note that the ploidy of the cell does not change, even though the number of chromatids has doubled (in humans, 46 chromosomes and 92 chromatids). There is now twice as much DNA.

> **Key Concept**
>
> In autosomal cells, division results in two genetically identical daughter cells. In germline cells, the daughters are *not* equivalent.

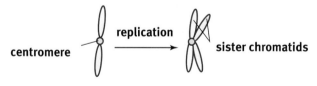

Figure 4.2

G$_2$ Stage (Postsynthetic Gap)

This is the final stage before actual cell division; think of it as quality control. We have already duplicated the DNA, and now we are just making sure that we have enough organelles and cytoplasm to make two daughter cells.

M Stage (Mitosis)

The mitotic stage consists of mitosis itself, along with cytokinesis. Mitosis is divided into four phases: prophase, metaphase, anaphase, and telophase. Cytokinesis is the splitting of the cytoplasm and organelles into the daughter cells.

Key Concept

Each chromatid is composed of a complete, double-stranded molecule of DNA. Sister chromatids are identical copies of each other. The term *chromosome* may be used to refer to either the single chromatid or the pair of chromatids attached at the centromere.

Key Concept

Mitosis

Prophase: chromosomes condense; spindles form

Metaphase: chromosomes align

Anaphase: sister chromatids separate

Telophase: new nuclear membranes form

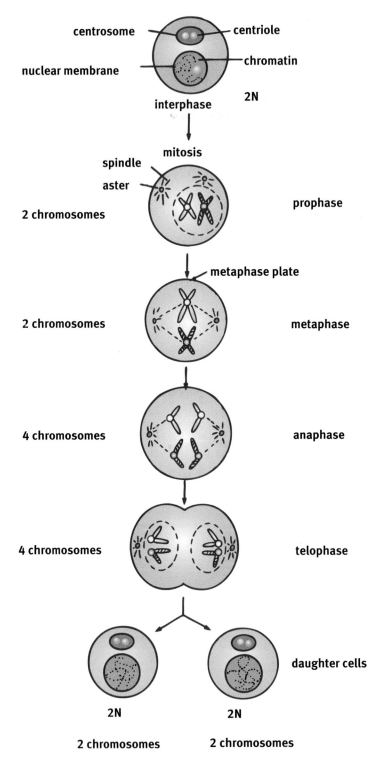

Figure 4.3

During interphase, individual chromosomes are not visible with light microscopy. They are in a less condensed form known as **chromatin**. Why would this be? During interphase, the DNA must be open so that we can transcribe genes from it and replicate it prior to cell division. During mitosis, however, it's preferable for the DNA to be tightly bound into chromosomes so that we don't lose any material during division.

The proper movement of our chromosomes depends on specialized subcellular organelles known as **centrioles.** These paired cylindrical organelles are outside the nucleus in a region known as the **centrosome** and are responsible for the correct division of the DNA. During prophase, the centrioles migrate to opposite poles of the cell and begin to form the **spindle fibers**, which are made from microtubules. Each of the fibers radiates outward from the centrioles, giving the chromosomes an attachment point for later separation during anaphase. These attachment points are known as **asters**. The asters extend toward the center of the cell to form a spindle apparatus. Subsequent shortening of this apparatus results in separation of sister chromatids.

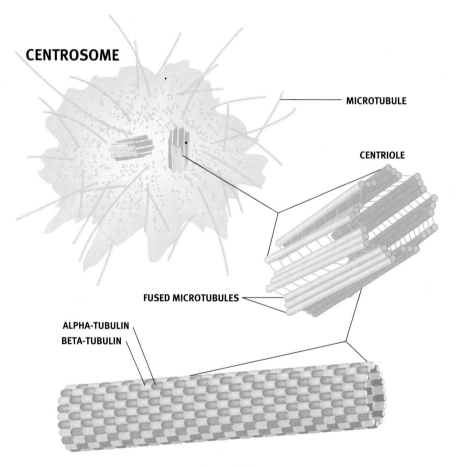

CENTROSOME

MICROTUBULE

CENTRIOLE

FUSED MICROTUBULES

ALPHA-TUBULIN
BETA-TUBULIN

Figure 4.4

Mitosis can be studied in four discrete phases, although the process itself is continuous. Indeed, we can watch certain types of quickly dividing cells undergo the entire mitotic process in about 20 minutes using nothing more than a light microscope. For the purposes of the MCAT, learn these phases and the major events in each, as they are definitely test-worthy.

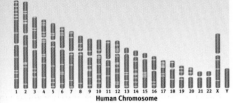

Human Chromosome

Prophase

The chromosomes condense, the centriole pairs separate and move toward opposite poles of the cell, and the spindle apparatus forms between them. The nuclear membrane dissolves, allowing spindle fibers to enter the nucleus, while the nucleoli become less distinct or disappear. Kinetochores, with attached kinetochore fibers, appear at the chromosome centromere.

Metaphase

The centriole pairs are now at opposite poles of the cell. The kinetochore fibers interact with the fibers of the spindle apparatus to align the chromosomes at the metaphase plate (equatorial plate), which is equidistant to the two poles of the spindle fibers.

Anaphase

The centromeres split, so that each chromatid has its own distinct centromere, thus allowing the sister chromatids to separate. The telomeres are the last part of the chromatids to separate. The sister chromatids are pulled toward the opposite poles of the cell by the shortening of the kinetochore fibers.

Telophase and Cytokinesis

The spindle apparatus disappears. A nuclear membrane re-forms around each set of chromosomes and the nucleoli reappear. The chromosomes uncoil, resuming their interphase form. Each of the two new nuclei has received a complete copy of the genome identical to the original genome and to each other. Cytokinesis occurs.

Cytokinesis

At the end of telophase, cytokinesis allows us to separate the cytoplasm and organelles so that each daughter cell has what it needs to survive on its own. Each cell undergoes a finite number of divisions before programmed death; for human somatic cells, this is usually between 20 and 50. After that, the cell can no longer divide without incorporating errors and will probably die without being replaced.

Some cells never undergo division (muscle and nerve), whereas others, such as cancer cells, escape this cycle and divide continuously. Indeed, unregulated cell division is one of the hallmarks of cancer.

Asexual Reproduction ★★★★☆☆

Asexual reproduction is the production of offspring from the genetic material of a single parent. It is similar to mitosis in eukaryotic cells in that the daughter cells will be genetically identical to their parents (other than random mutations that may arise during the process). We will briefly examine four different forms of asexual reproduction: **binary fission, budding, regeneration**, and **parthenogenesis**.

BINARY FISSION

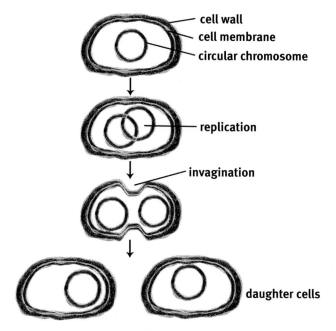

cell wall
cell membrane
circular chromosome

replication

invagination

daughter cells

Figure 4.5

This is a simple form of reproduction seen in prokaryotes (think bacteria). The circular chromosome attaches to the cell wall and replicates while the cell continues to grow in size. Eventually the plasma membrane and cell wall will begin to grow inward along the midline of the cell, to produce two equal daughter cells. This process also occurs in some simple eukaryotic cells. This process is simple so it can proceed rapidly; indeed, some strains of *Escherichia coli* can replicate every 20 minutes under ideal growth conditions. Some bacteria have plasmids of additional DNA that contribute to genetic diversity; however, this is an evolved adaptation and not the basis of binary fission.

BUDDING

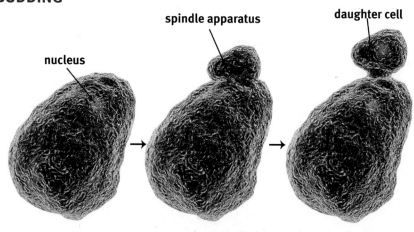

spindle apparatus

daughter cell

nucleus

Figure 4.6

Budding is *equal* replication followed by *unequal* cytokinesis. In other words, the daughter cell receives DNA identical to her parent's, but far less cytoplasm. The daughter cell may immediately break off or stay attached to the parent until it grows to full size. Budding takes place in several organisms, including hydra and yeast (both eukaryotes).

REGENERATION

One of the most fascinating topics in the entire animal kingdom is regeneration, in which an entire body part can be regrown. Lizards that lose their tails when threatened may regrow them, and annelid worms can regenerate anterior head segments. Regeneration primarily occurs in lower organisms and is accomplished by mitosis. Some animals have extensive capabilities; in fact, sea stars may reproduce their bodies from just an arm, so long as an area known as the central disk is intact. Higher organisms have more difficulty with this process, primarily due to nerve damage as central nervous system nerves do not regenerate. There are always exceptions; in humans for example, the liver exhibits extensive regenerative properties. In fact, it is now possible to perform liver transplants in which a piece of a living donor's liver is transplanted into a recipient. Both livers (or liver pieces) will grow back to the appropriate size, no worse for the wear!

PARTHENOGENESIS

Parthenogenesis is the process whereby an adult organism develops from an unfertilized egg. Many social insects (bees and ants) produce males via parthenogenesis. This process does not occur naturally in higher organisms, although it has been induced in the laboratory in rabbits. What does this mean in terms of the number of chromosomes that will be found in each cell? They will be haploid in number because only one parent contributed genetic material. The ability to think through key concepts such as this will help us when presented with new information on the MCAT.

Sexual Reproduction   ★★★★☆

The key difference in sexual reproduction that we are likely to be tested on for the MCAT is that the offspring are genetically unique. Each parent contributes one-half of the offspring's genetic material. The specialized sex cells that contribute to this process are known as **gametes** and they are produced through a process known as **meiosis**. Meiosis shares some similarities with mitosis. In both processes, for instance, genetic material must be duplicated. The differences between the two processes, however, are MCAT favorites. Mitosis results in two identical diploid ($2n$) daughter cells, whereas meiosis yields four different haploid (n) gametes; somatic cells undergo mitosis, whereas **gametocytes** undergo meiosis.

> **Key Concept**
>
> Binary fission results in two cells of equal size, whereas budding results in cells of unequal size. Both methods however, give rise to genetically identical cells.

> **Key Concept**
>
> The MCAT loves to test on the differences between mitosis and meiosis. Remember, the diploid number is maintained throughout mitosis, whereas the process of meiosis results in haploid cells.

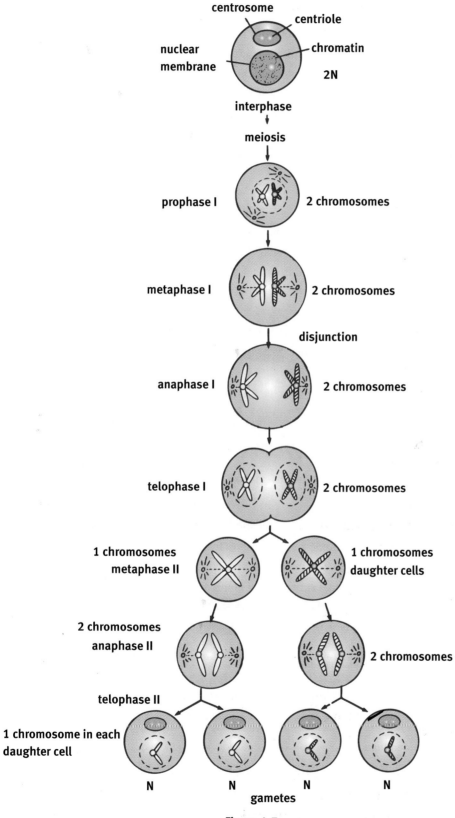

Figure 4.7

MEIOSIS

Whereas mitosis consists of one round of replication and division each, meiosis is composed of one round of replication followed by two rounds of division. Meiosis I (the first division) results in homologous chromosomes being separated, generating haploid daughter cells; this is known as the **reductional division**. Meiosis II (the second division) is similar to mitosis in that it results in the separation of sister chromatids, and is also known as the **equational division**. The result is four genetically unique haploid cells.

Prophase I

Although we begin the discussion with prophase, it's important for us to know that an interphase similar to that of mitosis duplicates homologous chromosomes in preparation for division. Homologous chromosomes code for the same genes; one is inherited from each parent. During prophase, the chromatin condenses into chromosomes, the spindle apparatus forms, and the nucleoli and nuclear membrane disappear. The first major difference between meiosis and mitosis occurs at this point. Homologous chromosomes come together and intertwine in a process called **synapsis**.

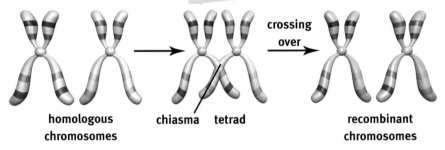

crossing over

homologous chromosomes · chiasma · tetrad · recombinant chromosomes

Figure 4.8

At this stage each chromosome consists of two sister chromatids, so each synaptic pair of homologous chromosomes contains four chromatids, and is therefore referred to as a tetrad. Chromatids of homologous chromosomes may break at the point of synapsis (**chiasma; pl: chiasmata**) and exchange equivalent pieces of DNA; this process is called **crossing over**. Note that crossing over occurs between homologous chromosomes and not between sister chromatids of the same chromosome (The latter are identical, so crossing over would not produce any change.) Those chromatids involved are left with an altered but structurally complete set of genes. Sister chromatids are no longer identical. Such genetic recombination can unlink linked genes, thereby increasing the variety of genetic combinations that can be produced via gametogenesis. Recombination among chromosomes results in increased genetic diversity within a species.

Metaphase I

Homologous pairs (tetrads) align at the equatorial plane, and each pair attaches to a separate spindle fiber by its kinetochore. Metaphase is the easiest to identify pictorially because the chromosomes are all neatly lined up on the metaphase plate. If you see a problem on the MCAT that asks you to identify stages of mitosis or meiosis, try to start with metaphase.

Anaphase I

Homologous pairs separate and are pulled to opposite poles of the cell. This process is called disjunction, and it accounts for a fundamental Mendelian law. During disjunction, each chromosome of paternal origin separates (or disjoins) from its homologue of maternal origin, and either chromosome can end up in either daughter cell. Thus, the distribution of homologous chromosomes to the two intermediate daughter cells is random with respect to parental origin. Each daughter cell will have a unique pool of alleles (genes coding for alternative forms of a given trait; e.g., yellow flowers versus purple flowers), from a random mixture of maternal and paternal origin.

Telophase I

A nuclear membrane forms around each new nucleus. At this point, each chromosome still consists of sister chromatids joined at the centromere. Are the cells haploid or diploid at this point? They are haploid; once homologous chromosomes separate, only the n number of chromosomes is left (23 in humans). There are still 46 chromatids: two per chromosome. Each chromatid within a pair, however, has the same origin (save for genetic recombination). The cell divides (by cytokinesis) into two daughter cells. Between cell divisions, there may be a short rest period, or interkinesis, during which the chromosomes partially uncoil.

Meiosis II

This second division is very similar to mitosis. Thus, we only need to learn the few salient differences between the two and we'll have a good grasp on both. We shouldn't do more work than is necessary for Test Day; instead, we should study efficiently, and this is a perfect example of how to do just that. First of all, meiosis II is not preceded by chromosomal replication. Let's go through the steps of meiosis II as a quick review. We'll see a couple more differences along the way.

Prophase II

The centrioles migrate to opposite poles and the spindle apparatus forms.

Metaphase II

The chromosomes line up along the metaphase plate. The centromeres divide, separating the chromosomes into pairs of sister chromatids.

Anaphase II

Sister chromatids are pulled to opposite poles by the spindle fibers.

Telophase II

A nuclear membrane forms around each new (haploid) nucleus. Cytokinesis follows and two daughter cells are formed. Thus, by the completion of meiosis II,

> **Key Concept**
>
> It is critical to understand how meiosis I is different from mitosis. The chromosome number is halved (reductional division) in meiosis I. The daughter cells have the haploid number of chromosomes (23 in humans). Meiosis II is similar to mitosis in that sister chromatids are separated from one another; therefore, no change in ploidy is observed.

> **Key Concept**
>
> | Mitosis | Meiosis |
> |---|---|
> | $2n \rightarrow 2n$ | $2n \rightarrow n$ |
> | Occurs in all dividing cells | Occurs in sex cells only |
> | Homologous chromosomes don't pair | Homologous chromosomes pair up at metaphase plate-forming tetrads |
> | No crossing over | Crossing over can occur |

Real World

four haploid daughter cells are produced per gametocyte. (In females, only one of these becomes a functional gamete.)

The random distribution of chromosomes in meiosis, coupled with crossing over in prophase I, enables an individual to produce gametes with many different genetic combinations. Thus, as opposed to asexual reproduction, which produces identical offspring, sexual reproduction provides the advantage of great genetic variability, which is believed to increase the capability of a species to evolve and adapt to a changing environment.

HUMAN SEXUAL REPRODUCTION

The haploid **sperm** and **ovum** fuse during fertilization to form a single-celled zygote in the **fallopian tubes**. These cells are produced by the **gonads**, which in both males and females are derived from the same embryological structure.

Male Reproductive Anatomy

In males, the primitive gonads develop into the **testes**. The testes have two functional components: the **seminiferous tubules** and the **interstitial cells** (**cells of**

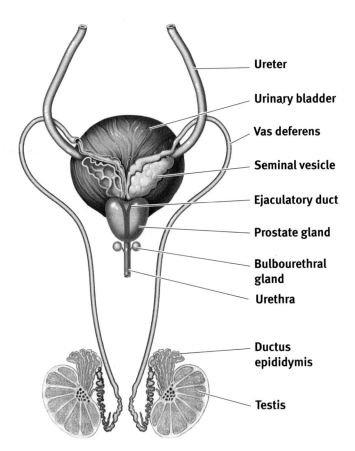

Figure 4.9

Leydig). Sperm are produced in the highly coiled seminiferous tubules, where they are nourished by **Sertoli cells**. The cells of Leydig secrete **testosterone** and other male sex hormones (**androgens**). The testes are located in the **scrotum**, which is an external pouch that hangs below the **penis** and maintains a temperature 2° to 4°C lower than the body. This temperature differential is essential to proper sperm production; if we think back to our chapter on enzymes, what might be true of enzymes that are testis-specific? Perhaps these enzymes function only at that lower temperature. This sort of critical thinking is exactly what we need on Test Day.

As sperm mature, they are passed to the **epididymis**. They gain motility in the form of a flagellum and are then stored until **ejaculation**. The maturation process of a sperm takes approximately 72 days from origination until ready for ejaculation. During ejaculation, sperm travel through the **ejaculatory duct** and **urethra**, and exit the body through the penis. In males, the reproductive and urinary systems share a common pathway; this is not the case in females.

As sperm passes through the reproductive tract, it is mixed with **seminal fluid**, which is produced through a joint effort by the **seminal vesicles**, **prostate gland**, and **bulbourethral gland**. The combination of sperm and seminal fluid is known as **semen**. The seminal vesicles contribute fructose to nourish sperm, and the prostate gland gives the fluid mildly alkaline properties so it will be able to survive the relative acidity of the female reproductive tract.

Spermatogenesis

Spermatogenesis, the formation of haploid sperm through meiosis, occurs in the seminiferous tubules. The diploid stem cells in males are known as **spermatogonia**

> **Mnemonic:**
>
> To remember the pathway of sperm from creation to ejaculation, think SEVEN UP:
>
> Seminiferous tubules
> Epididymis
> Vas deferens
> Ejaculatory duct
> (Nothing)
> Urethra
> Penis

> **Real World**
>
> Enlarged prostate glands are a common problem in older males. Because the prostate surrounds the urethra, classic symptoms of the condition are urinary frequency and urgency.

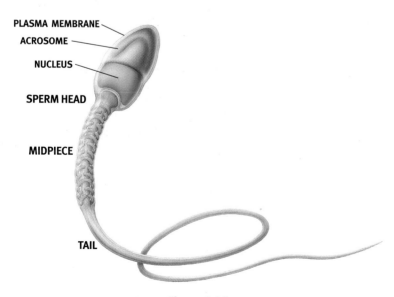

PLASMA MEMBRANE
ACROSOME
NUCLEUS
SPERM HEAD
MIDPIECE
TAIL

Figure 4.10

Key Concept

spermatogonia (2n)

↓

1° spermatocytes (2n)

↓ meiosis I

2° spermatocytes (n)

↓ meiosis II

spermatids (n)

↓

spermatozoa (n)

(sing: **spermatogonium**). In the process of differentiation, they replicate their genetic material and develop into diploid **primary spermatocytes**. The first meiotic division will result in haploid **secondary spermatocytes**, which then undergo meiosis II to generate haploid spermatids. The spermatids undergo maturation, to become **spermatozoa**. Spermatogenesis creates four functional sperm for each spermatogonium. A mature sperm is very compact. It consists of a head (containing the genetic material), a midpiece (to generate energy from fructose for motility), and a tail (for motility). What sort of organelles would we expect an abundance of in the midpiece? Since we're looking to create ATP, mitochondria would be our best bet. Each sperm head is covered by a cap known as an **acrosome**. This structure is derived from the Golgi apparatus and is necessary to penetrate the **ovum**. Once a male reaches sexual maturity (puberty), approximately 3 million sperm are produced per day.

Female Reproductive Anatomy

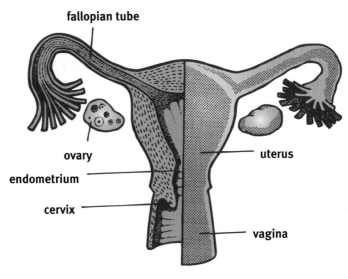

Figure 4.11

All of the female reproductive organs are internal, as opposed to external in the male. The gonads are known as **ovaries** and produce estrogen and progesterone (much more on this when we discuss the endocrine system in a later chapter). The ovaries are located below the digestive system in the pelvic cavity; each consists of thousands of **follicles**, which are multilayered sacs that contain, nourish, and protect immature ova. Between puberty and menopause, one egg per month will be released into the peritoneal sac, which lines the abdominal cavity. It then moves into the fallopian **tube**, or **oviduct**, which is lined with cilia to usher it along. The fallopian tubes are connected to the muscular **uterus**, which is the site of fetal development. The lower end of the uterus known as the **cervix** connects to the **vaginal canal**, where sperm is deposited during intercourse. The vagina is also the passageway through which childbirth occurs. The external female anatomy is known collectively as the **vulva**. As we mentioned earlier, unlike males, females have separate excretory and reproductive tracts.

Oogenesis

The production of female gametes is known as oogenesis. Although gametocytes undergo the same meiotic process in both females and males, there are some test-worthy differences to keep track of. First, there is no unending supply of stem cells analogous to spermatogonia in females. All the oogonia a woman will ever have are formed during fetal development. At birth, females have predifferenti-ated cells known as **primary oocytes**. These cells are $2n$ (like primary sperma-tocytes) and are actually frozen in prophase I. Once a woman reaches menarche, one primary oocyte per month will complete meiosis I, producing a **secondary oocyte** and a polar body. The division is characterized by unequal cytokinesis, which doles ample cytoplasm to one daughter (the secondary oocyte) and nearly none to the other (polar body). The polar body does not divide any further and never produces functional gametes. The secondary oocyte remains frozen in met-aphase II and does not complete the remainder of meiosis II unless fertilization occurs. Two cell layers surround oocytes: the **zona pellucida** and the **corona ra-diata**. Meiosis II is triggered when a sperm penetrates these layers with the help of acrosomal enzymes. The secondary oocyte undergoes the second division to split into a mature ovum and another polar body, which will eventually die. With respect to the scheme of meiosis we learned earlier, are four haploid daughter cells formed through oogenesis? Sort of. If the first polar body underwent equa-tional division, we'd have three polar bodies and one ovum as our final products. Although the ovum is the only functional gamete, all four would carry the haploid genetic material prescribed by theoretical meiosis. But, simply put, because its daughters would not be functional anyway, there is no productive reason for the first polar body to divide again. A mature ovum is a very large cell consisting of large amounts of cytoplasm and organelles.

Until menopause (usually between ages 45 and 55), women ovulate one second-ary oocyte approximately every 28 days. After menopause, the ovaries become less sensitive to their stimulating hormones (follicle-stimulating hormone [FSH] and luteinizing hormone [LH]) and eventually atrophy. So, if the ovaries contrib-ute to a negative feedback loop and are not responding to FSH and LH, what do we think will happen to the levels of these hormones? They will shoot sky-high because they have no estrogen and progesterone feedback (both of which are secreted by the ovaries). Profound physical and physiological changes usually accompany this process. We will discuss the complete interplay of FSH, LH, estrogen, and progesterone in a later chapter.

Key Concept

Remember that spermatogenesis in males is a 1:4 division, whereas in females oogenesis is 1:1.

Key Concept

1° oocyte (2n)

↓ meiosis I

2° oocyte (n)

↓ fertilization

↓ meiosis II

ovum (n)

Fertilization

Secondary oocytes are capable of being fertilized within 24 hours of ovulation. Sperm will usually survive for one to two days after ejaculation if the environment (uterine, in this case) is suitable. The fusion of these haploid cells, usually in the widest part of the fallopian tube, results in restoration of the diploid chromosome number and a cell known as a **zygote**.

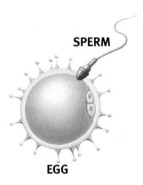

SPERM

EGG

Figure 4.12

How does fusion occur? Sperm cells secrete acrosomal enzymes to digest the corona radiata and penetrate the zona pellucida. Once the first sperm comes into direct contact with the secondary oocyte's cell membrane, it forms a tubelike structure known as the **acrosomal apparatus**, which extends to and penetrates the cell membrane. Its nucleus may then freely enter the ovum (no longer a secondary oocyte). After this process, the ovum undergoes a **cortical reaction**. Ca^{2+} ions are released into the cytoplasm, which in turn leads to the formation of the **fertilization membrane**. This membrane is impenetrable to other sperm; can we figure out why? To prevent multiple fertilizations. The release of Ca^{2+} also greatly increases the metabolic rate of the ovum and soon-to-be zygote.

Multiple Births

Monozygotic (Identical) Twins

Monozygotic twins develop when a single zygote splits into two. Because the genetic material is all the same, so, too, will be the offspring. If division is incomplete, conjoined twins may result in which the two offspring are physically attached at some point. Genetically identical offspring share the same genome and blood type.

Dizygotic (Fraternal Twins)

If two eggs are released in the same cycle, they may both be fertilized. Each zygote will implant in the uterine wall individually and develop a separate placenta, chorion, and amnion (although the placentas may fuse if the zygotes implant close to one another). Fraternal twins are no more genetically similar than any other pair of siblings.

Conclusion

We have taken a look at how cells produce more of themselves: one of the key tenets of the Cell Theory from Chapter 1. We first examined mitosis, which results in genetically identical daughter cells. We then moved on to asexual reproduction, which similarly results in genetically identical offspring. A variety of processes exist for asexual reproduction, including binary fission, budding, parthenogenesis, and regeneration. Sexual reproduction gives rise to genetically unique offspring and requires specialized cells known as gametes. Their fusion results in a zygote whose development will be discussed in Chapter 5. The generation of these cells requires a process known as meiosis, which is similar to mitosis but has several test-worthy differences. Finally, we discussed the anatomy of the male and female reproductive tracts. We will revisit these topics when we discuss the endocrine system, as well as in the next chapter, when we discuss fetal development.

CONCEPTS TO REMEMBER

☐ Reproduction is necessary for propagation of a species.

☐ Mitosis involves one round of DNA replication and one round of cellular division. Daughter cells are genetically identical.

☐ Asexual reproduction results in organisms that are genetically identical, thus severely limiting diversity in the species.

☐ Asexual reproduction is primarily used by lower organisms such as prokaryotes, yeasts, and hydra, and in certain circumstances, by some animals.

☐ Sexual reproduction provides for the combination of two genomes, resulting in genetically unique offspring.

☐ The generation of specialized sex cells for sexual reproduction is known as gametogenesis.

☐ Meiosis is a process similar to mitosis but consists of one round of replication followed by one round of division. Thus, the daughter cells are unique and haploid.

☐ The male reproductive and excretory tracts share some common structures.

☐ Females are born with all their gametes already existing as primary oocytes.

☐ Twinning can occur and result in monozygotic (genetically identical) or dizygotic (fraternal; genetically distinct) twins.

Practice Questions

1. Which of the following is the correct sequence of the development of a mature sperm cell?

   A. 1° spermatocyte → spermatid → 2° spermatocyte → spermatozoan

   B. 1° spermatocyte → 2° spermatocyte → spermatid → spermatozoan

   C. Spermatogonium → 1° spermatocyte → 2° spermatocyte → spermatozoan

   D. 1° spermatocyte → 2° spermatocyte → spermatogonium → spermatid

2. Which of the following correctly pairs the stage of development of an egg cell with the different periods in its life cycle?

   A. From birth to ovulation—prophase II

   B. At ovulation—meiosis I

   C. At ovulation—meiosis II

   D. At fertilization—meiosis I

3. Some studies suggest that in patients with Alzheimer's disease there is a defect in the way the spindle apparatus attaches to the kinetochore fibers. At which stage of mitotic division would you expect to see this problem?

   A. Prophase

   B. Metaphase

   C. Anaphase

   D. Telophase

4. If you wanted to incorporate a fluorescently labeled adenine into one of the two daughter cells that would arise as a result of mitosis, at which stage of cell development should you add in the nucleotide?

   A. G_1

   B. G_2

   C. M

   D. S

5. According to the endosymbiont hypothesis, mitochondria are bacterial descendants because they formed as a result of a eukaryotic cell engulfing a prokaryotic cell. Based on this, what type of division would you expect to see in mitochondria?

   A. Binary fission

   B. Mitosis

   C. Budding

   D. Regeneration

6. Upon ovulation, the oocyte is released into the

   A. fallopian tube.

   B. follicle.

   C. abdominal cavity.

   D. uterus.

7. Cancer cells are cells in which mitosis has gone wild. If a cure were found that could target only cancer cells without affecting normal cells, at which point in the cell cycle would the treatment effectively prevent cancer cell division?

   A. During the S stage

   B. During prophase

   C. During metaphase

   D. All of the above could work.

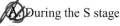

8. Which of the following INCORRECTLY pairs the term with its definition?

    A. Scrotum—location of the testes
    B. Epididymis—site of sperm maturation
    C. Vas deferens—tube connecting the epididymis to the prostate
    D. Semen—composed of seminal fluid and sperm

9. During which phase of the meiotic cycle does the cell have a diploid number of chromosomes?

    A. In the beginning of prophase I
    B. At the end of anaphase I
    C. At the end of telophase II
    D. Both A and B.

10. Which of the following does NOT contribute to genetic variability?

    A. Random fertilization of a sperm and an egg
    B. Independent assortment of homologous chromosomes
    C. Crossing over between homologous chromosomes during meiosis
    D. The interkinesis that occurs during telophase I

11. Which of the following statements correctly identifies a key difference between mitosis and meiosis?

    A. In metaphase of mitosis and metaphase of meiosis I, replicated chromosomes line up in single file. *Not in meiosis I*
    B. During anaphase of mitosis and anaphase of meiosis I, homologous chromosomes separate, but sister chromatids remain attached. *not in mitosis*
    C. At the end of telophase of mitosis and the end of telophase of meiosis I, the daughter cells are identical to the parent cell. *FALSE*
    D. During metaphase of meiosis I, homologous pairs of replicated chromosomes line up.

12. The chromosome number of an offspring produced via parthenogenesis would be

    A. diploid.
    B. haploid.
    C. 2 N.
    D. Both A and C.

13. Which of the following is true regarding prophase?

    A. The chromosomes separate and move to opposite poles of the cell.
    B. The spindle apparatus disappears.
    C. The chromosomes uncoil.
    D. The nucleoli disappear.

14. Which of the following INCORRECTLY pairs the term with its definition?

    A. Seminal vesicles—secrete sperm
    B. Urethra—the tube through which sperm is expelled from the body
    C. Seminiferous tubules—initial site of sperm formation
    D. Interstitial cells—produce testosterone and other androgens

Small Group Questions

1. Colchicine binds to tubulin and prevents its assembly into microtubules while cytochalasins bind to the ends of actin filaments and prevent their elongation. What effect would these substances have on cell division in animal cells?

2. In terms of biological diversity, would mitosis or meiosis be more important?

3. The evolutionary success of organisms depends on reproduction. Some organisms reproduce asexually while others reproduce sexually. What environmental conditions would favor sexual reproduction? What environmental conditions would favor asexual reproduction?

Explanations to Practice Questions

1. B

Diploid cells called spermatogonia differentiate into primary spermatocytes, which undergo the first meiotic division to yield two haploid secondary spermatocytes. These undergo a second meiotic division to become immature spermatids. The spermatids then undergo a series of changes leading to the production of mature sperm, or spermatozoa. The only answer that correctly identifies the sequence of development of a mature sperm cell is seen in (B).

2. B

From the time of birth until a few hours before ovulation, all egg cells are arrested at the prophase stage of meiosis I. These cells are referred to as primary oocytes. At ovulation, the egg cell has completed meiosis I and is now a haploid cell called a secondary oocyte. When a sperm penetrates the outer layers of the secondary oocyte, it undergoes meiosis II to become a mature ovum. The nucleus of the ovum fuses with the sperm to form a diploid zygote; if fertilization does not occur, the secondary oocyte will not undergo meiosis II. (B) is therefore the correct answer.

3. B

The spindle apparatus interacts with the kinetochore fibers in order to align the chromosomes on the equatorial plate during metaphase. (B) is therefore the correct answer.

4. D

In order to insure that the labeled adenine will be incorporated into the DNA of one of the daughter cells, we have to insert the nucleotide when the DNA of the parent cell replicates. As such, when each chromosome is replicated, one of the chromatids will include the labeled nucleotide. When the cell undergoes mitosis, only one of the daughter cells will contain the labeled adenine. The chromosomes are replicated during the S stage, where the *S* stands for *synthesis*. After replication, the chromosomes consist of two identical sister chromatids held together at a central region called the centromere. However, in our case, because we only added one labeled nucleotide, only one of the chromatids will contain it. Therefore, although the DNA sequence will be identical and the two chromatids will behave the same, we can easily distinguish one from the other. (D) correctly identifies the developmental stage at which we should include the labeled adenine to transfer it to only one of the new daughter cells.

5. A

Since mitochondria are bacterial descendents and possess their own DNA, we would expect them to divide in the same fashion as any other prokaryote. As such, we would expect mitochondria to divide through binary fission, a simple form of asexual reproduction. In binary fission, the chromosome replicates, and a new plasma membrane grows inward along the midline of the cell, dividing it into two equally sized cells, each one containing a duplicate of the parent chromosome. (A) is therefore the correct answer.

6. C

This subtle point about ovulation eludes most students and remains hard to believe until the organs are examined in anatomy class in medical school. The ruptured ovarian follicle releases an oocyte into the abdominal cavity, close to the entrance of the fallopian tube. With the aid of beating cilia, the oocyte is drawn into the fallopian tube, through which it travels until it reaches the uterus. If it is fertilized (in the fallopian tube), it will implant in the uterine wall. If fertilization does not occur, it will be expelled along with the uterine lining during menstruation. (C) is therefore the correct answer.

7. D

The question is asking us to determine at which point in the cell cycle we can prevent or at least lower the number of cells undergoing mitosis. One idea would be to prevent DNA synthesis during the S stage of the cell cycle. Without the DNA being replicated, the daughter cells would not be identical, with half having a normal diploid number of chromosomes, and half having zero DNA (nonviable daughter cells). Another idea would be preventing the mitotic cycle from occurring altogether in prophase by preventing spindle apparatus formation, or preventing the nuclear membrane from dissolving, etc. Similarly, a treatment that would act on cells in the metaphase stage of the cell cycle would also interfere with the mitotic cycle. Therefore, any of the three solutions presented in the answer choices would be a viable option, making (D) the correct answer.

8. C

The surest way to answer this question is to go through each answer choice and determine which one is false. Glancing at the answer choices, we notice that (A), (B), and (D) all correctly pair the terms with their respective definitions. In (C), however, there is an error. The vas deferens is the tube that connects the epididymis to the ejaculatory duct. The prostate, on the other hand, secretes a milky fluid that protects the sperm from the acidic environment of the female reproductive tract. Sperm first mix with this alkaline fluid before reaching the epididymis. (C) is therefore the correct answer.

9. D

Although this concept is sometimes difficult to grasp, it is important to be aware of each stage of the meiotic cycle. The first part of meiosis, meiosis I, begins with prophase I where crossing over occurs. Homologous pairs are lined up in metaphase I and pulled apart, leaving the sister chromatids intact in anaphase I. This concept is easily missed—each daughter cell at the end of telophase I thus contains two sister chromatids in each chromosome, but is considered to be haploid because these cells do not contain a full genetic complement, but rather two copies of half a complement. These sister chromatids are then pulled apart during meiosis II. Therefore, during both prophase and anaphase I, the cell will be diploid. It is not until after telophase I that the cell becomes haploid. At any stage after telophase I, the cell is haploid. At the end of telophase II, four distinct daughter cells, each containing n number of chromosomes, are present. The correct answer therefore is (D).

10. D

To safest way to answer this question correctly is to go through each answer choice and eliminate the ones that contribute to genetic variability. The random fertilization of a sperm and an egg, the independent assortment of homologous chromosomes, and crossing over between homologous chromosomes during meiosis all contribute to genetic variability during sexual reproduction. Interkinesis refers to the fact that, during telophase I, chromosomes partially uncoil before entering meiosis II. It has no impact on genetic variability, making (D) the correct answer.

11. D

Glancing at the answer choices, we notice that they all mention metaphase, anaphase, or telophase of either mitosis or meiosis I, so let's quickly review the major differences between these two cell division cycles. In metaphase of mitosis, replicated chromosomes line up in single file; during anaphase, sister chromatids separate and move to opposite poles of the cell; finally, at the end of telophase, the two daughter cells are identical to each other and the parent cell. In metaphase I of meiosis, homologous pairs of replicated chromosomes line up; during anaphase I, the homologous chromosomes separate but sister chromatids remain attached; at the end of telophase I, the two daughter cells are distinct from each other and the parent cell because crossing over occurred during prophase I. From the given choices, only (D) correctly identifies a key difference between mitosis and meiosis.

12. B

Parthenogenesis is the development of an unfertilized egg into an adult organism. Because the organism develops from a haploid egg, all of its cells will be haploid. This process occurs naturally in certain lower organisms such as bees, ants, and salamanders. (B) is therefore the correct answer.

13. D

In prophase, the chromatin condense into chromosomes, the spindle apparatus forms, and the nucleoli and nuclear membrane disappear. (D) matches a process that occurs during prophase and is thus the correct answer.

14. A

The safest way to answer this question correctly is to go through each answer choice and determine which one gives an incorrect definition of the respective term. Starting with (A), we notice an error right away: The seminal vesicles produce and secrete seminal fluid, not sperm. Sperm are produced by the seminiferous tubules, as stated in (C). The seminal vesicles secrete a fructose-rich fluid that serves as an energy source for the highly active sperm. (A) is therefore the correct answer.

5

Embryology

"Is it a boy or a girl?" is one of the most common questions asked of pregnant women, probably second only to "When are you due?" The suspense of the baby's sex never fails to excite family and friends, although only half of all bets are won. For centuries, members of the elder generations have offered advice and suggestions on how to predict the outcome, or even plan it. "Dangle a needle over your belly by a thread. Does it swing side-to-side or in circles?"

For the modern mom-to-be, needle dangling doesn't carry the same credibility as technological advances like ultrasonography. Ultrasonography is performed by placing a probe that emits high-frequency sound waves near the tissue to be examined. Early pregnancies are often better detected through transvaginal ultrasounds, in which a probe is safely placed inside the birth canal. Older, larger pregnancies are easily viewable by transabdominal sonography. The probe transduces a photo onto a computer screen that can be measured to determine gestational age, screen for multiple pregnancies or anomalies, or determine the baby's sex. Obstetricians look for three to four parallel lines to indicate an early vulva and labial folds in female fetuses and the presence of a developing scrotal sac in males.

So how early can eager grandparents place their bets? All embryos are female by default—that is, for a male fetus to develop, it must undergo not only masculinization, but also defeminization. These processes occur (or don't) around six to eight weeks postfertilization. Don't expect any answers before 16 to 17 weeks, though, because ultrasonography equipment is not yet advanced enough to give immediate answers. Human childbirth has existed for a couple of million years, whereas these techniques don't date back even a hundred. We'll stay tuned, though; who knows what will be possible in another century?

In this chapter, we'll follow the development of a unicellular, dependent zygote to an autonomously breathing baby. We'll examine how its cells divide and the way they differentiate. How the fetus connects to its mother is of great importance to us, and we'll discuss that along with an overview of the stages of pregnancy and childbirth.

Early Developmental Stages ★★★★☆☆

CLEAVAGE

The zygote takes a whirlwind ride within its first few days of existence. After fertilization in the fallopian tubes, the newly formed, single-celled entity must change both its name and address to continue to develop. In the process of moving to the uterus for implantation, it undergoes rapid mitotic cell divisions in a process called **cleavage**. The first cleavage officially creates an embryo, as it nullifies one of the

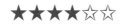

zygote's defining characteristics, unicellularity. Although several rounds of mitosis occur, the total size of the embryo remains unchanged during the first few divisions. Imagine wanting to make a nice steak dinner for a couple of study buddies. Using a kitchen cleaver, we could cut up a few pieces. Does this mean we now have more steak? No, we have more pieces but the same total amount of steak. Similarly, by dividing into progressively smaller cells (remember, these divisions are rapid, so there really isn't time for enlargement in between), the cells increase two ratios: the nuclear to cytoplasmic ratio and the surface area to volume ratio. Thus, the cells achieve increased area for gas and nutrient diffusion relative to overall volume. There are two types of cleavage: **indeterminate** and **determinate**. Indeterminate cleavage results in cells that can still develop into complete organisms.

Bridge

Monozygotic twins have identical genomes because they both originate from indeterminately cleaved cells of the same embryo.

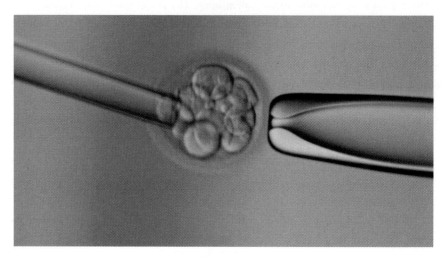

Figure 5.1

Determinate cleavage results in cells whose fates are, as they sound, determined; in other words, they are committed to **differentiating** into a certain type of cell. Think back to that steak dinner. After one cut, the beef is still versatile and can give us more than one kind of steak. But after several cuts, we begin to determine the final platter, be it filet mignon or New York strip.

For the MCAT, we should be aware of a few key time points in our embryo's development. The first, second, and third cleavages occur at 32, 60, and 72 hours postfertilization, respectively. At this point, our eight-celled embryo has completed its journey to the uterus.

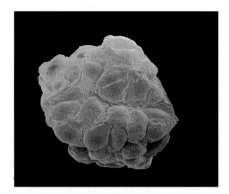

Figure 5.2

Several divisions later, the embryo becomes a solid mass of cells knows as a **morula**. That name is derived from the Latin word for *mulberry*, which might help us grasp what an embryo at this stage looks like. Next up is **blastulation**, which forms the similarly named **blastula**. Blastulas are characterized by the presence of a hollow, fluid-filled inner cavity known as a **blastocoel** (see Figure 5.3). The mammalian blastula is known as a **blastocyst** and consists of two noteworthy cell groups: the **trophoblast** and **inner cell mass**. The trophoblast cells surround the blastocoel and give rise to the chorion, whereas the inner cell mass protrudes into the blastocoel and gives rise to the organism itself.

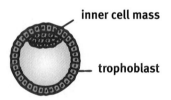

Figure 5.3

IMPLANTATION

Everything we've talked about so far happened as our zygote (and then embryo) free-wheeled its way down the fallopian tube and into the uterus. For development to continue, the blastocyst must settle down in its new home—the uterine wall. During blastulation (five to eight days postfertilization), the blastocyst implants in the **endometrium**, which has been prepared in anticipation. Specifically, the steroid hormone **progesterone** promotes proliferation of the (endometrial) mucosal layer to help the embryo implant. In addition, embryonic cells secrete enzymes that strategically burrow into the endometrial lining to allow for implantation. This is a key step, as it forms a connection to maternal circulation for nutrient and gas exchange. Implantation is like planting a tree. As we plant a seed (embryo) into the ground (endometrium), we'll want to make sure that the soil is fertile, as progesterone does to the endometrium. We'll also need a shovel to plant the seed in the ground, the same way that proteolytic enzymes allow the embryo to settle into the uterine wall. As the tree grows, it generates roots (like the **placenta**) that allow for gas and nutrient exchange with the soil (endometrium).

Mnemonic

Remember that an embryo with a "blasted-out" cavity is a blastula.

Real World

Sometimes, the blastula implants itself outside of the uterus, a situation referred to as an ectopic pregnancy. Over 95% of ectopic pregnancies occur in the fallopian tube (also known as the oviduct). Ectopic pregnancies are generally inviable because the narrow fallopian tube is not an environment in which an embryo can properly grow. If the embryo does not spontaneously abort, the tube may rupture, and a considerable amount of hemorrhaging may occur.

GASTRULATION

Once the cell mass implants, it can begin further developmental processes such as **gastrulation**, the generation of three distinct cell layers. Much of our developmental knowledge comes from the study of other organisms. In sea urchins, gastrulation begins with a small invagination in the blastula. Cells continue moving toward the invagination, resulting in elimination of the blastocoel. Imagine blowing up a beach ball but leaving the seal open. Now, as we begin to push down on a specific point, it will begin to form a two-layered cup just like our newly formed **gastrula**. The air escaping the beach ball can be likened to the loss of the blastocoel. The inner cell layer (inside of the cup and the spot to which we applied pressure) is known as the **endoderm**. The outer cell layer (and outside of the beach ball) is the **ectoderm**. The cavity created by the deep invagination is known as the **archenteron**, which later develops into the gut. The opening of the archenteron is called the **blastopore**. In **deuterostomes**, such as humans, the blastopore develops into the anus. In **protostomes**, it develops into the mouth.

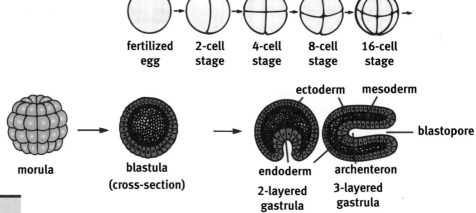

fertilized egg · 2-cell stage · 4-cell stage · 8-cell stage · 16-cell stage

morula · blastula (cross-section)

ectoderm · mesoderm · blastopore · endoderm · archenteron · 2-layered gastrula · 3-layered gastrula

Figure 5.4

Eventually some cells will also migrate into the area between the ectoderm and endoderm, generating a third cell layer known as the **mesoderm**. These primary germ layers are one of the most commonly tested MCAT topics. Knowing the structures to which they give rise will almost certainly translate into a point or two on Test Day. From the outermost to the innermost embryonic layer, they develop into:

Ectoderm—integument (including the epidermis, hair, nails, epithelium of the nose, mouth, and anal canal), lens of the eye, and the nervous system

Mesoderm—musculoskeletal system, circulatory system, excretory system, gonads, muscular and connective tissue coats of the digestive and respiratory systems

Endoderm—epithelial linings of digestive and respiratory tracts (lungs, too), and parts of the liver, pancreas, thyroid, bladder, and distal urinary and reproductive tracts

---

Mnemonic

How can we remember the blastopore's fate in protostomes versus deuterostomes? Let's think about any time we have been around toddlers or babies. When asked about their bodily habits, parents will often describe them euphemistically in terms of "number one" or "number two." Deuterostomes starts with *deu*, which sounds like *duo*, meaning *two*. Thus, in deuterostomes, the blastopore develops into the anus, associated with "number two." *Proto*– means *before*, so what comes way before the anus in the alimentary tract? The mouth.

Mnemonic

How can we keep track of our three germ layers? The ectoderm is the "attracto"-derm. These are systems and organs that attract us to other people: their looks, their eyes, and their smarts. The mesoderm is the "means"-o-derm. This is how we get from place to place in the world, and how constituents get from place to place in the body. Bone, muscle, heart, and blood vessels all allow us to do this. Finally, the endoderm is easy to remember because it gives rise to the "endernal" organs; these include parts of the long tube that runs from the mouth to the anus (digestive tract) and the organs attached to it (accessory organs of digestion). The endodermal layer also gives rise to the lungs.

WHAT ARE EMBRYONIC STEM CELLS?

Embryonic stem (ES) cells are derived from the portion of a very early stage embryo that would eventually give rise to an entire body. Because ES cells originate in this primordial stage, they retain the "pluripotent" ability to form any cell type in the body.

CELL FATE

Less than a week after a human egg is fertilized, the developing embryo contains about 100 to 150 cells that have yet to differentiate. The embryo is a hollow ball, called a blastocyst, consisting only of an outer cell mass, which in a pregnancy would later form the placenta, and an inner cell mass (ICM), which would become the fetus. Inside a womb, these cells would continue multiplying, beginning to specialize by the third week. The embryo, called a gastrula at this stage, would contain three distinctive germ layers whose descendants would ultimately form hundreds of different tissue types in the human body.

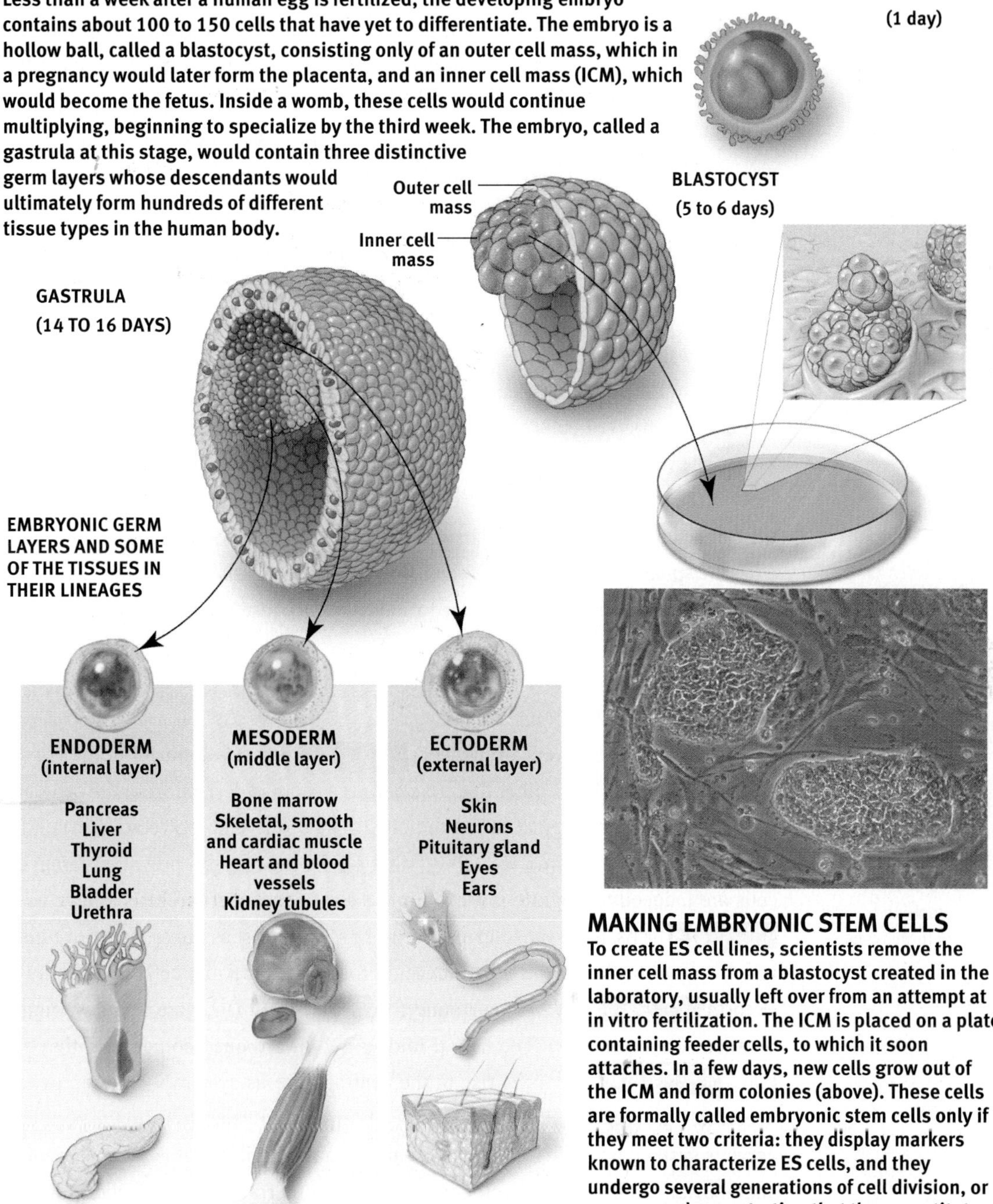

FERTILIZED EGG
(1 day)

BLASTOCYST
(5 to 6 days)

Outer cell mass

Inner cell mass

GASTRULA
(14 TO 16 DAYS)

EMBRYONIC GERM LAYERS AND SOME OF THE TISSUES IN THEIR LINEAGES

ENDODERM
(internal layer)

Pancreas
Liver
Thyroid
Lung
Bladder
Urethra

MESODERM
(middle layer)

Bone marrow
Skeletal, smooth and cardiac muscle
Heart and blood vessels
Kidney tubules

ECTODERM
(external layer)

Skin
Neurons
Pituitary gland
Eyes
Ears

MAKING EMBRYONIC STEM CELLS

To create ES cell lines, scientists remove the inner cell mass from a blastocyst created in the laboratory, usually left over from an attempt at in vitro fertilization. The ICM is placed on a plate containing feeder cells, to which it soon attaches. In a few days, new cells grow out of the ICM and form colonies (above). These cells are formally called embryonic stem cells only if they meet two criteria: they display markers known to characterize ES cells, and they undergo several generations of cell division, or passages, demonstrating that they constitute a stable, or immortalized, cell line.

Figure 5.5

You may wonder why the kidneys derive from mesodermal cells if they are contained in the abdomen. Aren't they internal organs? Well, yes, but they're not really in the abdomen. They're completely external to the gut sac (also known as the peritoneum), making them retroperitoneal organs. We won't need such detail until we get to medical school, so let's just remember "different cavity, different germ layer."

In Chapter 4, we discussed that all somatic cells in an organism contain the same DNA. They all have the same genome, so how can they differentiate to carry distinct functions? Primarily, it is by selective transcription of the genome; in other words, only the genes necessary in the eye are turned on in the eye. Imagine our seventh-grade school binder. It had five tabbed subjects: Algebra, English, Science, History, and Spanish. When we went to History class, we used only the History portion of our binder. In Spanish class, we only used the Spanish section. It's not that the other sections disappeared, but rather that we didn't need our Algebra notes to conjugate reflexive verbs.

Selective transcription is often related to the concept of induction, which is the ability of a certain group of cells to influence the fate of other nearby cells. This process is mediated by chemical substances called inducers that are passed from the organizing cells to the responsive cells. These chemicals are responsible for processes such as the guidance of neuronal axons (which is no easy feat considering that some go from the spinal cord all the way to our pinky toes). The tabs we used to organize our seventh-grade binders were similar to inducers, because they told us where to file away papers from each class.

NEURULATION

Once the three germ layers are formed, **neurulation,** or development of the nervous system, can begin. Remember that the nervous system is derived from the ectoderm. How, then, do cells originating on the outer part of the embryo (ectoderm) end up inside the final organism? Recalling what we learned in the previous paragraph, cells are induced to migrate inward. First, a rod of mesodermal cells known as the **notochord** forms along the long axis of the organism (just as our spinal cord runs up and down our back). These cells induce a group of ectodermal cells to slide inward to form **neural folds,** which surround a **neural groove** (imagine a valley running between two mountains). The neural folds grow toward one another until they fuse into a **neural tube** that gives rise to the central nervous system. At the tip of each neural fold are **neural crest cells**. These cells migrate outward to form the peripheral nervous system, including the sensory ganglia, autonomic ganglia, adrenal medulla, and Schwann cells. Finally, ectodermal cells will migrate over the neural tube and crests to cover the rudimentary nervous system.

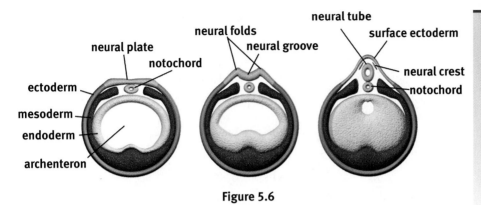

neural plate · notochord · neural folds · neural groove · neural tube · surface ectoderm · neural crest · notochord · ectoderm · mesoderm · endoderm · archenteron

Figure 5.6

Fetal Respiration

★★★★☆☆

We've mentioned that nutrient and gas exchange with maternal circulation is an important and necessary part of fetal development. This is taken care of by two specialized structures: the **placenta** and the **umbilical cord**, which develop in the weeks after fertilization. The placenta is primarily formed from an extra-embryonic membrane called the **chorion**, which, as we mentioned earlier, develops from trophoblast cells. Just like the umbilicus cord that connects astronauts to their space shuttles and provides them with oxygen, the human umbilical cord and vessels provide attachment to the chorion and nutrition for the fetus. The other three extra-embryonic membranes that we should be aware of are the **allantois, amnion,** and **yolk sac**. The allantois is surrounded by the amnion, which is a thin, tough membrane filled with **amniotic fluid** that serves as a shock absorber during pregnancy and labor (the same way our car's airbags lessen the impact of a collision). Moving outward, we come to the yolk sac, the site of early blood vessel development. Finally, the outermost embryonic layer is the chorion, which completely surrounds the other membranes, providing an added level of protection. **Chorionic villi** eventually grow into the placenta and support maternal–fetal gas exchange. Last but not least, the umbilical cord is surrounded by a jellylike matrix and is the initial connection of the fetus to the mother.

Key Concept

Although the fetus obtains its nutrients and oxygen from the mother, there is no actual mixing of the blood. Instead, the placenta allows for the close proximity of the fetal and maternal bloodstreams so that diffusion can occur between them.

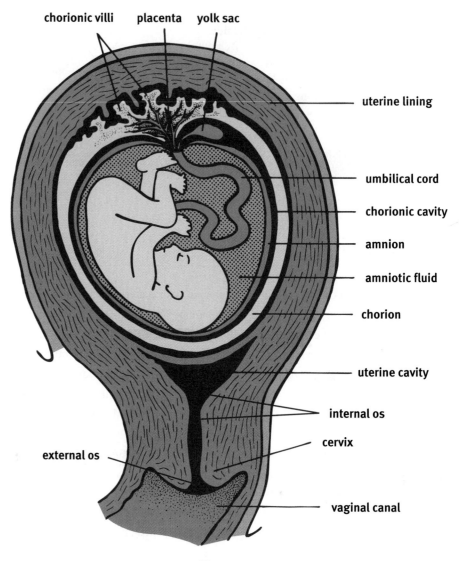

chorionic villi   placenta   yolk sac

uterine lining

umbilical cord

chorionic cavity

amnion

amniotic fluid

chorion

uterine cavity

internal os

cervix

external os

vaginal canal

Figure 5.7

Key Concept

Remember, gas exchange in the fetus occurs across the placenta. Fetal lungs do not function until birth.

Now that we have discussed the structural features of the organs of fetal development, we can examine how they function. The placenta is the organ where nutrient, gas, and waste exchanges occur. It is crucial that there be no mixing of maternal and fetal blood, as they may have different blood types. The simplest way to move nutrients and waste products would be diffusion; in fact, this is how water, glucose, amino acids, and inorganic salts are transferred. We should recall, though, that diffusion requires a gradient. So in order for oxygen to diffuse from mother to fetus, there must be a higher P_{oxygen} in maternal blood than in fetal blood. In addition to an oxygen gradient, fetal blood cells are equipped with **fetal hemoglobin** (**Hb-F**), which exhibits a greater affinity for oxygen than does maternal (adult) hemoglobin, known as Hb-A. Fetal hemoglobin's increased affinity makes it even more favorable for oxygen to diffuse away from maternal hemoglobin. Waste materials and carbon dioxide move in the opposite direction.

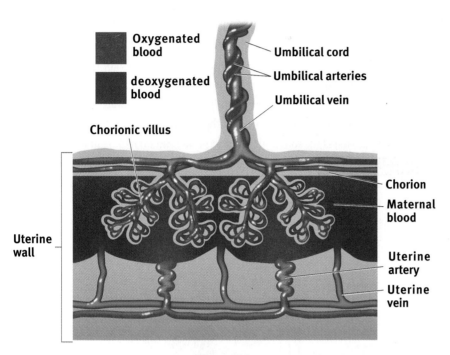

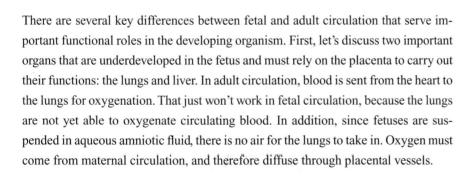

Figure 5.8

Key Concept

Consider what the fetal Hb–O$_2$ dissociation curve would look like compared with an adult's. For fetal Hb to "steal" oxygen from the maternal/adult Hb, it must demonstrate a higher affinity for O$_2$, which shifts the curve left (see Chapter 9).

The placental barrier also serves another function: immune protection. Remember that the fetus is immunologically naïve because it lacks both experience and exposure, defense-strengthening tools on which immune systems depend. Many foreign particles and bacteria are generally too large to cross the placental barrier by diffusion, but unfortunately, viruses (e.g., HIV, rubella), alcohol, and toxins (e.g., cocaine and other illicit drugs) are not. In addition, the placenta qualifies as an endocrine organ because it produces progesterone.

Fetal Circulation ★★★★★☆

There are several key differences between fetal and adult circulation that serve important functional roles in the developing organism. First, let's discuss two important organs that are underdeveloped in the fetus and must rely on the placenta to carry out their functions: the lungs and liver. In adult circulation, blood is sent from the heart to the lungs for oxygenation. That just won't work in fetal circulation, because the lungs are not yet able to oxygenate circulating blood. In addition, since fetuses are suspended in aqueous amniotic fluid, there is no air for the lungs to take in. Oxygen must come from maternal circulation, and therefore diffuse through placental vessels.

How do we keep blood away from the lungs? Two fetal shunts reroute blood within the heart. The first is called the **foramen ovale** and connects the right and left atria, with the intent that blood entering the right atrium from the superior vena cava will flow into the left atrium instead of the right ventricle, so that it can eventually be pumped out of the aorta into systemic circulation. Now, there must be some incentive for the blood to travel from the right atrium to the left, and in this case it's a pressure differential. Where is the pressure higher? The right atrium, because blood will travel spontaneously down the pressure gradient. This gradient is reversed in adults, so the foramen ovale must be shut after birth for the adult heart to function properly. We must remember, though, that the valve separating the right atrium and ventricle isn't closed shut, so not all blood will be immediately sent to the left side. The **ductus arteriosus** is present to shunt leftover blood from the pulmonary artery to the aorta. It works for the same reason that the foramen ovale does: the pressure in the right fetal heart is higher than that in the left.

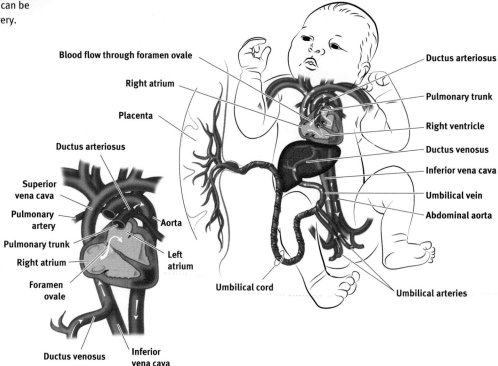

Figure 5.9

The liver is also underdeveloped, and would not be able to fully carry out its adult tasks in utero (detoxification, sugar storage, and balance, etc.) Actually, the liver's to-do list is long, which means that any blood supply that travels toward it would be put toward completing those various tasks. Since the placenta is plenty capable of pitching in during gestation, blood returning from the placenta via the umbilical vein is rerouted to the inferior vena cava via the **ductus venosus**. It's not that the fetal liver doesn't need oxygen; in fact, it needs a lot. But to prevent it from stealing oxygen designated for the rest of the body, the liver has its own reserves from arteries leaving the heart.

Speaking of shunts and vessels, we should be clear on what kind of blood the umbilical arteries and veins carry. Just like all other arteries that take blood *away* from the heart, the umbilical arteries carry blood *away* from the fetus. And just like all other veins that carry blood *toward* the heart, the umbilical veins carry blood *toward* the fetus. The best way to remember which kind of blood each carries is to recall which way the blood travels in each vessel, and to use that pathway to deduce what kind of blood is flowing. The fetus would return blood to the placenta only if all the oxygen in it were used up. Thus, the umbilical arteries carry deoxygenated blood. Similarly, the only kind of blood that the fetus wants from the placenta is oxygenated blood, so it must be the case that the umbilical veins carry oxygenated blood.

Gestation ★★★☆☆

Human pregnancy lasts an estimated 266 days, which are divided into three trimesters. As a general rule, the larger the animal, the longer the gestational period and the fewer the offspring. For example, elephants usually have one calf and gestate for 22 months (almost two years). Mice have 10 to 12 offspring per litter and gestate for only 20 days—quite a difference! Maybe their seemingly unparalleled fertility led to the old wives' tale that elephants are afraid of mice.

Although we don't need to know every detail of gestation for the MCAT (the way we will have to in medical school), there are some key developmental events with which we should be familiar.

FIRST TRIMESTER

During the first weeks, the major organs begin to develop. The heart begins to beat at approximately 22 days, and soon afterward the eyes, gonads, limbs, and liver start to form. By five weeks, the embryo is 10 mm in length and by week six, it has grown to 15 mm. The cartilaginous skeleton begins to harden into bone by the seventh week (see Chapter 6). By the end of eight weeks, most of the organs have formed, the brain is fairly developed, and the embryo is referred to as a fetus. At the end of the third month, the fetus is about 9 cm long.

SECOND TRIMESTER

During the second trimester, the fetus undergoes a tremendous amount of growth. It begins to move around in the amniotic fluid, its face appears human, and its toes and fingers elongate. By the end of the sixth month, the fetus measures 30 to 36 cm long.

THIRD TRIMESTER

The seventh and eighth months are characterized by continued rapid growth and further brain development. During the ninth month, antibodies are transported by highly selective active transport from the mother to the fetus for protection against foreign matter, in preparation for life outside the womb. The growth rate slows and the fetus becomes less active, as it has less room to move about.

Real World

Advances in medicine have allowed babies to be born as early as 24 weeks, which is far short of a normal 39. There is a chance that these neonates may survive, although there are often severe complications as fetal development is not complete at 24 weeks. These problems are most apparent in the respiratory system due to insufficient surfactant production; more on this in Chapter 8.

Birth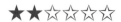

Vaginal childbirth is accomplished by rhythmic contractions of uterine smooth muscle, coordinated by prostaglandins and the peptide hormone oxytocin. Birth consists of three basic phases. First, the cervix thins out and the amniotic sac ruptures, which is commonly known as the *water breaking*. Next, strong uterine contractions result in the birth of the fetus. Finally, the placenta and umbilical cord are expelled. These are often referred to as *afterbirth*.

Conclusion

Our chapter has taken us through the rapid development of a single-celled zygote to the birth of a full-fledged baby. What normally takes nine months, we have accomplished in only a few pages!

Adult structures that arise from embryonic germ layers are of special importance to us because they are commonly tested on the MCAT. How about the rest of it? From the first cleavage to the last uterine contraction, we should simply extract the main structures and highlights of embryonic development in addition to the differences between fetal and adult physiology. Now that we are familiar with prenatal development, we'll move on to discuss adult organ systems in the next few chapters. Keep an eye out for Chapters 8 and 9 (adult circulatory and respiratory systems), which we can use as reference points for studying fetal physiology.

CONCEPTS TO REMEMBER

- ☐ The zygote undergoes several rapid divisions which ultimately result in determinate cleavage.

- ☐ Indeterminate cleavage allows for the generation of identical twins.

- ☐ Implantation of the embryo into the endometrium is necessary for proper and successful growth.

- ☐ Gastrulation is the generation of three primary germ layers: ectoderm, endoderm, and mesoderm.

- ☐ Each of the primary germ layers gives rise to specific organs and structures. This is an exceedingly important topic to be familiar with for Test Day success.

- ☐ The development of the nervous system is known as neurulation and occurs during gastrulation.

- ☐ Fetal respiration is carried out at the placenta and not in the developing lungs.

- ☐ Fetal circulation contains 3 shunts: the ductus venosus, the foramen ovale, and the ductus arteriosus, which serve to bypass blood from the liver and lungs.

- ☐ Gestation consists of 3 trimesters of 3 months each; certain key developmental milestones are reached during each trimester.

- ☐ Vaginal childbirth is accomplished by coordinated and rhythmic contractions of uterine smooth muscle.

Practice Questions

1. Which of the following developmental stages has the greatest nuclear-to-cytoplasmic material ratio?

   A. Eight-cell zygote
   B. Morula
   C. Blastula
   D. Archenteron

2. Which of the following associations is INCORRECT?

   A. Endoderm—thyroid
   B. Endoderm—lens of the eye
   C. Ectoderm—nails
   D. Mesoderm—kidneys

3. Which of the following changes does NOT occur immediately after birth?

   A. The infant begins to produce adult hemoglobin.
   B. Resistance in the pulmonary arteries decreases.
   C. Pressure in the left atrium increases.
   D. Pressure in both the inferior vena cava and the right atrium increases.

4. During which period is a teratogen most likely to affect brain development during gestation?

   A. First trimester
   B. Second trimester
   C. Third trimester
   D. At birth

5. From which of the following germ layers does the notochord form?

   A. Ectoderm
   B. Mesoderm
   C. Endoderm
   D. Archenteron

6. The influence of a specific group of cells on the differentiation of another group of cells is referred to as

   A. neurulation.
   B. indeterminate cleavage.
   C. determinate cleavage.
   D. induction.

7. Which of the following structures is NOT formed from the endoderm?

   A. Pancreas
   B. Lining of the respiratory tract
   C. Circulatory system
   D. Liver

8. Which of the following is true regarding fetal hemoglobin?

   A. It continues to be produced for a few months after birth.
   B. It can be found in small quantities in the mother's blood during pregnancy.
   C. It has a greater affinity for oxygen than adult hemoglobin.
   D. It can help transport vitamins across the maternal capillaries to fetal blood.

9. Which of the following may be found in the mother's bloodstream?

    A. hCG
    B. Fetal white blood cells
    C. CO_2 produced by fetal cells
    D. Two of the above

10. Which of the following INCORRECTLY pairs the fetal circulation shunt with its function?

    A. Ductus venosus—bypasses the liver
    B. Ductus venosus—bypasses the pulmonary veins
    C. Ductus arteriosus—directs blood from the pulmonary artery to the aorta *True*
    D. Ductus arteriosus—prevents blood from entering the lungs *True*

11. Which of the following blood vessels do NOT contain deoxygenated blood? *which contain O_2?*

    A. Fetal umbilical artery
    B. Adult pulmonary arteries
    C. Fetal umbilical vein
    D. Superior vena cava

12. Which of the following statements is FALSE?

    A. In fetal circulation, blood is oxygenated in the placenta.
    B. A small amount of blood reaches the fetal lungs.
    C. After birth, the blood pressure in the right atrium decreases.
    D. In fetal circulation, the blood delivered via the aorta has a higher partial pressure of oxygen than the blood that was delivered to the lungs.

13. Which of the following changes to fetal circulation occurs after birth?

    A. Increased left atrial pressure coupled with decreased right atrial pressure causes the foramen ovale to close.
    B. The ductus venosus degenerates over time, completely closing three months after birth.
    C. The infant starts to produce adult hemoglobin.
    D. All of the above.

14. The placenta releases all of the following hormones EXCEPT

    A. progesterone.
    B. IH.
    C. hCG.
    D. estrogen.

Small Group Questions

1. What would happen if a mammalian embryo failed to produce sufficient amounts of human chorionic gonadotropin (hCG) in early pregnancy?

2. Compare and contrast fetal and adult circulation.

3. Why can the allantois be considered an adaptation to terrestrial life?

Explanations to Practice Questions

1. C

The question is asking us to determine the developmental stage with the greatest nuclear-to-cytoplasmic material ratio. During the series of rapid mitotic divisions known as cleavage, the number of cells increases dramatically without a corresponding increase in the amount of cytoplasm. As such, a high ratio of nuclear-to-cytoplasmic material will be found at the stage with the greatest amount of cells. From the given choices, the stage with the greatest number of cells is the blastula. (C) is therefore the correct answer.

2. B

In order to answer this question, it could be useful to quickly review the embryonic layers. The ectoderm gives rise to the integument (the epidermis, hair, nails, and epithelium of the nose, mouth, and anal canal), the lens of the eye, and the nervous system. The endoderm gives rise to the epithelial linings of the digestive and respiratory tracts and parts of the liver, pancreas, thyroid, and bladder. Finally, from the mesoderm arise the musculoskeletal system, the circulatory system, the excretory system, and the gonads. Therefore, the only incorrect association can be found in (B), since the lens of the eye is derived from the ectoderm.

3. D

The safest way to answer this question is to review all the answer choices and eliminate the ones that do occur immediately after birth. When a baby is born, she can finally breathe air, and thus no longer needs fetal hemoglobin to extract oxygen from her mother's blood. Right away, the infant begins to produce adult hemoglobin. Because she starts breathing, resistance in the pulmonary vessels decreases, which causes an increase in blood flow through the lungs. Along with it, as normal blood circulation

begins, the foramen ovale snaps closed and the ductus arteriosus and ductus venosus constrict, the pressure in the left atrium increases. So far, we can eliminate (A), (B), and (C). However, when blood flow through the umbilical cord stops, the blood pressure in the inferior vena cava decreases, causing a decrease in the pressure in the right atrium. (D) states the exact opposite of this, making (D) the correct answer.

4. A

The question is basically asking us when exactly during human pregnancy the brain develops. During the first weeks of gestation, the major organs begin to develop, among them the brain. This explains why it is so dangerous when women who do not know they are pregnant consume alcoholic drinks; even a small amount of alcohol in the first trimester can harm the embryo's brain development, possibly leading to fetal alcohol syndrome. (A), first trimester, is thus the correct answer.

5. B

A rod of mesodermal cells, called the notochord, develops along the longitudinal axis just under the dorsal layer of ectoderm. Through inductive effects from the notochord, the overlying ectoderm starts bending inward and forms a groove on the dorsal surface of the embryo. The dorsal ectoderm will eventually pinch off and develop into the spinal cord and brain. (B) is therefore the correct answer.

6. D

The influence of a specific group of cells on the differentiation of another group of cells is termed *induction*. For example, the eyes are formed through a constant back-and-forth game of induction from the brain on the ectoderm and the ectoderm on the brain, each one influencing the other at different stages of development, until, little by little, all the parts of the eye are formed. (D) is therefore the correct answer.

7. C

Before looking at the answer choices, let's quickly review the different structures that arise from the endoderm. The endoderm is responsible for the differential development of the epithelial linings of the digestive and respiratory tracts (including the lungs), parts of the liver, pancreas, thyroid, and bladder. From the answer choices, the only structure that is not formed from the endoderm is the circulatory system. In fact, the circulatory system is formed from the mesoderm, making (C) the correct answer.

8. C

The main points to remember about fetal hemoglobin are that it has a higher affinity for oxygen than adult hemoglobin, and it stops being produced at birth, when the infant can breathe on its own and is capable of making adult hemoglobin. Therefore, the correct answer is (C).

9. D

The bloodstreams of the mother and fetus are not directly connected. Large macromolecules and cells cannot cross the placental barrier. However, smaller molecules such as ethanol, drugs, and hormones can cross the placenta. Thus, the mother may have detectable hCG in her blood, but fetal white blood cells should not be found in her bloodstream. CO_2 released during fetal respiration diffuses through the placenta into maternal circulation, so fetal CO_2 would also be found in maternal blood. (D) is therefore the correct answer.

10. B

Glancing at the answer choices, we notice that they can be divided into two groups: half mention the ductus venosus, while the others mention the ductus arteriosus. Let's quickly review the function of each of these shunts in fetal circulation. Since the liver is not yet formed and not yet ready to break down toxins, blood must be shunted away from it. This is accomplished via the ductus venosus,

allowing blood to bypass the liver before converging with the inferior vena cava. In addition, because the fetus obtains oxygen from the mother's blood, a shunt exists to divert blood away from the undeveloped fetal lungs. The ductus arteriosus directs blood from the pulmonary artery to the aorta, in this way preventing blood from entering the lungs. Therefore, from the given (A), (C), and (D) correctly pair the shunt with its respective function. Only (B) is false, and therefore the answer we are looking for.

11. C

Let's begin by looking at the two adult blood vessels and deciding what type of blood they carry, since adult circulation can seem more familiar than fetal circulation. The pulmonary arteries carry blood from the right ventricle to the lungs, taking deoxygenated blood from the body to the lungs where it can be oxygenated. Similarly, the superior vena cava brings blood from the upper body, such as the head and the brain, and thus contains deoxygenated blood. This leaves choices (A) and (C). In fetal circulation, the umbilical artery carries blood from the infant's body to the placenta, which means that the blood is deoxygenated. By contrast, the umbilical vein carries blood from the placenta to the fetus, and therefore contains oxygenated blood. (C) is thus the correct answer.

12. D

Let's attack this question by going through each answer choice and eliminating the ones that are true. (A) states that in fetal circulation, blood is oxygenated in the placenta. This is a true statement. In the fetus, the lungs do not oxygenate blood as they do in adult circulation. However, a small amount of blood must and does reach the pulmonary circulation to nourish the developing lungs. Therefore, we can eliminate (B). Next, (C) states that at birth, the blood pressure in the right atrium decreases. Indeed, when the umbilical blood flow stops, the blood pressure in the inferior vena cava decreases, causing a decrease in the pressure in the right atrium. We are left with (D). In fetal circulation, the blood delivered via the aorta will have a lower partial pressure of oxygen than the blood delivered to the lungs. This is because oxygenated and deoxygenated blood mix in the heart through the foramen ovale. Also, the deoxygenated blood bypasses the lungs through the ductus arteriosus, which allows blood to pass from the pulmonary arteries to the aorta. Thus, the blood in the aorta will have a lower oxygen content than the blood delivered to the lungs. (D) contains a false statement and is therefore the correct answer.

13. D

Let's answer this question by reviewing each answer choice and determining whether it is true. If we find two true statements, (D) must be the correct answer and we no longer have to read the third statement. Similarly, if we find one false statement, then (D) must be incorrect. (A) states that increased left atrial pressure coupled with decreased right atrial pressure causes the foramen ovale to close. This statement is true and important in the healthy development of an infant. If the foramen ovale, ductus arteriosus, and ductus venosus do not close soon after birth, this poses a problem that needs to be fixed through surgery or medication for the infant to thrive. Indeed, (B) must also be a true statement based on the previous explanation. The ductus venosus degenerates over time, and in most infants, is completely closed after three months. (D) must therefore be the correct answer, but let's quickly take a look at (C). The infant starts producing adult hemoglobin soon after birth, and by the end of the first year, very little fetal hemoglobin can be detected in blood. (D) is thus the correct answer.

14. B

During gestation, the placenta functions as an endocrine gland, producing the hormones progesterone, estrogen and human chorionic gonadotropin (hCG), all of which are essential for maintaining a pregnancy. From the given choices, the only hormone that is not released by the placenta is luteinizing hormone (LH), which is secreted during the normal menstrual cycle by the anterior pituitary to stimulate ovulation. (B) is therefore the correct answer.

The Musculoskeletal System

Populations affected by large disasters or traumatic events like wars or earthquakes often serve as fodder for unique medical discoveries. These discoveries may result from conditions of a disaster itself or from the subsequent recovery period. Furthermore, those conditions may be instantaneous (e.g., painful injury) or created over several years (e.g., a change in diet due to famine). During World War II, Nazi Germany bombed London for 57 consecutive days in the beginning of what came to be known as the *Blitzkrieg*, or eight-month Lightning War. Victims of the Blitz, as it is known in London, included those afflicted with a specific set of symptoms: pain and swelling, with accompanying effects of depleted blood volume (shock, weakness, low blood pressure, and decreased urine output). Less obvious was acute kidney failure, which can lead quickly to death when untreated.

What caused the Blitz victims to suffer from these symptoms? Extreme physical trauma to muscles - namely, compression - destroys skeletal muscle tissue. This condition is called rhabdomyolysis (*rhabdo–* refers to the skeleton, *myo–* to muscle, and *–lysis* to breakdown). There are other causes of this extremely painful disorder, such as electric shock, alcohol withdrawal, tetanus, or even extreme physical exercise. The symptoms alert physicians to pinpoint myocardial infarction (heart attack) as the culprit, but if any injuries are documented, rhabdomyolysis is the next suspect.

The products of skeletal muscle dissolution, some of which are toxic, circulate in the blood until they are filtered out. Creatine kinase is one of these products; in fact, rhabdomyolysis is defined as a creatine kinase level five times the normal upper limit. Myoglobin is another. Much like hemoglobin, myoglobin uses heme to carry oxygen. It is not, however, housed within a red blood cell. Thus, an erythrocyte-free urine sample that tests positive for heme points compellingly toward rhabdomyolysis. Myoglobin oxygen reserves are just one of the specialized features of muscles, as we will see in this chapter. Muscles also have unique endoplasmic reticula (called sarcoplasmic reticula) and specialized cell membranes (sarcolemmas). Some muscle cells can even contract without nervous input. In the next few pages, we'll learn all about muscles and their interactions with the body, starting with the skeletal system.

Skeletal System ★★★★☆☆

From Chapter 5, we should recall that the skeleton is derived from the mesoderm (or "means-o-derm"). Two types of skeletons exist: **exoskeletons** and **endoskeletons**. 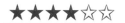 Exoskeletons encase whole organisms and are commonly are found in arthropods (e.g., shellfish and insects).

Mnemonic

Endo– means *within* (endoderm, endocytosis). *Exo–* means *outside of* (exocrine, exocytosis). We will see these roots in other chapters and should be sure to remember them for Test Day.

Vertebrates like us have **endoskeletons**. We should take a minute to think about the relative advantages of these systems. What would we like about exoskeletons? Like suits of armor, they protect entire organisms because they surround them completely. However, we can identify one major drawback. Organism growth requires shedding of the exoskeleton (picture lobsters and crabs). Our endoskeletons, on the other hand, are internal; thus, they don't protect our surfaces and organs as well as exoskeletons, but we don't need to shed them as we grow, either.

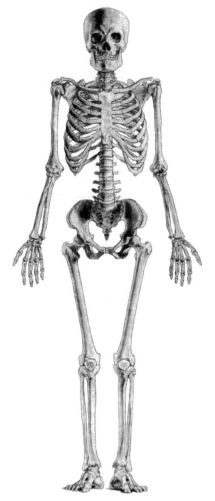

Figure 6.1

The components of our skeletal system are divided into **axial** and **appendicular** sections. The axial skeleton consists of the skull, vertebral column, and ribcage; it provides the basic central framework for the body. The appendicular skeleton consists of the arms, legs, and pelvic and pectoral girdles that are attached to the axial skeleton for stability. Our skeleton is built much like a skyscraper. The axial skeleton represents the steel beams that make up the basic core of the building and provide the overall shape. The appendicular skeleton includes the smaller beams and concrete, which also provide some structure but ultimately depend on the larger beams for attachment. Both skeleton types are eventually covered by other structures (muscle, connective tissue, and vasculature); similarly, our skyscraper would be fitted with carpets, windows, and lights that go over the steel.

The skeleton is created from two major components: **cartilage** and **bone**.

Cartilage ★★☆☆☆

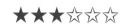

Back at summer camp, we probably often used pipe cleaners to make some of our arts and crafts projects. Cartilage is similar in that it is softer and more flexible than bone, which we might liken to a strong beam of wood. Cartilage consists of a firm (but elastic) matrix called **chondrin** that is secreted by cells called **chondrocytes**.

From our last chapter, we should recall that much of the fetal skeleton is made up of cartilage. This is highly advantageous, because fetuses need to grow in a cramped environment as well as pass lithely through the birth canal. During development (both pre- and postnatal), much of this cartilage will calcify into bone. Adults have cartilage only in body parts that need a little extra flexibility (external ear, nose, walls of the larynx and trachea, and joints). Degradation of this cartilage, usually in old age, can lead to medical issues like arthritis. Arthritis is painful because a lack of cartilage in joints leads bones to rub directly against one another. One last point we should keep in mind is that cartilage is relatively avascular (without blood and lymphatic vessels) and is not innervated. That's not to say it wouldn't hurt if a heated debate over endosymbiosis led to a punch in the nose! The pain would be transmitted through receptors in the skin and underlying tissue.

Bone ★★★★☆

Like our cartilage, bone is also comprised of connective tissue derived from embryonic mesoderm. Bone is much harder than cartilage, which is important because it must support our entire bodies. Although it is quite strong, it is also relatively lightweight. Consider that an average human femur is about 40 times as strong as concrete.

MACROSCOPIC BONE STRUCTURE

Bone's characteristic strength is derived from **compact bone**. It lives up to its name, as it is both strong and compact. The other type of bone structure is **spongy** or **cancellous** bone. Spongy bone is also well-named because it looks just like a kitchen sponge. Its lattice structure is visible under microscopy and consists of bony spicules (points) known as **trabeculae**. If we can imagine a honeycomb, then we know

---

Mnemonic

Simply remembering that the root *chondro*– relates to cartilage will clue us into both the material and the cells that make it up.

Real World

Nonarticular cartilage can grow and repair throughout life. This is why the noses and ears of many older individuals seem larger than the other features on the face.

Real World

An adult human has 206 bones. Over 100 of these are in the feet and hands.

Mnemonic

Hemo– and *hemato–* are word roots that mean *blood*. They are derived from the Ancient Greek *haima*. *Poiesis* means *to make*. Therefore, hematopoeisis is blood-making! Word roots can help us get through difficult vocabulary on Test Day.

exactly what trabeculae look like. These cavities are filled with **bone marrow**, which may be either **red** or **yellow**. Red marrow is filled with hematopoietic stem cells, which are responsible for generation of all the cells in our blood (see Chapter 9); yellow marrow is composed primarily of fat and is relatively inactive. When patients undergo bone marrow transplants, where do those transplanted cells come from? From a generous donor whose hip marrow was extracted using an extra long needle. Ouch!

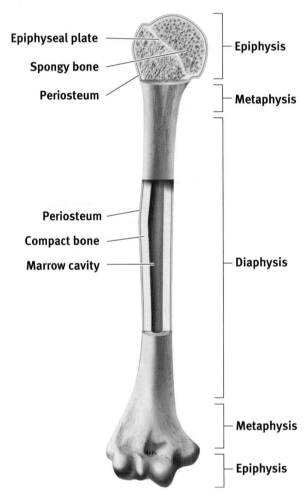

Figure 6.2

Real World

The epiphyseal plates seal due to the effects of sex hormones (testosterone in males and estrogen in females). Thus, growth continues through puberty until approximately age 25, when the process is complete, although most of the growth is done between the onset of puberty and age 18.

Bones in the appendicular skeleton are typical **long bones**, which are characterized by cylindrical shafts called **diaphyses** (singular: **diaphysis**) and dilated ends called **epiphyses** (singular: **epiphysis**). The peripheries of the epiphyses and diaphyses are both composed of compact bone, whereas their internal cores differ. Long bone diaphyses are full of marrow. The epiphyses, on the other hand, have a spongy bone core inside their compact bone sheath for more effective dispersion of force at the joints. Separating the epiphysis and diaphysis in each bone is an **epiphyseal plate**, which is a cartilaginous structure and the site of longitudinal growth. Finally, a fibrous sheath called the **periosteum** surrounds the long bone to protect it as well as serve as a site for muscle attachment. Some periosteum cells are capable of differentiating into bone-forming cells; a healthy periosteum is necessary for bone growth and repair.

MICROSCOPIC BONE STRUCTURE

In our last two sections, we mentioned that compact bone is strong but didn't yet discuss where that strength comes from. It comes from the **bone matrix**, which has both organic and inorganic components. The organic components include collagen, glycoproteins, and other peptides. The inorganic components include calcium, phosphate, and hydroxide ions that harden together to form hydroxyapatite crystals. Minerals such as sodium, magnesium, and potassium are also stored in bone.

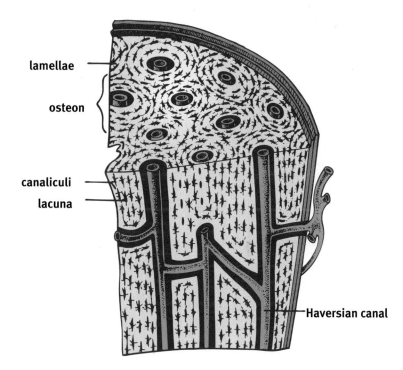

Figure 6.3

> **Key Concept**
>
> Bone appears to be rigid and static, but it is actually quite dynamic. It is both vascular and innervated, which is why it hurts so much to break one. In addition, bone remains in a vigorous equilibrium between construction and destruction, known as bone remodeling.

Strong bones require uniform distribution of inorganic material. The bony matrix is similarly ordered into structural units known as **osteons** or **Haversian systems**. Each of these osteons encircles a central microscopic channel known as a **Haversian canal**, surrounded by concentric circles of bony matrix called **lamellae**. Remember that tree stump next to your cabin at summer camp? The one on which you and your three-legged race partner engraved your undying love? The Haversian system is the center of the tree stump and the rings are the lamellae that surround it. These canals contain the blood vessels, nerve fibers, and lymph that keep the bone in peak condition. The rings in a tree are not touching; rather, they are spaced out a bit. So,

> **Mnemonic**
>
> Just as all things cartilage started with *chondro–*, all things bone start with *osteo–*.

too, are the lamellae in our bone. Interspersed within the matrix are spaces called lacunae, which house mature bone cells known as osteocytes.

These osteocytes are involved in bone maintenance. Each of the lacunae is interconnected by canaliculi, which are little canals that allow for exchange of nutrients and wastes between them and the Haversian canals.

BONE FORMATION (OSSIFICATION)

We mentioned previously that most of the bones in the body are created by the hardening of cartilage. This process is known as endochondral ossification (*endo-* means *within*, *chondro-* means *cartilage*), and it is responsible for the formation of most of the long bones in the body. Bones may also be formed through intramembranous ossification, in which undifferentiated embryonic connective tissue (mesenchymal tissue) is transformed into, and replaced by, bone.

BONE REMODELING

We now can introduce our last two players on the scene: osteoclasts and osteoblasts. Let's head back to summer camp one more time. On rainy days, we were stuck inside with building blocks. We'd build a large castle, only to have it knocked down by another, less imaginative child who wanted to use the same blocks to build a fortress. We could knock the fortress down and rebuild a slightly different castle, but it would just get knocked down again by someone else. The construction and destruction would continue in a never-ending cycle. Similarly, osteoblasts *build* bone and osteoclasts *resorb* bone. These processes together contribute to the constant maintenance of bone. During bone reformation, essential ingredients like calcium and phosphate are obtained from the blood. During bone resorption (breakdown), these ions are released into the bloodstream. Endocrine hormones like parathyroid hormone and calcitonin are involved in the remodeling process, as well as other compounds such as vitamin D. The old adage, "Use it or lose it," has its place here, because bone remodeling is affected by exercise and use.

Key Concept

Osteo*blasts* build bone; osteo*clasts* destroy or resorb bone.

Real World

Osteoporosis is the most common bone disease in the United States. It is thought to be the result of increased osteoclast resorption and some concomitant slowing of bone formation, both of which lead to loss of bone mass. Estrogen is believed to help prevent osteoporosis by stimulating osteoblast activity.

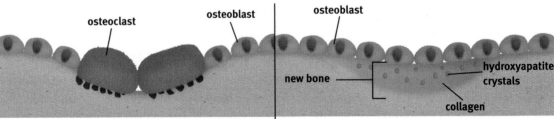

DEGRADATION: Osteoclasts release enzymes that dissolve bone, releasing calcium into the bloodstream.

REFORMATION: Osteoblasts build new bone using both organic and inorganic materials.

Figure 6.4

Joints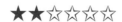

Before we leave the skeletal system, we need to discuss how the 206 bones in the adult body articulate with one another. Like bone and cartilage, joints are also made of connective tissue and come in two major varieties: **movable and immovable.** Movable joints work like door hinges and allow for bones to shift relative to one another (think knees and elbows). These joints are strengthened by **ligaments,** which are pieces of fibrous tissue that connect bones to one another, and consist of a **synovial capsule** that encloses the actual **joint cavity** (**articular cavity**). Since all of these structures are solid, we use **synovial fluid** to ease the movement of one structure over the other. Synovial fluid is a lubricant and works just like the oil with which we grease our car's pistons. The **articular cartilage** that we mentioned previously also contributes to the joint by coating the articular surfaces of the bones, so that impact is restricted to the lubricated joint cartilage, rather than to the bones. Immovable joints (e.g., in the skull) consist of bones that we would not want to move relative to one another; imagine a brace that we use to join two pieces of wood so that they are held in fixed positions. We definitely want our skull to be fixed in place, as it is protects our brain, the repository of all our Test Day knowledge!

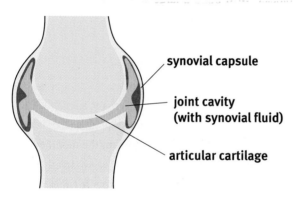

Figure 6.5

Now that we have introduced the basic structure of our skyscraper (skeleton), we want to start filling the floors of our building. Let's begin with muscles, which exist in three varieties: **skeletal**, **smooth**, and **cardiac**.

Skeletal Muscle

A great way to relieve some MCAT stress is to take a leisurely walk outside in the sunshine. This is achieved by skeletal muscle, which is innervated by the **somatic** nervous system. Muscles are intricate in their design but are ultimately made up of repeating units (like a polymer in chemistry). We'll start small and build up to a whole muscle.

The basic contractile unit of a muscle is the **sarcomere**. These sarcomeres are then put together end to end to build **myofibrils**.

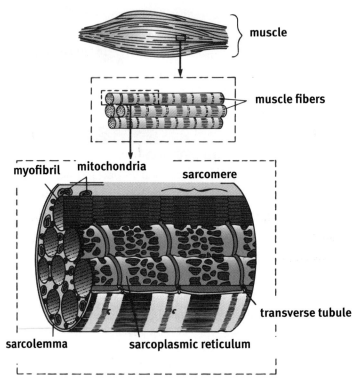

Figure 6.6

Myofibrils are surrounded by a covering known as the **sarcoplasmic reticulum** (SR; a modified endoplasmic reticulum that contains a great deal of Ca^{2+}). Outside the sarcoplasmic reticulum, we arrive at the **sarcoplasm**, the modified cytoplasm in these cells. As we reach the cell membrane (**sarcolemma**), we finally have a complete cell. Many myofibrils can be contained within each **myocyte** (muscle cell). Most cells are multinucleate due to the fusion of several embryonic uninucleate cells. These nuclei are usually found at the cell periphery. What we refer to as a "muscle" is simply a parallel arrangement of many of these myocytes. The sarcolemma is capable of propagating an action potential. A system of **T-tubules** is connected to the sarcolemma and oriented perpendicularly to the myofibrils, allowing for ions to flow.

When skeletal muscle is viewed microscopically, it is striated, appearing as if it has stripes. This is due to the alignment of Z-lines (which we'll discuss in a second) and their increased density relative to other structures. Skeletal muscle consists of **red** and **white** fibers. Red muscle fibers (also known as slow twitch) have a high **myoglobin** content and primarily derive their energy aerobically. Myoglobin is a protein similar to hemoglobin, but consists of a single polypeptide chain. It binds oxygen more tightly than hemoglobin. We will discuss the functional consequence of this in Chapter 9. White fibers (fast twitch) are anaerobic and have much less myoglobin. Based on what we learned in Chapter 3 and the way in which these cells derive their energy, which cells would we expect to be mitochondria-rich and which -poor? Red fibers are mitochondria-rich because they derive energy aerobically, and white fibers are mitochondria-poor because they do not use an electron transport chain. White fibers can contract more rapidly, but are also easier to fatigue.

The Sarcomere ★★★★☆

STRUCTURE

Before we move into the actual contraction of muscles, let's take a moment to really dissect the sarcomere, which we should recall is the basic unit of the muscle fiber. Sarcomeres are made up of **thick** and **thin** filaments. The thick filaments are organized bundles of **myosin**, whereas the thin filaments are made up of **actin** along with two other proteins, **troponin** and **tropomyosin**.

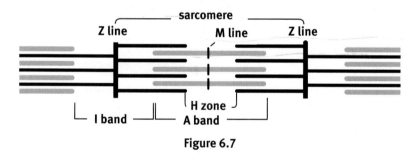

Figure 6.7

> ### Mnemonic
>
> *Myosin*, the "thicker" word, is composed of thick filament. *Actin*, the "thinner" word, is composed of thin filament. We can also remember that *troponin* and *tropomyosin*, both of which start with *t*, are associated with *acTin*, rather than myosin.

Let's return to our biologist's toolbox (which is getting to be large at this point) and pull out our handy-dandy electron microscope to visualize some muscular micro-anatomy. **Z-lines** define the boundaries of each sarcomere (and are responsible for the striated nature of skeletal and cardiac muscles). The **M-line** runs down the center of the sarcomere. The **I-band** is the region containing exclusively thin filaments whereas the **H-zone** exclusively contains thick filaments. Much as we used *thick* and *thin* to remember the association with myosin and actin, respectively, we can note that the letter *I* is thinner and the letter *H* thicker to help us remember which filament type each refers to (actin or myosin) on Test Day. The **A-band** contains the thick filaments in their entirety, including any overlap with thin filaments. During contraction, the H-zone, I-band, and distance between Z-lines all become smaller, whereas the A-band's size remains constant.

> ### Key Concept
>
> Z-lines, I-band, and H-zone—all of these get smaller or closer together during contraction because they are defined relative to one another. The A-band remains constant because it is defined as the total length of the thick fibers ("A"ll of the thick fibers), regardless of state of contraction.

CONTRACTION

Contraction of muscle requires a series of coordinated steps that are repeated to induce further shortening. As we examine each step, let's keep the key players in mind, one of which we saw in previous chapters and will continue to see: ATP.

Initiation

A good MCAT study session should involve a midnight ice cream break. When do we decide we're ready for it? Hunger pangs from our stomach are a pretty good message that we need a snack. The nervous system will send this signal via a **motor neuron**. This signal will travel down the neuron until it reaches the **nerve terminal (synaptic bouton)**, where the release of neurotransmitter (e.g., acetylcholine) into the **synapse** results in contraction of the muscle due to binding of the neurotransmitter to its receptor on the muscle. This connection point between nerve and muscle is aptly named the **neuromuscular junction**. If enough acetylcholine binds to the muscle cell, the muscle will be depolarized (action potential generation) and the sarcolemma's permeability will increase.

Shortening of the Sarcomere

Now that our muscle has its signal, how do we get it to contract in a coordinated fashion? The action potential generated at the neuromuscular junction will be conducted along the sarcolemma and T-system and then transmitted into the muscle fiber itself. If we recall that the sarcoplasmic reticulum is full of Ca^{2+} and electrically responsive to depolarization, we can predict that this will result in the massive release of calcium ions from the SR. Calcium will bind to troponin, causing tropomyosin to shift, and exposing the **myosin binding sites** on actin. Muscle cells need calcium the same way that we need a ticket to board an airplane. With our calcium ticket, we're allowed to pass through security (tropomyosin shift), exposing the gates (myosin binding sites) that allow us to get to our destination (actin and myosin binding that result in movement).

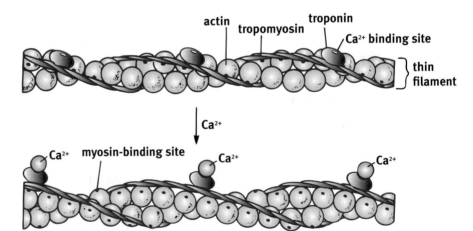

Figure 6.8

The free globular heads of the myosin molecules move toward and bind the exposed sites on actin. The newly formed actin–myosin cross bridges then allow actin to pull on myosin, which draws the thin filaments to the center of the H-zone and shortens the sarcomere (see Figure 6.9).

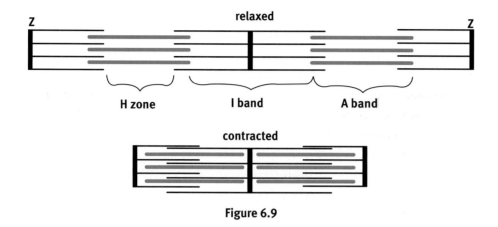

Figure 6.9

ATPase activity in the myosin heads provides the energy for the power stroke and results in dissociation of actin from myosin. The myosin then resets itself by binding another molecule of ATP and is free to bind another actin molecule.

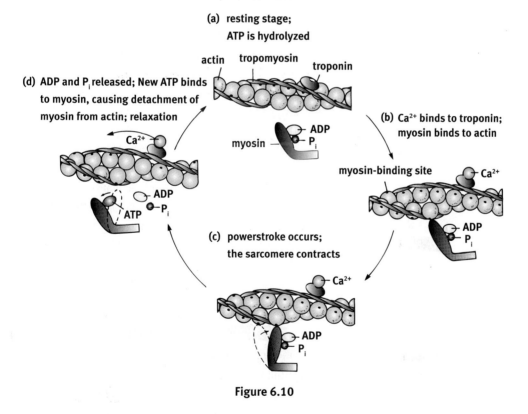

Figure 6.10

Relaxation

Once the SR's receptors are no longer stimulated, calcium levels will fall. The SR tightly controls intracellular calcium, so that muscles are contracted only when necessary. The products of ATP hydrolysis that were released from the myosin head during the power stroke leave room for a new ATP molecule to bind,

Key Concept

ATP is required for both the contraction and release of muscle fibers.

MCAT Expertise

Why do muscle fibers contract in an all-or-none fashion? Because they are innervated by neurons whose basic signal is an action potential, which is an all-or-none phenomenon. The ability to relate organs' interactions with one another is critical for MCAT success.

allowing for dissociation of myosin from the thin filament. Once the myosin and actin disconnect, the sarcomere can return to its original width. Without calcium, the myosin-binding sites will be covered by tropomyosin and prevent contraction. After death, ATP is no longer produced. Myosin heads cannot detach from actin, making it impossible for muscles to relax. This is known as rigor mortis.

STIMULUS AND MUSCLE RESPONSE

With any luck, we all have study buddies who won't actually throw a punch if we disagree on endosymbiosis. Could that punch break a nose? Power is directly related to how much force we generate from the muscle. Let's take a quick look at how stimulation is coupled to muscle response.

Stimulus Intensity

Muscle cells (like nerves with action potentials) exhibit what is known as an **all-or-none** response; either they respond completely or not at all. To respond, stimuli must reach a **threshold value**. For example, imagine a long car trip with an annoying sister. It might be fun (maybe just to see what happens) to poke her in the arm. At first nothing will happen; she'll just ignore it. After several pokes, an annoyance threshold will be attained, and she'll turn around and retaliate (complete response).

The strength of this individual response by a muscle fiber cannot be adjusted because the only options are all or nothing. Rather, muscles control overall force by the number of fibers they recruit to respond. Maximal response occurs when all fibers are stimulated to contract simultaneously. Instead of a single punch (one contraction or simple twitch), perhaps this sister is so annoyed that she ends up initiating a no-holds-barred throwdown once the car is stopped (maximal response).

Tonus refers to muscles in a constant state of low-level contraction. It is essential for some voluntary and involuntary muscles.

Simple Twitch

A simple twitch is the response of a single muscle fiber to a brief stimulus at or above the threshold. It consists of a **latent period, contraction period, and relaxation period**. The latent period is the time between reaching threshold (enough pokes) and onset of contraction (getting punched). It is during this time that the action potential spreads along the muscle and allows for Ca^{2+} to be released from the SR. After this period, the muscle will be unresponsive to stimuli. This is known as the **refractory period**, of which there are two types: **absolute** and **relative**. During the absolute refractory period, no amount of stimulus (sister-poking) will generate a response because the muscle is restoring its resting potential. During the relative period, the muscle can still be activated, but a higher than normal stimulus is required.

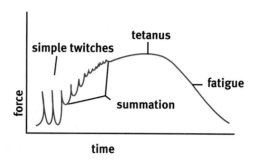

Figure 6.11

Summation and Tetanus

If we expose our muscle fibers to frequent and prolonged stimulation, they will have insufficient time to relax. The contractions will begin to combine, becoming stronger and more prolonged. This is known as **frequency summation**. If we continue to poke our sister often, her punches back will come closer and closer together and become stronger. Eventually, the contractions may become so frequent that there is no time for the muscle to relax. This is known as **tetanus** and is stronger than a simple muscle fiber twitch. Prolonged tetanus will result in muscle fatigue.

Smooth Muscle ★★★☆☆☆

Smooth muscle is responsible for involuntary action and is controlled by the **autonomic nervous system**. It is found in the digestive tract, bladder, uterus, blood vessel walls, and many other locations. Smooth muscle cells have single centrally placed nuclei. Just like skeletal muscle, they contain actin and myosin, but those fibers are not organized in a striated fashion. Smooth and skeletal muscles also contract in the same way. However, smooth muscle is capable of longer and more sustained contractions. Moreover, it can contract without nervous system input, which is known as **myogenic activity**.

Cardiac Muscle ★★★☆☆☆

Our last type of muscle is **cardiac muscle**. This is the hydraulic lift that allows the elevators and transport systems to travel up and down inside the skyscraper (which we will learn more about in Chapter 9). Cardiac fibers' characteristics are a conglomerate of the properties of smooth and skeletal muscle. They are primarily uninucleate and involuntary like smooth muscle, but are striated like skeletal muscle. Like both other types of muscle, calcium is required for contraction. Cardiac muscle may also exhibit myogenic activity. Knowing the basic differences between muscle types may translate into quick points on Test Day.

Table 6.1. Muscle Types

Smooth Muscle	Cardiac Muscle	Skeletal Muscle
• Nonstriated	• Striated	• Striated
• 1 nucleus per cell	• 1–2 nuclei per cell	• Multinucleated cells
• Involuntary/Autonomic nervous system	• Involuntary/Autonomic nervous system	• Voluntary/Somatic nervous system
• Smooth continuous contractions	• Strong forceful contractions	• Strong forceful contractions

Energy Reserves

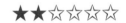

CREATINE PHOSPHATE

Muscles require energy in order to function. Muscles can generate ATP from several sources: fatty acids, glycogen, and glucose (recall Chapter 3 and see Chapter 7). In addition, energy can be derived from a high-energy compound known as **creatine phosphate**. During times of plenty, we store away creatine phosphate by transferring a phosphate from ATP to creatine. This process can be reversed during muscle use to rapidly generate ATP from ADP. It is advantageous to have creatine phosphate reserves because they allow for immediate creation of ATP that would otherwise need to be formed from glycolysis or the TCA cycle.

$$\text{Creatine} + \text{ATP} \leftrightarrow \text{creatine phosphate} + \text{ADP}$$

MYOGLOBIN

If we think back to Chapter 3, we learned that we could generate more energy by aerobic rather than anaerobic metabolism. However, what was absolutely required? Oxygen. Myoglobin, which is found in muscle and similar in function to hemoglobin, binds oxygen and holds on to it (more tightly than hemoglobin). As exercising muscles run out of oxygen, we can use myoglobin's reserves to keep aerobic metabolism going. Once we exhaust these reserves, we'll have to ferment the remaining pyruvate to regenerate NAD+ and start glycolysis again.

Key Concept

Skeletal Muscle

- Striated
- Voluntary
- Somatic innervation
- Many nuclei per cell
- Ca²⁺ required for contraction

Cardiac Muscle

- Striated
- Involuntary
- Autonomic innervation
- 1–2 nuclei per cell
- Ca²⁺ required for contraction

Smooth Muscle

- Nonstriated
- Involuntary
- Autonomic innervation
- One nucleus per cell
- Ca²⁺ required for contraction

Bridge

Remember that the lactic acid from fermentation can be converted back into energy-producing intermediates once sufficient levels of oxygen become available. This process occurs in the liver and is known as the Cori cycle (Chapter 3).

Connective Tissue ★★☆☆☆

Connective tissue is rightly named in that its purpose is to bind and support other tissues. Much as we might use nails and glue and screws to bind the floors of our skyscraper together, connective tissue holds the body together.

Connective tissue is composed of a sparsely scattered population of cells contained in an amorphous ground substance that may be liquid, jelly-like, or solid. Loose connective tissue is found throughout the body. It attaches epithelium to underlying tissues and is the packing material that holds organs in place. It contains proteinaceous fibers of three types: **collagenous fibers**, which are composed of collagen and have great tensile strength (think nails and screws); **elastic fibers**, which are composed of elastin and endow connective tissue with resilience (think of glue which can expand and contract in building joints); and **reticular fibers**, which are branched, tightly woven fibers that join connective tissue to adjoining tissue. There are two major cell types in loose connective tissue: **fibroblasts**, which secrete substances that are components of extracellular fibers, and **macrophages**, which engulf bacteria and dead cells via phagocytosis (recall Chapter 1).

Dense connective tissue is connective tissue with a high proportion of collagenous fibers. The fibers are organized into parallel bundles that give the fibers great tensile strength, just like the woven steel cable bundles that hold up the Golden Gate Bridge in San Francisco. Dense connective tissue forms **tendons**, which attach muscle to bone, and **ligaments**, which hold bones together at the joints.

> ### Mnemonic
> We have already seen the root *lig–* in ligaments which connect bone to bone. We also see it in DNA *ligase*, which joins parts of the sugar phosphate backbone in DNA. Again, word roots will help us with unfamiliar vocabulary on the MCAT.

Muscle-Bone Interactions ★★★☆☆

Just as the multiple systems in our skyscraper must interact, locomotion depends on interactions between the skeletal and muscular systems. If a given muscle (including associated joints) is attached to two bones, contraction of the muscle will cause only one of the two bones to move. The end of the muscle attached to the stationary bone is called the **origin**; in limb muscles it corresponds to the **proximal** end. The end of the muscle attached to the bone that moves during contraction is called the **insertion**; in limb muscles, the insertion corresponds to the **distal** end.

Often, our muscles work in antagonistic pairs; one relaxes while the other contracts. Such is the case in the arm, where the biceps and triceps work antagonistically. When we move our hand toward our shoulder, the biceps contract and the triceps relax; when we move our hand down again, the biceps relax and the triceps contract (see Figure 6.12). We should take a moment to discuss why this antagonism occurs. We spent a good bit of time discussing muscle contraction, but haven't yet mentioned muscle elongation. It's because muscles don't have an elongation function; the contraction of the antagonistic muscle will lengthen the paired muscle (e.g., biceps contracts, triceps elongates). Note that elongation is different from relaxation. All muscles can relax when the myosin heads and actin are unbound. There are also **synergistic** muscles, which assist the principal muscles during movement.

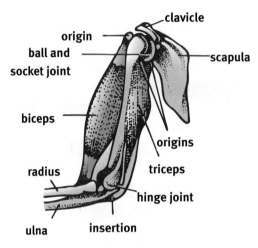

Figure 6.12

Muscles also may be classified by the type of movements they coordinate. A **flexor** muscle will contract to decrease the angle of a joint (e.g., the biceps will flex the elbow joint), whereas an **extensor** muscle will contract to straighten the joint (e.g., the action of the triceps on the elbow). An **abductor** moves a part of the body away from the body's midline; an **adductor** moves a part of the body toward the midline.

Conclusion

This chapter introduced us to two organ systems that work in close concert with one another. We began our discussion with the skeletal system, focusing on bone's properties and functions. A brief foray into joints led us to discuss the muscular system in greater detail. Striated muscles (skeletal and cardiac) have defined sarcomeres, whereas smooth muscle does not. Cardiac and smooth muscles are under involuntary control, whereas skeletal muscle usage is voluntary. Muscle contraction depends on the presence of ATP and calcium, and multiple energy reserves are available to replenish muscles when necessary. We concluded our chapter with a discussion on the interactions between muscle and bone, as they work together to allow us movement.

CONCEPTS TO REMEMBER

☐ Cartilage, bone, ligaments, and tendons are all connective tissues. Muscle is contractile tissue.

☐ Cartilage is made by chondrocytes and serves as a flexible building medium.

☐ Bones may be either compact or spongy. The type depends on the location and specific purpose of the bone.

☐ Compact bone is filled with bone marrow, which may be red or yellow. Red marrow is important for hematopoeisis.

☐ Bones consist of both organic and inorganic components. Complex microscopic anatomical structures (e.g., Haversian canals) allow for bones to receive nutrients for the organic components.

☐ Joints are the juxtaposition of two or more bones. They may be movable or immovable and are often associated with a cartilaginous lining.

☐ Muscles may be divided into three major categories: skeletal, cardiac, and smooth.

☐ The sarcomere is the basic functional unit of all muscle.

☐ Contraction of muscle occurs in an all-or-none fashion analogous to the action potential of a neuron. Increased force is due to increased muscle fiber recruitment, not the increase of force of any one individual fiber's contraction.

☐ The interaction of muscles and bones is what allows for locomotion. Muscles are often paired antagonistically such that one lengthens while the other contracts.

Practice Questions

Questions 1, 2, and 3 are based on the following diagram.

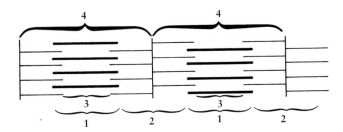

1. During muscle contraction, which of the following regions decrease(s) in length?

   A. 2 only

   B. 3 only

   C. 4 only

   D. 2, 3, and 4

2. Region 1 refers to

   A. the thick filaments only.

   B. the thin filaments only.

   C. the A band.

   D. the I band.

3. Which region represents one sarcomere?

   A. 1

   B. 2

   C. 3

   D. 4

4. With which of the following molecules does Ca^{2+} released from the sarcoplasmic reticulum bind?

   A. Myosin

   B. Actin

   C. Troponin

   D. Tropomyosin

5. Which of the following cells is correctly coupled with its definition?

   A. Osteoblasts—bone cells involved in the secretion of bone matrix

   B. Osteoclasts—immature bone cells

   C. Osteocytes—multinucleate cells actively involved in bone resorption

   D. Chondrocytes—undifferentiated bone marrow cells.

6. You are looking at a right leg X-ray of a child whose right femur has slowed its growth and is below the average length for a child of this age. To which region of the bone should you pay particular attention to see if there are any abnormalities?

   A. Diaphysis

   B. Epiphyses

   C. Epiphyseal plate

   D. Periosteum

7. Which of the following INCORRECTLY pairs the type of fiber with its definition?

   A. Red fibers—slow-twitching

   B. Red fibers—high levels of myoglobin

   C. White fibers—fast-twitching

   D. White fibers—high levels of myoglobin

8. When the knee moves back and forth as a person walks, what keeps the surfaces of the leg bones from rubbing against each other?

   A. The articular cartilage

   B. The epiphyses

   C. The periosteum

   D. A sheath of smooth muscle

9. When a muscle fiber is subjected to very frequent stimuli

    A. an oxygen debt is incurred.

    B. a muscle tonus is generated.

    C. the contractions combine in a process known as summation.

    D. the threshold value is reached.

10. In order to facilitate the process of birth, the infant's head is somewhat flexible. This flexibility is given in part by the two fontanelles, which are soft spots of connective tissue on the infant's skull. With time, these fontanelles will ossify through a process known as

    A. endochondral ossification.

    B. intramembranous ossification.

    C. resorption.

    D. longitudinal growth.

11. When a muscle is attached to two bones, usually only one of the bones moves. The part of the muscle attached to the stationary bone is referred to as

    A. origin.

    B. proximal.

    C. distal.

    D. insertion.

12. Which type of muscle is always multinucleated?

    I. Cardiac muscle

    II. Skeletal muscle

    III. Smooth muscle

    A. I only

    B. II only

    C. III only

    D. I and II only

13. Which type of muscle has myogenic activity?

    I. Cardiac muscle

    II. Skeletal muscle

    III. Smooth muscle

    A. I only

    B. II only

    C. III only

    D. I and III only

14. Red bone marrow is involved in erythrocyte function, whereas yellow bone marrow

    A. is involved in leukocyte formation.

    B. is involved in draining lymph.

    C. is involved in spicule formation.

    D. contains adipose tissue.

15. Which of the following statements regarding the periosteum is INCORRECT?

    A. The periosteum serves as the site of attachment of bone to muscle.

    B. Cells of the periosteum differentiate into osteoblasts.

    C. The periosteum is a fibrous sheath that surrounds long bones.

    D. None of the above.

Small Group Questions

1. Contrast the ways by which chondrocytes and osteocytes are nourished.

2. Explain how rigor mortis occurs.

Explanations to Practice Questions

1. D

We are given a diagram of a sarcomere and asked to determine which regions shorten during muscle contraction. Glancing at the answer choices, we notice that we are only interested in regions 2, 3, and 4. Region 2 refers to the I band, formed only of thin actin filaments. During muscle contraction, the I band reduces in size as the thick filaments overlap the thin filaments. Region 3 refers to the H zone, formed only of thick myosin filaments. During contraction, this region also decreases in length as the thin filaments overlap the thick filaments. Finally, region 4 on the diagram refers to the area between the Z lines, which defines the boundary of a single sarcomere. During muscle contraction, as the sarcomere shortens, the Z lines come closer together, so region 4 also decreases in length. As such, all of these three regions decrease in length during muscle contraction, making (D) the correct answer.

2. C

Looking at the diagram, we notice that region 1 contains both thick and thin filaments overlapping one over the other. This region refers to the A band and is measured from one end to the other of the thick filaments. This is also the only portion of the sarcomere that does not change length during muscle contraction. (C) is the correct answer.

3. D

One sarcomere is represented by the area between two vertical lines, referred to as the Z lines. In addition, the Z lines anchor the thin filaments. In the diagram, a sarcomere is therefore defined by region 4, making (D) the correct answer. The sarcomere is also the contractile unit in striated muscle cells.

4. C

Calcium is released from the sarcoplasmic reticulum into the sarcoplasm. It binds the troponin molecules on the thin filaments, causing the strands of tropomyosin to shift, thereby exposing the myosin-binding sites on the filaments, as can be seen in the diagram. (C) is the correct answer.

5. A

Let's quickly define each one of the four cells discussed in the answer choices. Osteoblasts are bone cells involved in the secretion of bone matrix, as (A) states. Osteoclasts are large, multinucleated cells involved in bone resorption. Osteocytes are mature osteoblasts that eventually became surrounded by their matrix and whose primary role is bone maintenance. Finally, chondrocytes are cells that secrete chondrin, an elastic matrix that makes up cartilage. Only (A) couples the type of cell with its definition and is therefore the correct answer.

6. C

This question is basically asking us where exactly longitudinal growth occurs in bones. The most likely site of abnormalities in this child's femur is the epiphyseal plate, a disk of cartilaginous cells separating the diaphysis from the epiphysis. The epiphyseal plate is the site of longitudinal growth. (C) is thus the correct answer.

7. D

Glancing at the answer choices, we realize that our task is to characterize the two types of fibers, red and white. Red fibers are slow-twitching fibers that have high levels of myoglobin and many mitochondria. They derive their energy from aerobic respiration and are capable of sustained vigorous activity. In general, marathon runners have more red fibers. White fibers, on the other hand, are fast-twitching fibers and contain lower levels of myoglobin and fewer mitochondria. Because of their composition, they derive more of their energy anaerobically and fatigue more easily. Short distance runners usually have more white fibers. From the given choices, the only one that incorrectly pairs the type of fiber with its characteristic is (D).

8.   A

The articular surfaces of the bones are covered with a layer of smooth articular cartilage. In addition, the joints contain a clear, viscous liquid called synovial fluid, which lubricates the surfaces that glide past each other, preventing the bones from rubbing. (A) is therefore the correct answer.

9.   C

When a muscle fiber is subjected to very frequent stimuli, the muscle cannot fully relax. The contractions begin to combine, becoming stronger and more prolonged. This is known as frequency summation. (C) therefore is the correct answer.

10.   B

The question is basically asking us for the name of the ossification process which occurs in the skull. This is known as intramembranous ossification, where mesenchymal cells directly create bone matrix, as stated in (B).

11.   A

The part of the muscle that is attached to the stationary bone is referred to as the origin, as (A) indicates. In limb muscles, the origin corresponds to the proximal end. The part of the muscle that is attached to the bone that moves during contraction is called the insertion. In limb muscles, this corresponds to the distal end.

12.   B

The only type of muscle that is always multinucleate is skeletal muscle, making (B) the correct answer. Cardiac muscle may contain one or two centrally located nuclei, so statement I is incorrect. Smooth muscle, on the other hand, only has one centrally located nucleus.

13.   D

Myogenic activity refers to the ability of a muscle to contract reflexively without nervous stimulation. Smooth and cardiac muscle both possess myogenic activity because they can contract reflexively without stimulation. (D) is therefore the correct answer.

14.   D

Yellow marrow is inactive and largely infiltrated by adipose tissue, making (D) the correct answer.

15.   B

The periosteum is a fibrous sheath that surrounds long bones, and is the site of attachment to muscle tissue. Choices (A) and (C) are therefore true statements about the periosteum and can be eliminated. Let's take a look at (B). Cells of the periosteum do not differentiate into osteoblasts. (B) is thus the correct answer.

7

Digestion

In the connoisseurial world of coffee consumers, no coffee is rarer or more prized than Kopi Luwak, also known as Civet coffee. Only one thousand pounds of this exquisite bean are released into the world's coffee market each year. It sells for an astonishing $160 to $600 per pound! High-end cafés that are able to procure a small quantity for their customers may charge between $50 and $100 per cup of this luxurious brew. You might be wondering what could possibly be so special about these beans to justify (or at least explain) the breathtaking prices. We can assure you that it is nothing close to what you might be thinking. No, it's not the variety of the bean itself, or the growing conditions, or anything related to the process of roasting or brewing the beans. Brace yourself, and hold your nose, because you're about to go where you would have least expected.

In the native language of Indonesia, where this coffee originates, *kopi* means *coffee* and *luwak* is the local name given to the Asian Palm Civet, a cat-sized mammal native to southeast Asia and southern China. Its diet consists of fruits such as mango and rambutan, palm flower sap, small insects, and even small mammals. It also happens to enjoy perfectly ripe red coffee cherries (berries). The civets eat the cherries, and as they pass through their digestive tracts, the flesh surrounding the coffee beans is digested but the beans themselves are not, because civets lack the enzymes necessary for digesting the hard beans. Since the beans are not digested, they pass through the intestinal tract and are defecated. At this point, we are forced to acknowledge the truth of the saying, "One's trash is another's treasure," for the defecated beans are collected, washed (thank goodness for small things!), and lightly roasted, at which point they are ready for market.

Those who drink Civet coffee insist that it is not for mere shock value that they do so; rather, they claim that the digestive enzymes in the civet's gut penetrate into the hard bean and break down the proteins that are responsible for the bitter flavor normally present in coffee. As a result of these enzymatic activities, they claim, the "processed" beans yield a brew that is sweeter, richer, and altogether unique—and worth every dollar spent. We don't know about you, but we will stick to our large half-caf, low-fat, no-foam soy vanilla lattés, thank you very much.

As we continue our survey of organ systems, we come to the digestive system. Although this chapter is brief, it is jam-packed with information we can use to our advantage on Test Day. As with our previous reviews of other organ systems, we will start with a basic anatomical overview of the organs of digestion (including accessory organs) and then move on to discuss how these organs function to provide overall nutrition to the organism. This structure–function approach will keep us focused on the most important information for Test Day. The digestive system allows us to take in complex compounds in the foods that we eat and drink, and reduce them to smaller, simpler compounds that can be absorbed from the gut, transported to the tissues by the circulatory system, and used by the cells for energy, growth, development, maintenance, and other essential activities.

We have already imagined the system of beams and concrete in a skyscraper as analogous to the musculoskeletal system of the human body. Let's continue with this imagery by considering the manner in which bulk supplies are brought into a city office building and subsequently broken down into smaller units for distribution and use. Many large buildings have a loading dock where pallets of supplies are received. Certainly, this office building will receive deliveries of supplies such as pens, pencils, and paper in bulk, but no one office worker is going need 100 pens or 5,000 sheets of paper in a single day. Instead, the distribution center (which we might consider the digestive system of this building) will break these large bulk shipments down to the amounts that can then be used by the people working inside the building. Indeed, once broken down into the smaller units, the pens and paper and toner for the copiers will even be transported from the loading dock and distribution center (the building's gut) to all the different offices, departments, and building inhabitants through the elevators, hallways, and staircases, which we might characterize as the building's circulatory system.

The foodstuffs that we eat, and from which we derive nutrition, are made of carbohydrates, proteins, and fats, along with vitamins, minerals, and water. The large organic molecules are the bulk shipments we receive into our body, but these must be broken down into smaller units in our digestive system for the cells of our body to use and benefit from the energy stored in our food. For example, the glucose molecules that are the substrate of cellular respiration (see Chapter 3) originate from the carbohydrates in our diet. These carbohydrates (called *polysaccharides*) must first be digested into monomeric forms (called *monosaccharides*) and then absorbed from the digestive system into the circulatory system by which they are delivered to the tissues and cells of the body.

Key Concept

The individual molecules that the body can absorb will be discussed in detail later in the chapter. The big picture to keep in mind is that all foodstuffs are broken down to simple sugars, amino acids, and fatty acids.

Anatomical Considerations

The sort of digestion that we considered in Chapter 3, such as glucose breakdown, and the digestion of compounds within lysosomes is a form of **intracellular digestion**. We are now concerned with **extracellular digestion**, which occurs outside the cells' borders. In humans, digestion occurs within the lumen of the **alimentary canal**, as it does for all mammals. This canal is actually "outside" the body in that the space contained within it is outside cell borders: between the mouth and anus is one long continuous tube, sectioned off by sphincters. One could argue that the difference between humans and cannoli is minimal, except, of course, that cannoli are much more delicious.

The human digestive tract, as alluded to earlier, has specialized sections with different functional roles. The most basic functional distinction is that between digestion and absorption. Digestion involves the breakdown of food into its constituent organic molecules: lipids (fats) into free fatty acids, starches (carbohydrates) into monosaccharides, and proteins into amino acids. Digestion can be subdivided into mechanical and chemical processes. Mechanical digestion is the physical breakdown of large food particles into smaller food particles, but does not involve the breakage of chemical bonds. Chemical digestion is the enzymatic cleavage of chemical bonds (e.g., the peptide bond of proteins or the glycosidic bond of starches). Absorption involves the transport of products of digestion from the digestive tract into the circulatory system for distribution to the body's tissues and cells. Our digestive tract begins with the **oral cavity**, followed by the **pharynx**, **esophagus**, **stomach**, **small intestine**, and **large intestine**. In addition, there are the salivary glands and accessory organs such as the **pancreas**, **liver**, and **gall bladder**.

Epithelium

If we were to look at our own body (using the microscope from the biologist's toolbox), we could see that our exterior surfaces (e.g., skin, tongue, inner eyelids, nasal cavities) as well as the interior surfaces we can't visualize directly (lungs, and gastrointestinal and urinary tracts) are covered with continuous sheets of epithelial cells. These constitute a first border and primary protection against the outside world. For this purpose, these cells are tightly joined and may also be ciliated. We will see examples of this ciliation in both this chapter and Chapter 8 when we discuss the respiratory system. In most of our body cavities (e.g., nasal cavities, inner eye lids, mouth, gastrointestinal tract), these epithelia are known as **mucous membranes**. Our skin and other epithelial linings help us by preventing fluid loss as well as by allowing for selective absorption of materials that our bodies require, especially in the digestive tract. Because we want to be sure that our epithelium doesn't escape from us (think cartoon characters being literally scared out of their skin), it is bound to a connective tissue layer known as the **basement membrane**. This sort of structure is analogous to the foundation a house is built on to give it stability. In the digestive tract, the epithelium that is attached to the basement membrane is replaced every few days, due to the harsh conditions (e.g., corrosive environments or extreme temperatures) to which the epithelium is exposed.

We can classify different epithelia according to the number of layers they have and the shape of their cells. You shouldn't worry too much about remembering all the types for the MCAT, as that will be a medical school focus. Instead, you should know that there are different types and that they can serve different purposes. Let's start with layers. **Simple** refers to one layer, **stratified** means multiple layers, and

Key Concept

Although all of these tissue types have epithelium, we should be careful not to confuse this with their embryological origin. In adults, epithelia are developed from all three germ layers. The epithelium of the skin is derived from ectoderm; the epithelium of blood vessels is derived from mesoderm; the epithelium of the GI tract is derived from endoderm.

pseudostratified means that it looks like multiple layers due to differences in cell height, but it is really just one.

Turning to shape, cells may be **cuboidal**, **columnar**, and **squamous**. We can think of the first two using the root of the word. Cuboidal cells look like the sugar cubes we might put in our coffee (one lump or two?), whereas columnar cells look like the columns of buildings. Squamous cells are scalelike, much as we might see on a snake or lizard. In fact, Squamata is the name of the order of scaled reptiles that includes snakes and lizards. Now that we have the basic definitions out of the way and know the names of the structures in digestion, let's examine Figure 7.1 and take a walkthrough of the digestive system. As we do, if we ever get lost, we can just glance back at our figure to become reoriented. One critical point that we should consider with each organ in this system is its role in digestion.

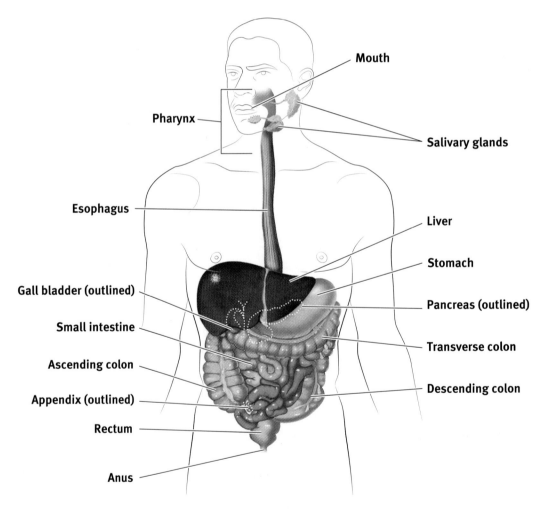

Figure 7.1

Oral Cavity

It all starts here. We might think about the mouth as the loading dock in our office building where boxes of supplies are taken in. The mouth can carry out both **mechanical** and **chemical digestion**. Mechanical digestion in the mouth, in a process called **mastication**, involves the breaking up of large food particles into smaller particles by using the teeth, tongue, and lips—much as workers on the loading dock will begin to unpack the larger boxes from the truck. This is an important first step in the digestion process. What would be the advantage in doing this, since the chemical bonds in the food are not broken? For a hint, think back to our discussion of the early stages of embryology when the cell divided rapidly after fertilization. The cells increased their surface area to volume ratio to allow for greater gas and nutrient exchange across the cell membrane. The results of mastication are similar: mechanical digestion increases the surface area of the food particles for more efficient chemical digestion.

Chemical digestion through enzymatic activity (those enzymes from Chapter 2 keep making an appearance) allows for breakage of the chemical bonds that store the actual food energy (remember ATP?). The salivary glands in our mouth secrete saliva, which aids mechanical digestion by moistening and lubricating the food. If you have ever swallowed a cracker or tortilla chip too fast, and experienced painful scratching as it moved down your esophagus, you know that saliva is important. In addition, saliva (secreted from the salivary glands in response to nervous system signals that sense the presence of food in the oral cavity) contains **salivary amylase**, also known as **ptyalin**, and **lipase**. Ptyalin is capable of hydrolyzing starch into smaller sugars (maltose and dextrin), whereas lipase catalyzes the hydrolysis of lipids. The amount of chemical digestion that occurs in the mouth is minimal, though, because the food does not stay in the mouth for long. Our muscular **tongue** will then form the food into a **bolus** that is forced back to the pharynx and swallowed.

Pharynx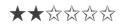

The pharynx is the cavity that leads from the mouth and nose to the esophagus. You might also recognize that the pharynx has a connection to the larynx, which is a part of the respiratory tract. How can we prevent food from getting into the respiratory tract? We make use of our **epiglottis**, which folds down and covers the trachea during swallowing (see also Chapter 8). Failure of this mechanism can lead to choking.

> **Key Concept**
>
> The chemical digestion of carbohydrates is initiated in the mouth but is completed in the small intestine. Salivary amylase (active in the mouth) and pancreatic amylase (active in the small intestine) have the same function.

> **Real World**
>
> If you chew on a plain cracker long enough without swallowing, the cracker will start to taste sweet as salivary amylase begins to hydrolyze the complex carbohydrates (starches) in the cracker into disaccharides such as maltose. These compounds interact with receptors on our taste buds, leading to the sensation of sweetness. The next time you take an MCAT study break, you should feel free to try this experiment, not only to provide you with brain power in the form of maltose and dextrin that your cells can convert to glucose, but also to drive home an MCAT concept: Digestion . . . sweet!

Esophagus

The esophagus serves as the connection from the mouth to the stomach, much as there might be a conveyer system to move supplies around the loading dock in our office building. The esophagus is a muscular tube that starts out with striated muscle and transitions into smooth muscle in the thorax. What does this mean in terms of control? The majority of the esophagus (and most of the rest of the gastrointestinal tract, for that matter) is under involuntary control through the autonomic nervous system. Only the upper third of the esophagus, with its striated skeletal muscle, is under voluntary motor control. You can initiate a swallow, but the continuation of that muscular contraction in the form of **peristalsis** is involuntary. At no point is the involuntary nature of peristalsis more evident than when the direction of contraction reverses. Try as you might, there is no stopping a digestive system that insists on expelling its contents through the same oral cavity by which those contents entered the system.

The swallow initiated in the muscles of the oropharynx continues into the smooth muscles of the esophagus as the progressive contractions known as peristalsis. These contractions form waves that continue throughout the gastrointestinal tract and push the food through the tube. The bolus doesn't just fall down the esophagus with a passive reliance on gravity; rather, it is actively pushed, propelled, and squeezed from one region of the digestive tract to the next. This is most evidenced by the fact that if you eat or drink something while hanging upside down, the food or drink are moved against gravity into your stomach rather than falling or flowing out of your mouth and/or nose. As the bolus approaches the stomach, a muscular ring known as the **lower esophageal sphincter (cardiac sphincter)** opens to allow the passage of food.

Stomach

Recall from Chapter 3 that we have three main energy sources: carbohydrates, proteins, and fats. The chemical digestion of carbohydrates and fats is initiated in the mouth. No mechanical or chemical digestion takes place in the esophagus (except for the continued enzymatic activity initiated in the mouth by the salivary enzymes). Now we come to our first major site of digestion. Let's turn to the stomach and see what it can do.

We might not think of our stomach as a storage organ, but it has a capacity of about two liters (think of that bottle of soda you might drink while studying for the MCAT) and is muscular. In humans, the stomach is located on the right side of the upper abdomen under the diaphragm (see Chapter 8). You are probably already aware that the stomach uses acid and enzymes to digest food in a fairly harsh environment.

Real World

Weakness in the lower esophageal sphincter can lead to classic heartburn after eating. As food and acid reflux into the lower esophagus, irritating the less protected mucosa, pain receptors are stimulated. The location of the sphincter, right behind the heart, leads to this common misnomer.

So what would we expect of the mucosa here? It is quite thick, to protect the stomach from autodigestion.

The stomach mucosa contains the **gastric glands** and the **pyloric glands**. The gastric glands respond to signals from the brain, which are activated by the sight, taste, and smell of food. Just as our mouth waters when we see a meal, so, too, do our gastric glands. These glands are composed of three cell types: **mucous cells**, **chief cells**, and **parietal cells**. The function of the mucous cells is simple to remember: They produce the mucus that protects the muscular wall from the harshly acidic (pH 2) and proteolytic environment of the stomach (which, as muscle, is made of protein).

Gastric juice is the combination of secretions from the other two cell types in the gastric glands. The chief cells, which are the "chiefs" of digestion in the stomach, secrete **pepsinogen**, which is the zymogen form of the proteolytic enzyme **pepsin** (recall zymogens from Chapter 2). Pepsin will digest proteins by cleaving peptide bonds near aromatic amino acids, resulting in short polypeptide fragments. Parietal cells secrete **hydrochloric acid (HCl)**, a strong acid that serves many purposes. We know that zymogens must be activated, and HCl does that for pepsin. Pepsin, which is most active at pH 2 (maintained by the HCl concentration), is unique among human enzymes, most of which are active in neutral to slightly basic pH ranges (i.e., the pH of blood). The acid also kills most harmful bacteria (with the exception of *Helicobacter pylori*, the infection of which is usually asymptomatic but can cause inflammation and ulcers) and breaks down the intracellular glue that holds food together.

Now let's turn our attention to the pyloric glands. These glands secrete **gastrin**, which is a hormone. Gastrin induces our stomach to secrete more HCl and to mix the contents of the stomach. This produces an acidic, semifluid mixture known as **chyme**. The combined mechanical and chemical digestive activities of the stomach result in a significant increase in the surface area of the food particles (now unrecognizable as food) so that when the chyme reaches the intestines, the absorption of nutrients from it can be maximized.

You should remember for Test Day that *the stomach is primarily a site of digestion, not absorption*. There are certain substances (e.g., alcohol, aspirin) that can be directly absorbed, but for our purposes we should think of the stomach as a digestive site.

Real World

Zöllinger-Ellison syndrome is a rare disease resulting from a gastrin-secreting tumor (gastrinoma). Typically, this tumor is found in the pancreas. As we would suspect, the excess gastrin leads to excessive HCl production. Not surprisingly, one of the most common reports of Zöllinger-Ellison syndrome is the presence of intractable ulcer disease.

Small Intestine

Food leaves the stomach through the **pyloric sphincter**, entering the duodenum of the small intestine. Now we come to the exciting part. The bulk supplies received at the loading dock have been partially broken down, but are still not ready for distribution throughout the building (circulatory system). More digestion (breaking down) must take place. Indeed, the bulk of chemical digestion, as well as most absorption, occurs in the small intestine. Let's see how.

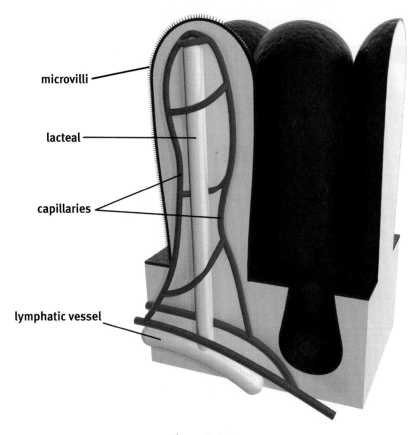

microvilli

lacteal

capillaries

lymphatic vessel

Figure 7.2

The small intestine is divided into three sections: **duodenum**, **jejunum**, and **ileum**. The small intestine is quite long (six meters), and to further maximize the surface area available for absorption, a specialized microanatomy is in place. The surface of the inner wall of the small intestine is covered in projections called **villi** (from the Latin for *shaggy hair*), each of which is covered in its own set of **microvilli**. This has the overall effect of increasing the relative surface area to over 300 square meters, thereby dramatically increasing the absorptive capabilities of the small intestine. Bacteria reside throughout the small intestine and assist with its digestive and absorptive functions. In Figure 7.3, we see bacteria (green) lining the duodenum wall. There are actually over 400 different species of bacteria residing in the gut!

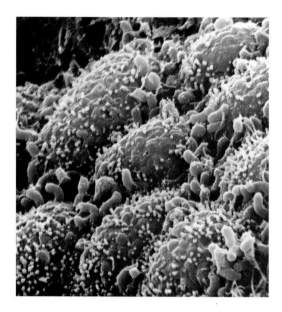

Figure 7.3

DIGESTIVE FUNCTIONS

Simple to remember for the MCAT, most *d*igestion occurs in the *d*uodenum; note that both start with a *d*. At this point, the accessory organs of digestion become necessary, because the enzymes and other compounds secreted by the accessory organs (liver, gall bladder, and pancreas) are key to successful digestion. As chyme enters the duodenum, it triggers the release of hormones that lead to secretions from the small intestine itself, as well as from the accessory organs of digestion.

Pancreatic juice is a complex mixture of several enzymes in a bicarbonate (basic) solution. As we mentioned in Chapter 2, this bicarbonate helps to neutralize acidic chyme as well as provide an ideal working environment for each of the digestive enzymes. The enzymes produced by the pancreas are most active around pH 8.5. Pancreatic juice contains enzymes that can digest all three types of nutrients: carbohydrates, fats, and proteins. Pancreatic amylase, which breaks down large polysaccharides into small disaccharides, is responsible for carbohydrate digestion. The pancreatic peptidases (**trypsinogen**, **chymotrypsinogen**, **elastinogen**, and **carboxypeptidase**) are released in their zymogen form, but once activated, are responsible for protein digestion. Enterokinase, produced by the small intestine, is the master switch. It activates trypsinogen to trypsin, which can then activate the other zymogens. Finally, the pancreas secretes **lipase**, which is capable of breaking down fats to free fatty acids.

Bile is a complex fluid made up of bile salts, bile pigments, and cholesterol. It is produced by the liver and stored in the gall bladder. The gall bladder releases bile into the duodenum by way of the bile duct in response to the hormone **cholecystokinin (CCK)**, which is released by the small intestine in response to the movement of chyme out of

Key Concept

Intestinal and pancreatic enzymes are key to proper digestion and absorption. Only the monomeric form of the organic compounds (i.e., monosaccharides, monopeptides, and free fatty acids) can be absorbed by the gut. Without the pancreatic and intestinal enzymes, the compounds in the chyme couldn't be further broken down, which would prevent their absorption in the small intestine. They would pass through to the large intestine, where they would be digested by the bacterial flora (e.g., lactose used as substrate for cellular respiration in *E. coli*) or expelled by the body in the feces.

Bridge

Just as we saw that cholesterol served a positive function in mediating membrane fluidity, here again we see a good effect of cholesterol: serving as the substrate to make bile salts.

Real World

Although the gall bladder stores bile, it isn't completely necessary for life. High-fat diets commonly result in formation of stones or sludge within the gall bladder or cystic duct. If this blockage cannot be cleared, the gall bladder may have to be removed. This is known as a cholecystectomy. The bile will now no longer be stored in the gall bladder, but will be released from the liver directly into the duodenum. This may present problems if a person ingests a high-fat meal and the liver cannot keep up with demand for bile.

the stomach and into the intestines. The pH of bile is between 7.5 and 8.8; so, like the pancreatic juice, it is alkaline, to help neutralize the acidity from the stomach.

Bile salts, made from cholesterol, are not enzymes and therefore do not directly impact chemical digestion (the enzymatic cleavage of chemical bonds). However, they serve an important role in the mechanical digestion of fats and ultimately facilitate the chemical digestion of lipids. If we think back to Chapter 1, where we learned about the phospholipid bilayer, we can understand how bile salts work. Like phospholipids, bile salts have a hydrophobic and hydrophilic region. This allows them to serve as a bridge between aqueous and lipid environments. In fact, bile salts are much like the common soaps and detergents we use to wash our hands, clothes, and dishes. In the small intestine, they serve a key function by allowing fat to be emulsified. An emulsification is a mixture of two immiscible liquids. Because chyme is aqueous, without bile, fats would spontaneously separate out of the mixture, forming two layers (aqueous and lipid) just as oil and vinegar salad dressing separate into two layers. Without bile to **emulsify** the dietary fats and cholesterol into **micelles**, we would be unable to keep it in solution (where the water-soluble pancreatic lipase is found). In addition, these micelles expose more of the surface of the fats to the actions of lipase. The bottom line is that we need both bile and lipase. Bile gets the fats into the solution and increases the surface area by placing them in micelles (mechanical digestion). Then, lipase can come in to hydrolyze the ester bonds holding the lipids together (chemical digestion). A common trend is emerging: Systems throughout the body use increased surface area to increase the efficiency of different processes.

We now understand the importance of the accessory organs through their production of enzymes and compounds essential for both mechanical and chemical digestion in the small intestine. But what about the small intestine itself? Chyme in the duodenum causes the small intestine to release disaccharidases (**maltase, lactase**, and **sucrase**), **peptidases** (including **dipeptidases**), **enterokinase, secretin**, and **CCK**. The first three are enzymes that can digest disaccharides (e.g., lactase breaks down lactose into a galactose and a glucose). Peptidases break down proteins (or peptides, as the name implies). Dipeptidases cleave the peptide bond of dipeptides to release monopeptides (free amino acids). **Secretin** is a hormone that causes pancreatic juice to be exuded from the pancreas. Finally, **CCK**, also a hormone, stimulates the release of both pancreatic juice and bile. We can see that the small intestine itself is capable of digesting carbohydrates and proteins. In fact, the enzymes secreted by the small intestine are collectively called the brush border enzymes because they act upon their dimeric substrates at the brush border where the monomeric products will be absorbed. If you are having trouble remembering all these compounds when studying for Test Day, refer to Table 7.1 at the end of the chapter.

As with all organ systems, there are mechanisms of control in the digestive system. For example, bile release is tied to the level of fat ingested. If you have a very fatty meal (say, a double burger with cheese and a large order of french fries), the duodenum will release the hormone **enterogastrone** to slow the movement of the chyme and allow a greater time to digest the fat. Furthermore, the autonomic nervous system can exert control over the digestive system. The parasympathetic division is involved in stimulation (rest and digest) and the sympathetic is involved in inhibition (fight or flight) of digestive activities. The fact that so often we feel sleepy and lethargic (as many people call it, food coma) after eating a big meal is due, in part, to parasympathetic activity. On the other hand, if your lovely picnic in the woods were disrupted by a large grizzly bear, your sympathetic division would kick into high gear, and suddenly, digesting that cookie you had just eaten wouldn't be at the top of your body's priority list. Your sympathetic system would decrease blood flow to the digestive organs and decrease their activity.

ABSORPTIVE FUNCTIONS

Up to this point, we have only discussed the breakdown (digestion) of the food. We haven't discussed how the nutrients (i.e., the organic molecules, vitamins, and minerals) are taken up by the body for use. The absorptive processes mostly occur in the jejunum and ileum. Let's examine the absorption of each class of nutrients separately.

We'll start with carbohydrates and amino acids. Simple sugars (e.g., glucose, galactose) and amino acids are absorbed by active transport and facilitated diffusion into the epithelial cells lining the gut. Then, they move across the epithelial cell into the intestinal capillaries. Because blood is constantly passing by the epithelial cells in the capillaries, carrying the carbohydrate and amino acid molecules away from them, a concentration gradient is established such that the capillary blood has a lower concentration of these molecules than the epithelial cells. Thus, the simple carbohydrates and amino acids diffuse from the epithelial cells into the capillaries. The absorbed molecules then go to the liver via the **hepatic portal circulation**.

What about fats? Small fatty acids will follow the same process as carbohydrates and amino acids by diffusing directly into the intestinal capillaries. Let's stop and think for a minute: why don't they need transporters? They are nonpolar, so they can easily traverse the cellular membrane. Larger fats, glycerol, and cholesterol move separately into the intestinal cells but then re-form into triglycerides (think back to Chapter 3). The triglycerides and esterified cholesterol molecules are packaged into insoluble **chylomicrons** and, rather than entering the bloodstream, they enter the lymphatic circulation through **lacteals,** small vessels that form the beginning of the lymphatic system. These lacteals converge and enter the venous circulation through the lymphatic duct in the neck region (the thoracic duct).

Chylomicrons are processed directly in the bloodstream into low-density lipoprotein (LDL), the so-called "bad" cholesterol). Because this occurs right in the bloodstream,

Key Concept

Most fat bypasses the liver. This means it directly enters the circulation without first-pass metabolism. The liver has moderate control over the levels of sugar and protein in the blood because the absorbed carbohydrates and amino acids are first directed to hepatic portal circulation before being released to the rest of the body. Fats aren't subject to such restrictions.

Mnemonic

HDL is Healthy. LDL is Less healthy.

LDL in excess can lead to atherosclerosis. LDL molecules are taken up by the liver, where they can be repackaged into high-density lipoprotein (HDL, "good" cholesterol), very low-density lipoprotein (VLDL), or more LDL.

NEW ROLES FOR FAMILIAR ACTORS

POPULAR DESCRIPTIONS of atherosclerosis correctly cast low-density lipoprotein (LDL) as "bad" and high-density lipoprotein (HDL) as "good." Yet these particles (*shown in cutaway views*) fulfill their roles in more ways than scientists once thought.

Lipoproteins transport cholesterol in the bloodstream. LDLs truck it from the liver and intestines to various tissues, which use it to repair membranes or produce steroids. HDLs haul cholesterol to the liver for excretion or recycling. The classic view of how atherosclerosis develops implies that excess LDL promotes the condition by accumulating on vessel walls. More recent work shows that it accumulates *within* vessel walls, where its components become oxidized and altered in other ways; the altered components then incite an inflammatory response that progressively—and dangerously—alters arteries.

Physicians also generally explain HDL's protective effects as deriving from its removal of cholesterol from arteries. HDL certainly does that, but new findings indicate it can also combat atherosclerosis by interfering with LDL oxidation. —*P. L.*

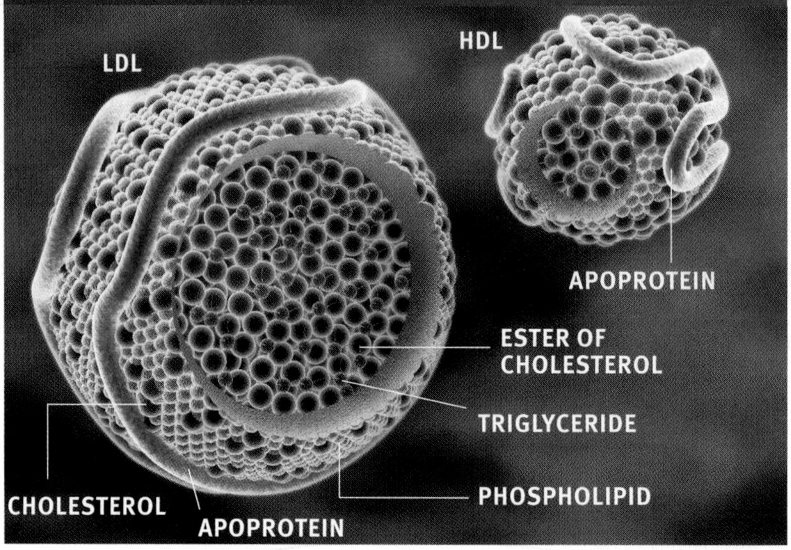

Figure 7.4

You do need to know for Test Day the different mechanisms of vitamin absorption. We can categorize vitamins as either fat- or water-soluble. Because there are only four fat-soluble vitamins (A, D, E, and K), we can memorize them, knowing that anything else we might come across on Test Day (e.g., B vitamins or vitamin C) must be water-soluble. Failure to digest fat properly, which would subsequently inhibit its proper absorption, may lead to a deficiency of the fat-soluble vitamins, which are normally absorbed alongside the fats. The water-soluble vitamins are absorbed, along with water, amino acids, and carbohydrates, across the endothelial cells and pass directly into the plasma of the blood.

Large Intestine

The final part of the gastrointestinal tract is the large intestine. It is primarily involved in water absorption, although the overall water balance in the body is controlled by the kidneys. The large intestine is, well, larger than the small intestine in terms of diameter. However, it is only 1.5 meters long, and therefore shorter than the small intestine in overall length. The large intestine is divided into three major sections: the **cecum**, **colon**, and **rectum**. The cecum is simply a pocket with no outlet that connects the small and large intestines and contains the **appendix**. The appendix is a tiny structure that was once thought to be **vestigial**, although recent evidence has suggested that it may have a role in warding off certain bacterial infections. Inflammation of the appendix (appendicitis) is a medical emergency; in fact, it is the most common reason for an unscheduled surgery in the United States.

Table 7.1. Digestive Enzymes

Nutrient	Enzyme	Site of Production	Site of Function	Function
Carbohydrates	Salivary amylase (Ptyalin)	Salivary glands	Mouth	Hydrolyzes starch to maltose
	Pancreatic amylase	Pancreas	Small intestine	Hydrolyzes starch to maltose
	Maltase	Intestinal glands	Small intestine	Hydrolyzes maltose to two glucose molecules
	Sucrase	Intestinal glands	Small intestine	Hydrolyzes sucrose to glucose and fructose
	Lactase	Intestinal glands	Small intestine	Hydrolyzes lactose to glucose and galactose
Proteins	Pepsin (secreted as pepsinogen)	Gastric glands	Stomach	Hydrolyzes specific peptide bonds
	Trypsin (secreted as trypsinogen)	Pancreas	Small intestine	Hydrolyzes specific peptide bonds Converts chymotrypsinogen to chymotry
	Chymotrypsin (secreted as chymotrypsinogen)	Pancreas	Small intestine	Hydrolyzes specific peptide bonds
	Carboxypeptidase	Pancreas	Small intestine	Hydrolyzes terminal peptide bond at carboxyl end
	Aminopeptidase	Intestinal glands	Small intestine	Hydrolyzes terminal peptide bond at amino end
	Dipeptidases	Intestinal glands	Small intestine	Hydrolyzes pairs of amino acids
	Enterokinase	Intestinal glands	Small intestine	Converts trypsinogen to trypsin
Lipids	Bile*	Liver	Small intestine	Emulsifies fat
	Lipase	Pancreas	Small intestine	Hydrolyzes lipids

*Note that bile is NOT an enzyme.

Key Concept

Although the large intestine reabsorbs massive amounts of water, it is the kidneys that actually regulate total body water.

The colon is responsible for absorbing water and salts (e.g., sodium chloride) in the undigested material from the small intestines. The colon acts as a recycling system, sifting through the processed food and pulling those last little bits of nutrients out of the remaining waste products. Too little or too much water absorption can cause diarrhea or constipation, respectively.

Finally, the rectum serves as a storage site for **feces**, much as the office workers would temporarily store trash and waste before it is removed from the office building. Feces consist of indigestible material, water, bacteria (*E. coli*, etc.), and certain digestive secretions that aren't reabsorbed (enzymes and bile). The **anus** is the opening through which wastes are eliminated, and consists of two sphincters: the **internal** and **external** anal sphincters. The external sphincter is under voluntary control (somatic), but the internal sphincter is under involuntary control (autonomic). Do you remember which embryonic structure gives rise to the anus in humans? It's the blastopore (see Chapter 5 for more details).

Conclusion

In this chapter, we have reviewed a lot of information about the digestive system that we can use to our advantage on Test Day. We began with an overview of the anatomy, keeping in mind that the system is designed to carry out extracellular digestion. Considering all our foodstuffs are made up of fats, proteins, and carbohydrates, these compounds have to be broken down to their simplest molecular forms before they can be absorbed and distributed to the tissues and cells of the body. As we moved through the gastrointestinal tract, we discussed whether each organ was a site of absorption, digestion, or both. We spent a good bit of time discussing each of the enzymes involved in digestion and its specific purpose. Absorption primarily occurs in the jejunum and ileum, where transport across the epithelial cells is slightly different depending on the compound. Finally, we discussed the large intestine and its three sections and its role in water and salt absorption, as well as its role in the temporary storage of waste products. Although the amount of information about the digestive system may seem overwhelming, these concepts are relatively simple and a systematic approach (think charts, tables, or flash cards) to managing this information will spell Test Day success for you.

CONCEPTS TO REMEMBER

☐ Digestion consists of two processes: mechanical and chemical. Mechanical breaks the food into smaller pieces, whereas chemical breaks the actual bonds in food molecules.

☐ The mammalian digestive tract is a one-way system that begins with the mouth and ends at the anus. Several accessory organs of digestion are attached.

☐ The stomach is responsible for digestion through the use of enzymes and HCl that is secreted by the parietal cells.

☐ The epithelium of the stomach is protected from damage by mucous that is secreted from mucous cells.

☐ Pancreatic juice contains bicarbonate that helps neutralize the acidic chyme after it leaves the stomach. Bile also contributes to this effect.

☐ The enzymes in pancreatic juice and from the duodenum are capable of digesting all three classes of foods: carbohydrates, proteins, and fats.

☐ Bile is required for the proper digestion and absorption of fats, as they must be emulsified for these processes to occur.

☐ Vitamins are also absorbed. They may be either fat- or water-soluble. The fat-soluble vitamins are A, D, E, and K.

☐ The large intestine consists of three sections: the cecum, colon, and rectum.

☐ Although the large intestine reabsorbs water, its primary function is not to regulate total body water. Rather, it absorbs water so that feces are semisolid by the time they reach the rectum. Salts and some vitamins (e.g., vitamin K, which is produced by bacteria in the large intestine) may also be absorbed.

Practice Questions

1. Which of the following associations between the type of gastric cell or gland and its secretions is correct?

   A. Mucous cells—HCl
   B. Chief cells—pepsinogen
   C. Parietal cells—mucus
   D. Pyloric glands—gastric juice

2. Which of the following is NOT part of the small intestine?

   A. Ileum
   B. Cecum
   C. Jejunum
   D. Duodenum

3. In an experiment, enterokinase secretion was blocked. As a direct result, levels of all of the following enzymes were affected EXCEPT

   A. trypsin.
   B. aminopeptidase.
   C. chymotrypsin.
   D. carboxypeptidase.

4. Which of the following INCORRECTLY pairs the digestive hormone with its function?

   A. Trypsin—hydrolyzes specific peptide bonds
   B. Lactase—hydrolyzes lactose to glucose and galactose
   C. Pancreatic amylase—hydrolyzes starch to maltose
   D. Lipase—emulsifies fats

5. Where are proteins digested?

   A. Mouth and stomach
   B. Stomach and large intestine
   C. Stomach and small intestine
   D. Small intestine and large intestine

6. Which of the following choices INCORRECTLY pairs a digestive enzyme with its site of secretion?

   A. Sucrase—salivary glands
   B. Carboxypeptidase—pancreas
   C. Trypsin—pancreas
   D. Lactase—intestinal glands

7. You are looking at a CT scan of the abdomen of a child who presented to you with various symptoms, including projectile vomiting. You notice a constriction in the digestive system that prevents food from reaching the small intestine. Which structure is the most likely site of the problem?

   A. Cardiac sphincter
   B. Pyloric sphincter
   C. Cecum
   D. Rectum

8. All of the following processes occur in the mouth EXCEPT

   A. moistening of food.
   B. bolus formation.
   C. chemical digestion of starch.
   D. chemical digestion of proteins.

9. The two graphs below show the relative activities of two enzymes in solutions of varying pH. Which of the following choices correctly identifies the two enzymes?

1.

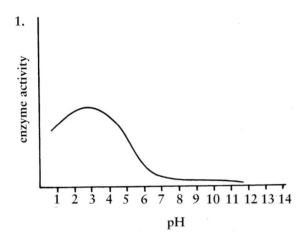

2.

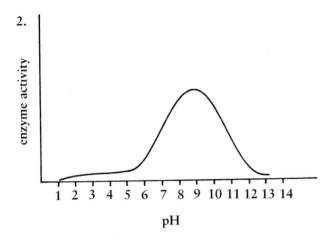

    A. 1—chymotrypsin; 2—pepsin
    B. 1—pepsin; 2—chymotrypsin
    C. 1—bile; 2—lactase
    D. 1—carboxypeptidase; 2—enterokinase

10. Which of the following choices correctly illustrates the course that a piece of bread takes through the digestive tract?

    A. Mouth → trachea → esophagus → cardiac sphincter → stomach → pyloric sphincter → small intestine → large intestine → rectum → anus

    B. Mouth → pharynx → esophagus → cardiac sphincter → stomach → pyloric sphincter → small intestine → large intestine → rectum → anus

    C. Mouth → pharynx → esophagus → pyloric sphincter → stomach → cardiac sphincter → small intestine → large intestine → rectum → anus

    D. Mouth → pharynx → esophagus → cardiac sphincter → stomach → pyloric sphincter → small intestine → large intestine → anus → rectum

11. The epiglottis is to the trachea as the lower esophageal (cardiac) sphincter is to the

    A. stomach.
    B. heart.
    C. small intestine.
    D. liver.

12. Which of the following choices correctly pairs the nutrient with its site of absorption?

    A. Chylomicrons—lacteals
    B. Amino acids—large intestine
    C. Vitamins A and E—stomach
    D. Cholesterol—ascending colon

13. Starch is hydrolyzed into maltose by

    A. salivary amylase.
    B. maltase.
    C. pancreatic amylase.
    D. both A and C.

14. The intestinal capillaries transport nutrients from the intestines to the

    A. large intestine.

    B. liver.

    C. kidney.

    D. heart.

15. Which of the following choices INCORRECTLY pairs a digestive enzyme with its site of secretion?

    A. Pancreatic amylase—pancreas

    B. Aminopeptidase—stomach

    C. Enterokinase—intestinal glands

    D. Maltase—intestinal glands

16. Which of the following INCORRECTLY pairs a digestive enzyme with its function?

    A. Sucrase—hydrolyzes sucrose to glucose

    B. Carboxypeptidase—hydrolyzes the terminal peptide bond at the amino end

    C. Trypsin—hydrolyzes some peptide bonds and converts chymotrypsinogen to chymotrypsin

    D. Lactase—hydrolyzes lactose to glucose and galactose

Small Group Questions

1. Why do you suppose the monosaccharide glucose is circulated in the blood of humans rather than a disaccharide, such as sucrose, which is the transport sugar found in plants?

2. How does the stomach protect itself from its own acidic environment?

3. In the digestive system, some enzymes are secreted as inactive precursors that are later converted to their active forms. Why might this occur?

Explanations to Practice Questions

1. B

The surest way to answer this question correctly is to analyze each answer choice. (A) is false because mucous cells secrete mucus. (B) is true, because chief cells do indeed secrete pepsinogen, the zymogen of the protein-hydrolyzing enzyme pepsin. (C) and (D) are indeed false, since parietal cells secrete hydrochloric acid, whereas the pyloric glands secrete gastrin. (B) is therefore the correct answer.

2. B

The small intestine is divided into three sections: the duodenum, the jejunum, and the ileum. Thus, the correct answer is (B) because the cecum is part of the large intestine.

3. B

Let's take a look at each one of the listed enzymes and eliminate the ones that are affected by enterokinase. Trypsin is the active form of trypsinogen, a zymogen activated by enterokinase, so we can eliminate (A). Aminopeptidase does not interact with enterokinase in any way, and therefore would not be affected by a blockage in enterokinase secretion. We can now select (B). For the sake of completion, let's take a look at the last two choices. Chymotrypsin is the active form of chymotrypsinogen, another pancreatic enzyme activated by enterokinase. Finally, carboxypeptidase is secreted as a zymogen and activated by trypsin, which, in turn, requires enterokinase to be activated from its zymogen form, trypsinogen. (B) is therefore the correct answer.

4. D

The best way to answer this question is to look at each answer choice and determine if the association is false. Looking at (A), we can decide right away that it is a correct association, because trypsin does indeed hydrolyze specific peptide bonds. (B) is also true: Lactase hydrolyzes lactose to glucose and galactose. Next, we can eliminate (C) because it is true that pancreatic amylase hydrolyzes starch to maltose. We are left with (D), which must be false. The function of lipase is to hydrolyze lipids; bile salts emulsify fats. (D) is therefore the correct answer.

5. C

Protein digestion begins in the stomach, where pepsin (secreted as pepsinogen) hydrolyzes specific peptide bonds. Protein digestion continues in the small intestine as trypsin (secreted as trypsinogen), chymotrypsin (secreted as chymotrypsinogen), carboxypeptidase, aminopeptidase, and dipeptidase hydrolyze specific parts of the peptide. (C) is therefore the correct answer.

6. A

Let's take a look at each choice in part and determine which one contains a false association. Starting with (A), we notice a mistake right away. Sucrase is secreted by the intestinal glands, not the salivary glands. Its function is to hydrolyze glucose to fructose. Glancing at the other choices, we confirm once more that (A) is the correct answer.

7. B

The question is basically asking us to identify the structure that would prevent food from reaching the small intestine. Because the child presents with projectile vomiting, we can assume that food reached the stomach but cannot continue its course to the intestine. The structure that regulates the passage of chyme from the stomach to the small intestine is called the pyloric sphincter, and is the most likely site of the patient's problem. (B) is thus the correct answer.

8. D

The mouth has an important role in digestion, because it is the first part of the digestive tract to interact with food. Several things happen in the mouth as we eat. First, the mouth (the teeth and tongue, specifically) churns the food into small pieces, a process called mechanical digestion. The salivary glands produce saliva, which helps moisten the food. With the help of the tongue, a bolus is formed that will then be swallowed and sent through the esophagus to the stomach. Only one type of chemical digestion occurs in the mouth: the chemical digestion of starch to maltose, a process initiated by salivary amylase (ptyalin). (D) is therefore the correct answer as the chemical digestion of protein begins in the stomach.

9. B

The question gives us two graphs and asks us to identify the type of enzyme that each one represents based on how the enzyme's activity changes as a function of pH. Looking at the first graph, we notice that the enzyme has maximal activity at a relatively low pH (3–4). It must be an enzyme that functions in an acidic environment, most likely in the stomach. The second graph portrays an enzyme whose optimal activity occurs at a high pH (9.5). It must correlate to an enzyme that works in a basic environment, such as the small intestine. Our task now is to select the answer choice which pairs the first graph to a gastric enzyme, and the second graph to a small intestinal enzyme. (B) matches our prediction, and is therefore the correct answer. Pepsin is secreted in the stomach and works best in an acidic pH, whereas chymotrypsin acts in the small intestine at a basic pH.

10. B

In the mouth, teeth chew the bread into smaller particles and salivary amylase digests some of the starch (the major component of bread) into maltose. The bread bolus is then propelled through the pharynx and esophagus, entering the stomach through the cardiac sphincter. There is no chemical digestion of starch in the stomach, so after a couple of hours, the chyme will pass through the pyloric sphincter and enter the small intestine. In the small intestine, pancreatic amylase hydrolyzes starch into maltose, whereas maltase, sucrase, and lactase hydrolyze various disaccharides into their respective monosaccharides. Most of the monosaccharides (i.e., glucose, fructose, and galactose) are absorbed into the circulatory system through the intestinal wall. Finally, the piece of bread will finish its course through the large intestine and the rectum, and will eventually be expelled through the anus. The only choice that correctly identifies all of the different segments of the digestive tract is (B).

11. A

The epiglottis is a small flap that covers the trachea during swallowing; in a way, it is a switch that ensures food and air travel through different passageways. The lower esophageal (cardiac) sphincter controls the passage of food into the stomach and prevents anything from getting out of the stomach. The correct answer therefore is (A).

12. A

Glancing at each choice, we realize that only chylomicrons are correctly paired with their site of absorption. Large fatty acids and glycerol, which combine to form triglycerides, along with phosphoglycerides and cholesterol, are packaged into protein-coated droplets called chylomicrons. The chylomicrons are then absorbed into tiny lymph vessels within the villi called lacteals, which lead to the lymphatic system. (A) is therefore the correct answer.

13. D

Starch is hydrolyzed to maltose by two different enzymes: salivary amylase (secreted by the salivary glands) in the mouth and pancreatic amylase (secreted by the pancreas) in the small intestine. (D) is therefore the correct answer

14. B

The intestinal capillaries transport nutrients from the intestines to the liver, where they get processed, repackaged, and distributed. (B) is therefore the correct answer.

15. B

Let's take a look at each choice to determine which one contains a false association. (A) can be eliminated because pancreatic amylase is indeed secreted by the pancreas (as the name indicates). (B) is a red flag; aminopeptidase is secreted by the intestinal glands. Although this means that (B) is the correct answer, for the sake of completion, let's check the last two choices. It is true that both enterokinase and maltase are secreted by the intestinal glands, so (C) and (D) can be eliminated.

16. B

Let's quickly analyze each choice and determine which one contains a false association. Sucrase does indeed hydrolyze sucrose to galactose, a process that occurs in the small intestine; we can eliminate (A). Carboxypeptidase on the other hand, is an enzyme that hydrolyzes a terminal peptide bond at the carboxy terminal, as the name indicates. (B) is therefore false, and the correct answer. Glancing at the other two answers, we confirm that (C) and (D) are indeed true associations.

Respiration

8

Coughing. Fever. Shortness of breath. Hypoxia. All are symptoms of a type of hypersensitivity pneumonitis, which is also known as extrinsic allergic alveolitis (EAA). More specifically, they're symptoms of hot tub lung.

The first two names refer to alveolar inflammation caused by the inhalation of some substance that was not properly filtered out by nasal hairs and mucus. Hot tub lung is a specific form of EAA caused by the gram-positive *Mycobacterium avium*. That genus name might sound somewhat familiar; in fact, *M. avium*'s cousin is none other than *M. tuberculosis*! Although hot tub lung seems contagious by its mechanism of infection, it's not easily transmitted from one human to the next, the way tuberculosis is.

So what exactly *is* its mechanism of infection? Many of us see hot environments as inhospitable for bacterial growth, but let's remember that the number of bacterial *species* outnumbers animal species at least by the millions (even billions might be an underestimate). Surely there exist species that can survive in every environment on earth! Including those at 102°F, that is, the temperature at which most hot tubs are set. It just so happens that *M. avium* flourishes at this temperature. Bubbles at the hot water's surface burst, releasing nice warm mist into the air. That warm mist, unfortunately, might be full of *M. avium* waiting to make their new home. The happy, relaxed bathers who breathe these bacteria might be in for a long road of respiratory troubles.

Not all cases of hot tub lung are severe, but certainly none are enjoyable. They're often misdiagnosed as asthma or bronchitis, and sometimes treated with steroids. As mentioned earlier, hot tub lung falls in a category of hypersensitivities, which can potentially go away by themselves. As a result, antibiotic therapy is not always recommended. The best way to avoid hot tub lung is to make sure that the tub is being cleaned properly and routinely before entering it.

Hot tub lung is as aptly named as some other types of hypersensitivity pneumonitis: mushroom-worker's lung, cheese-washer's lung, and wine-grower's lung. The lesson here isn't to avoid hot tubs, mushrooms, cheese, and wine. It's that the lungs are essential, sensitive organs with delicate membranes that must be protected. Many types of stressors (pathogens, particles, or chemicals) can irritate them and cause respiratory distress. In this chapter, we'll look at the structure of the lungs and their precious membranes, along with the microanatomy of respiration. We'll also talk about respiratory volumes and how pulmonologists assess proper lung function. Last but not least, we'll preview gas exchange to prepare us for a discussion of gas transport in the next chapter.

Anatomy

Gas exchange occurs at the **lungs**. Air enters the respiratory tract through the **external nares** of the nose and then passes through the nasal cavity, where it is filtered through mucous membranes and nasal hairs. Just as the air that is brought into a building may be passed through a filtration system for cleaning, there are numerous cilia in the nasal pathway that trap particulate matter (such as dust) so that we don't breathe it into our lungs.

Next, air passes into the pharynx and the **larynx**. The pharynx serves as a tunnel between the mouth and esophagus through which food travels (Chapter 7), whereas the larynx is only a pathway for air. To keep food out of the respiratory tract, the opening of the larynx (glottis) is covered by the **epiglottis** during swallowing. From the larynx,

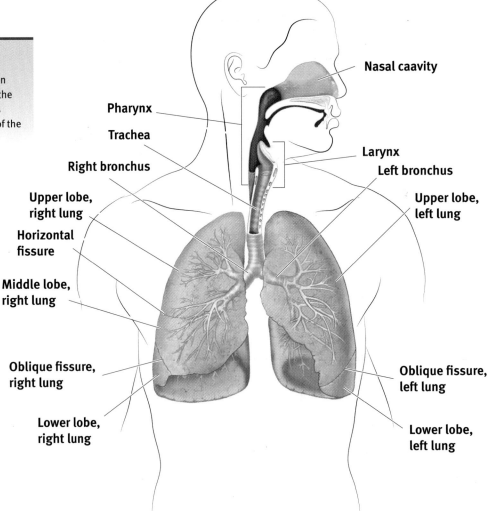

Figure 8.1

air passes into the cartilaginous **trachea** and then into the mainstem **bronchi** (one per side). These bronchi continue to divide into smaller structures known as **bronchioles** until they are tiny structures in which gas exchange occurs (the **alveoli**). This is analogous to a building's ventilation system, which will continue to divide into smaller and smaller tubes and pipes until we reach the vent in each individual room.

The bronchi and trachea also contain ciliated epithelial cells to catch material that may have made it past the initial check in the nose. Each alveolus is coated with **surfactant**, a detergent that lowers surface tension and prevents the alveolus from collapsing on itself. A network of capillaries surrounds each alveolus to carry oxygen and carbon dioxide. The branching and minute size of the alveoli allow for an exceptionally large surface area for gas exchange—approximately 100 m².

Ventilation

The lungs themselves are contained in the **thoracic cavity**, which, we will see in the next chapter, also contains the heart. They are separated from the organs of digestion by a muscle known as the **diaphragm** that is necessary for **inspiration**. Although breathing is controlled autonomically, the diaphragm is actually composed of skeletal muscle and is therefore under somatic control.

The chest wall forms one side of the thoracic cavity. Membranes known as **pleurae** (sing: **pleura**) surround each lung. The pleurae are a closed sac against which the lung grows. The surface adjacent to the lung is **visceral** and all other parts of the sac are **parietal** (see Figure 8.2). Imagine that we have a large, partially deflated balloon. Now, let's take our fist and push it against the balloon so that the balloon comes up and surrounds our hand. This is analogous to a lung and its pleurae. Our fist is the lung and the balloon represents both pleural layers. The side directly touching our fist is the visceral pleura, and the outer layer is the parietal pleura, which is

Bridge

The digestive system uses villi and microvilli to generate a similar advantage.

Real World

Pneumothorax is a common result of a penetrating injury to the chest. Air enters the intrapleural space, thereby increasing the intrapleural pressure and collapsing the lung. Pneumothorax is treated by inserting a needle and withdrawing air from the intrapleural space.

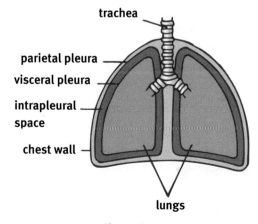

Figure 8.2

associated with the chest wall in real life. The space within the sac is referred to as the **intrapleural space**, which in our bodies contains a thin layer of fluid (imagine pouring a bit of water into the balloon before blowing it up). This fluid helps lubricate the two pleural surfaces. In addition, there is a pressure differential between the intrapleural space and the lungs. This difference is critical for proper respiration.

STAGES OF VENTILATION

Let's turn to the mechanics of ventilation. This might sound a lot like physics, and the process of ventilation is, in fact, grounded in physics. We can use pressure to do useful work in a system. Here, we are going to use pressure differentials between the lungs and intrapleural space to drive air into the lungs.

Inhalation

Inhalation is an active process. We use our diaphragm as well as the **external intercostal muscles** (layer of muscles between the ribs) to expand the thoracic cavity. As the cavity enlarges, the diaphragm flattens down and the chest wall moves out. Intrapleural volume increases. Can we predict what will happen to intrapleural pressure? From our understanding of Boyle's law, an increase in intrapleural volume leads to a decrease in intrapleural pressure.

Now we have low pressure in the intrapleural space. What about inside the lungs? The gas in the lungs is at atmospheric pressure, which is now higher than the pressure in the intrapleural space. We can see, then, that the lungs will expand as air is sucked in from a higher-pressure environment. What environment is this? The outside world. This mechanism is referred to as **negative-pressure breathing**, because the driving force is the lower (relatively negative) pressure in the intrapleural space compared with the lungs (alveoli). If we were curious, we would also predict that this pressure differential would affect how the heart fills, since it's also in the thoracic cavity (which we don't need to know for the MCAT, but will learn plenty about in medical school).

Exhalation

Luckily, exhalation does not have to be an active process. Simple relaxation will reverse the processes we discussed in the last paragraph. Let's see how. As the diaphragm and external intercostals relax, the chest cavity decreases in size (volume). What will happen to pressure in the intrapleural space? It will go up, again explained by Boyle's law. Now, pressure in the intrapleural space is higher than in the lungs, which is still at atmospheric level. So air will be pushed out, resulting in exhalation. During highly active tasks, we can speed this process up by using the **internal intercostal muscles**, which oppose the externals and pull the rib cage down, actively decreasing the volume of the thoracic cavity. Finally, we should recall that surfactant prevents the complete collapse of our alveoli during exhalation by reducing surface tension at the alveolar surface.

Bridge

Boyle's law says that the pressure and volume of gases are inversely related. This is the principle underlying negative-pressure breathing.

Real World

Emphysema is a disease characterized by the destruction of alveolar walls. This results in reduced elastic recoil of the lungs, making the process of exhalation extremely difficult. Most cases of emphysema are caused by cigarette smoking.

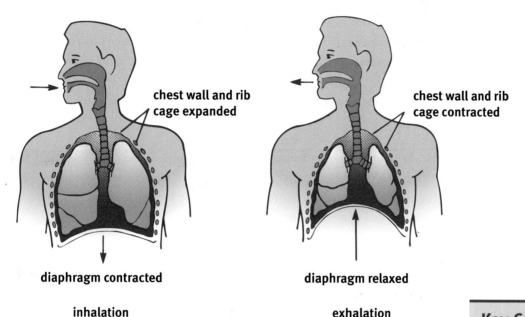

chest wall and rib cage expanded

chest wall and rib cage contracted

diaphragm contracted

diaphragm relaxed

inhalation

exhalation

Figure 8.3

CONTROL OF VENTILATION

Breathing requires input from our nervous control center, which we will examine in much more detail in a later chapter. Let's just briefly mention a few controls that are relevant to this discussion. Our ventilation is primarily regulated by neurons (**ventilation centers**) in the medulla oblongata that rhythmically fire to cause regular contraction of respiratory muscles. These neurons are primarily sensitive to carbon dioxide concentration. As the partial pressure of carbon dioxide rises, the respiratory rate will increase to counter it. How is carbon dioxide concentration measured? **Chemoreceptors** on the neurons' surfaces monitor changes in the blood's pH. Let's say that pH is decreased (increased proton concentration). Can we predict what will happen? The answer to this is a critically important MCAT concept that will be covered in great detail in Chapter 9.

We can, to a limited extent, control our breathing through the cerebrum. We can choose to breathe more rapidly or slowly; however, extended periods of hypoventilation would lead to increased carbon dioxide levels and an override by the medulla oblongata (which would jumpstart breathing). The opposite process (hyperventilation) would blow off too much carbon dioxide and inhibit ventilation (hopefully before we pass out!)

Lung Capacities and Volumes ★★★★☆☆

Certainly we can't pop our lungs out to measure air volumes, but pulmonologists (doctors who deal with the lungs and respiration) need to somehow assess lung

Key Concept

Inhalation and exhalation are different processes in terms of energy expenditure. Muscle contraction is required to create the negative pressure in the thoracic cavity that forces air in during inspiration. Expiration during calm states is entirely due to elastic recoil of the lungs and musculature. Of course, during more active states, the muscles can be used to force air out and speed the process of ventilation.

Key Concept

Although oxygen is necessary for life, it is primarily a response to rising CO_2 that drives ventilation. It is not until oxygen falls to a very low level that hypoxia would drive the ventilatory response.

capacities. One instrument used is a **spirometer**, which can measure the amount of air normally present in the lungs and the rate at which ventilation occurs. Note that we do not breathe all that rapidly when oxygen is abundant; a normal respiration rate is around 12 breaths per minute. On top of Mount Everest where there is only one third as much oxygen as at sea level, ventilation may increase to 80 to 90 times per minute!

Let's start with the largest measure and work our way down. **Total lung capacity** (**TLC**) in healthy human beings is about six to seven liters. Graphically, we can imagine two three-liter bottles: one for each lung. If we breathe in as much as possible, the total amount of air in our lungs at this point is the TLC.

Now let's say we breathe out until we cannot breathe out any more (i.e., we force out all air using our musculature). The total amount we forced out was the **vital capacity** (**VC**). This makes sense as it is the amount that we can actually (or vitally) use. The amount left over is the **residual volume** (**RV**). There will always be some air left over, because expelling it all would require lung collapse, which we definitely want to avoid. Now, if we were to add the VC and RV, what would we get as our answer? The TLC.

Of course, we don't always work at the extremes, which is what TLC, VC, and RV represent. Instead, we shallowly breathe only what we need, which may be a liter or so with each breath. This is known as the **tidal volume** (**TV**). It is analogous to the difference in level between the ocean's high tide (breathe in) and low tide (breathe out). The TV is not like the VC, which we had to force out. TV is the air that naturally comes out with exhalation. If we use respiratory muscles to push air out, the last bit of air that exits is the **expiratory reserve volume** (**ERV**). Because there is an expiratory reserve volume, there must also be an **inspiratory reserve volume** (**IRV**), which is the amount of extra air we can take in after a tidal breath. One last formula: What should the TV, ERV, and IRV sum to? The vital capacity, which is the total amount of gas that can be moved.

Key Concept

Remember that TLC = RV + VC and that VC = TV + ERV + IRV.

Let's take a look at Figure 8.4 to see these represented graphically.

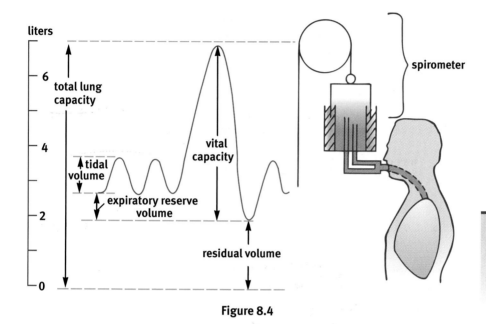

Figure 8.4

Gas Exchange ★★★★★★

Our last item for this chapter is the actual movement of gas in the lungs, which is, after all, their primary function. As we already mentioned, a network of pulmonary capillaries surrounds each alveolus. The capillaries bring deoxygenated blood from the pulmonary arteries, which stem from the right ventricle. As they approach, the single-celled alveolar layers allow for diffusion of carbon dioxide from the blood into the lungs and oxygen in the opposite direction. The oxygenated blood returns to the heart via the pulmonary veins. The driving force is the pressure differential of the gases. Since blood is deoxygenated as it enters, it has a relatively low partial pressure of oxygen and a relatively high pressure of carbon dioxide, facilitating the transfer of each down its respective concentration gradient. Since the gradient between the blood and air in the lungs is already present as the blood enters the lungs, no energy is required for gas transfer.  Although we will discuss this further in Chapter 9, it's worth mentioning that oxygen travels through the body using hemoglobin as its transporter.

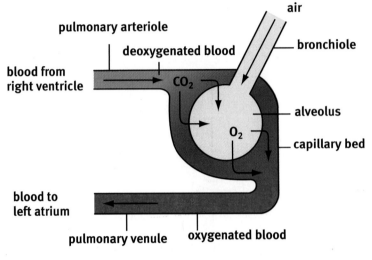

Figure 8.5

Now that we have mastered the respiratory system, let's take a break from MCAT studying and go skiing. How would our respiratory systems adjust on the slopes as we move to higher altitudes where there is less available oxygen? First, we can breathe more rapidly to try and increase gas exchange; second, we could make more red cells to carry the oxygen (polycythemia; see Chapter 9). In the long term, we could develop more blood vessels (vascularization), which would facilitate the distribution of a lower amount of oxygen to tissues; and finally, we can alter the binding dynamics of hemoglobin to oxygen. This will be a major point of discussion in Chapter 9. Now, let's exhale and get ready for the next chapter.

Conclusion

The functional unit of the lung is the alveolus just as the basic unit of muscle was the sarcomere. We learned that gas exchange across the lungs is a result of passive diffusion of carbon dioxide and oxygen down their concentration gradients. This diffusion is accomplished in the alveoli, which, when laid out, have an area of 100 m²! The actual process of breathing in and out is controlled by chemoreceptors in the ventilatory centers of the brain stem. Although we can voluntarily influence our breathing rate to a certain degree, our nervous system takes care of ventilation and gas concentrations in the body. Pressure gradients between the intrapleural space and lung provide the physical basis for ventilation. We literally suck air in from the atmosphere, because the pressure in the thoracic cavity during inspiration is lower than that in the outside world. Boyle's law is a key to understanding this process. The binding of oxygen to hemoglobin in the lungs is a concept that will be expanded on in the next chapter, as well as how altitude, pH, and chemicals may affect this binding.

CONCEPTS TO REMEMBER

☐ The alveolus is the basic unit of the lung and the site of gas exchange.

☐ The external nares and nasal cavity provide a method to both remove contaminants from air as well as humidify it before it reaches the lungs.

☐ The epiglottis provides a mechanism to prevent large material from entering the larynx and bronchi.

☐ The diaphragm and intercostal muscles are responsible for generating the negative pressure differential between each intrapleural space and its associated lung.

☐ Negative-pressure breathing is explained by Boyle's law and results in air literally being sucked into the lungs during inspiration.

☐ pH-sensitive chemoreceptors in the medulla oblongata control respiration rate.

☐ Measurement of lung volumes can be accomplished by using a spirometer. Deviations from standard values may indicate pathological conditions (e.g., increased TLC in emphysema).

☐ Total lung capacity is the sum of residual volume and vital capacity.

☐ Vital capacity is the sum of inspiratory reserve volume, tidal volume, and expiratory reserve volume.

☐ Gas exchange in the lungs is a passive process resulting from the large, preexisting concentration gradients of oxygen and carbon dioxide.

Practice Questions

1. All of the following facilitate gas exchange in the lungs EXCEPT

    A. thin alveolar surfaces.
    B. moist alveolar surfaces.
    C. differences in the partial pressures of O_2 and CO_2.
    D. active transport.

2. Which of the following associations between the two stages of respiration and the contraction of muscles is correct?

    A. Inhalation—diaphragm relaxes
    B. Inhalation—intercostal muscles relax
    C. Exhalation—diaphragm contracts
    D. Exhalation—intercostal muscles relax

3. What does negative-pressure breathing refer to?

    A. Breathing in low-oxygen conditions
    B. Breathing in low-pressure conditions
    C. Inhalation
    D. Breathing with use of a ventilator

4. The intrapleural space in the lungs is bounded by the

    A. visceral pleura and the parietal pleura.
    B. visceral pleura and the diaphragm.
    C. parietal pleura and the alveolar pleura.
    D. parietal pleura and the lungs.

5. Which of the following best describes the residual volume of the lungs?

    A. The amount of air normally inhaled and exhaled with each breath
    B. The maximum amount of air that can be forcibly inhaled and exhaled from the lungs
    C. The volume of air that can still be forcibly exhaled following a normal exhalation
    D. The volume of air that always remains in the lungs

6. The lungs can collapse from

    A. insufficient surfactant production.
    B. rupture of the parietal pleura.
    C. overproduction of surfactant.
    D. both A and B.

7. Which of the following mechanisms exist in the respiratory system to ensure that inhalation occurs rapidly and safely?

    A. The epiglottis covers the glottis to ensure that food does not enter the trachea during swallowing.
    B. The trachea and bronchi are lined by ciliated epithelial cells.
    C. The large surface area of the alveoli facilitates gas exchange.
    D. All of the above.

8. Which is the correct sequence of passagesways air travels through during inhalation?

   A. Pharynx → trachea → bronchioles → bronchi → alveoli

   B. Pharynx → trachea → lungs → bronchi → alveoli

   C. Larynx → pharynx → trachea → bronchi → alveoli

   D. Pharynx → larynx → trachea → bronchi → alveoli

9. Which of the following is generally a passive process?

   A. Inhalation

   B. Exhalation

   C. Gas exchange

   D. Both B and C

10. Total lung capacity is equal to the vital capacity plus the

   A. tidal volume.

   B. expiratory reserve volume.

   C. residual volume.

   D. inspiratory reserve volume.

Small Group Questions

1. Why are there more pulmonary veins than pulmonary arteries?

2. Would you expect the vital capacity of mountain dwellers to be greater or less than the vital capacity of people residing at sea level? What other physiological adaptations would you expect to observe in mountain dwellers?

Explanations to Practice Questions

1. D

Gas exchange in the lungs relies on passive diffusion of oxygen and carbon dioxide. This is accomplished easily because there is always a difference in the partial pressures of these two gases. In addition, the thin and moist alveolar surfaces allow for fast diffusion and gas exchange across their membranes. Therefore, (A), (B), and (C) can be eliminated. (D) is indeed the correct answer, since active transport is not needed in the gas exchange process in the lungs.

2. D

The muscles involved in ventilation are the diaphragm (which separates the thoracic cavity from the abdominal cavity,) and the intercostal muscles of the rib cage. During inhalation, the diaphragm contracts and flattens, while the external intercostal muscles contract, pushing the rib cage up and out. These actions cause an overall increase in the size of the thoracic cavity. During exhalation, both the diaphragm and the external intercostals relax, causing a decrease in the size of the thoracic cavity. Thus, the only correct association from the given answers is (D).

3. C

During inhalation, as the diaphragm and external intercostal muscles contract, the rib cage and chest wall are pushed up and out, and the thoracic cavity increases in volume. This volume increase, in turn, reduces the intrapleural pressure, causing the lungs to expand and fill with air. This process is referred to as negative-pressure breathing because air is drawn into the lungs by a vacuum. In contrast, positive-pressure breathing, as in a patient on a ventilator, occurs when air is forced into the lungs because the pressure is greater in the ventilator than in the lungs. (C) is therefore the correct answer.

4. A

The lungs are surrounded by two membranes: the visceral pleura and the parietal pleura. The parietal pleura surrounds the visceral pleura. The space between the pleurae is referred to as the intrapleural space and contains a thin layer of serous fluid. (A) is therefore the correct answer.

5. D

The residual volume is the volume of air that always remains in the lungs, and cannot be forcibly exhaled. (D) is thus the correct answer. (A) refers to the tidal volume, (B) defines the vital capacity, and (C) describes the expiratory reserve volume.

6. D

There are two major mechanisms in place to prevent the lungs from collapsing. First, the pleurae (visceral and parietal) surround and protect the lungs. An injury to the chest in which the parietal pleura is ruptured results in air getting into the intrapleural space, which can quickly cause the lungs to collapse, a condition known as pneumothorax. In addition, the alveoli are coated with a thin layer of surfactant, which reduces the high surface tension of the fluid lining the alveoli and prevents the lungs from collapsing during exhalation. As such, (A) and (B) are both true, making (D) the correct answer.

7. D

Several mechanisms exist to ensure that inhalation is rapid and poses no danger to the body. First, to prevent food particles from reaching the lungs, a flap of epiglottis covers the entrance to the trachea, called the glottis, during swallowing. Second, the trachea and bronchi are lined with ciliated epithelial cells, which filter and trap particles inhaled along with the air. Third, at the level of the alveoli, several mechanisms exist to ensure rapid inhalation: Thin, moist alveolar surfaces facilitate gas exchange, while lining of the alveoli with surfactant prevents lung collapse and also facilitates gas exchange. Based on this, (D) is the correct answer.

8. D

Air enters the respiratory tract through the external nares (nostrils) and travels through the nasal cavities. It then passes through the pharynx and into a second chamber called the larynx. Ingested food also passes through the pharynx on its way to the esophagus; to ensure that food does not accidentally enter the larynx, the epiglottis covers the larynx during swallowing. After the larynx, air goes to the trachea, which eventually divides into two bronchi, one for each lung. The bronchi branch into smaller and smaller bronchi, the terminal branches of which are referred to as bronchioles. The bronchioles are surrounded by clusters of alveoli. From the given sequences, only (D) correctly describes the sequence of the passages through which air travels.

9. D

Exhalation is generally a passive process involving elastic recoil of the lungs and relaxation of both the diaphragm and the external intercostal muscles (however, during vigorous exercise or forced expiration, active muscular contraction assists in expiration). Gas exchange is also a passive process; the gases diffuse down their partial pressure gradients. Inhalation, however, is an active process requiring contraction of the diaphragm and the external intercostals. (D) is thus the correct answer.

10. C

Total lung capacity is equal to the vital capacity (the maximum amount of air that can be forcibly inhaled and exhaled from the lungs) plus the residual volume (the air that always remains in the lungs, preventing the alveoli from collapsing). (C) is therefore the correct answer.

Cardiovascular System

As late as the 19th century, physicians adhered to the principle of health known as *humouralism*. No, this was not some strange hybrid of medicine and stand-up comedy. Humouralism was a theory of the makeup and functioning of the human body, developed by Greek and Roman physicians and philosophers, and adopted by Islamic physicians. It was dominant in medical thought and practice until it was ultimately displaced by modern medical research in the 1800s.

The humoral theory holds that the human body is composed of four fluids or substances called humors. These are black bile, yellow bile, phlegm, and blood. In the state of health, these four humors are in balance, but excess or deficiency of any one of them causes illness, disease, and even maladaptive personality characteristics. Over the course of a lifetime, the levels of each of the four humors would rise and fall in accordance with diet and activity, resulting in maladies reflective of the imbalance. Treatments were intended to restore the balance.

Furthermore, personalities came to be associated with each of the humors. Those who had an excess of phlegm were phlegmatic, which was associated with winter and characterized as wet and cold. Phlegmatic people were said to be calm, unemotional, and shy. Those who had an excess of blood were sanguine, which was associated with spring and characterized as wet and hot, and were said to be fun-loving, spontaneous, gregarious, but also prone to arrogance, indulgence, and even mania.

Perhaps one of the most well-known medical treatments associated with humouralism is the practice of bloodletting. Since many diseases were associated with an excess of blood, physicians (for nearly 2,000 years, mind you!) would rely on the withdrawal of significant amounts of blood from their patients to restore balance to the four humors. Methods for bloodletting were many and some were dramatic, including drawing blood from major veins in the arm or neck and puncturing arteries. Devices known as scarificators were developed to cut through to the superficial vessels. Most famously, leeches were used, especially in the early 19th century, to draw out the excess blood. In fact, in the early decades of the 1800s, hundreds of millions of leeches were used by European physicians; in the 1830s, France alone imported about 40 million leeches per year for medical treatments.

Now, before you start feeling superior to these "primitive" doctors and their "barbaric" medical practices, you should be aware that although the humoral theory has been completely discredited by modern medical research, some practices associated with humouralism are still being used, albeit based on very different medical understanding and for very different purposes. For example, new research has shown that medicinal leeches can be used effectively in microsurgery, where they help prevent blood coagulation, and in reconstructive surgery, where they help stimulate circulation to the reattached organ.

One of the most commonly tested MCAT topics is the cardiovascular system, which serves a variety of functions including the movement of respiratory gases, nutrients, and wastes. We will review the structures and functional anatomy of the cardiovascular system and then discuss blood and its functional components. Electrically excitable cells, whose connections we will outline, initiate and spread contractions throughout the heart. A quick recap of genetics and inheritance will help us understand ABO and Rh antigens, whose functional consequences we will also discuss. In addition, the ability of oxygen and carbon dioxide to bind to hemoglobin will be detailed, including a discussion of the factors that may affect this binding.

Anatomy of the Cardiovascular System

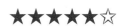

The cardiovascular system consists of a muscular four-chambered **heart**, **blood vessels**, and **blood.** In casual observation, we usually think and speak of the heart as a single pump, but actually it is two pumps connected in series (analogous to a circuit with two batteries in series). The right pump (the right heart) accepts deoxygenated blood returning from the body and moves it to the lungs by way of the pulmonary arteries for oxygenation. The left pump (the left heart) receives oxygenated blood from the lungs by way of the pulmonary veins and forces it out to the body through the aorta. The connections of the left and right heart to the systemic and pulmonary circulations, respectively, are commonly tested and easily learned MCAT topics. Each side of the heart is made up of two chambers: an **atrium** (pl. *atria*) and a **ventricle**. The atria are thin-walled, and you can think of them as the lobbies or waiting rooms for each side of the heart: Blood is received (from the body or from the lungs) in the atria before it is moved to the ventricles, which are more muscular because they do the actual work of pumping the blood out of the heart (to the body or the lungs).

We can follow the path of blood through the left and right sides of the closed cardiovascular circuit by picking any place within the circuit as our starting point. If we begin, say, in the left atrium with oxygenated blood, then we can follow the blood as it moves to the left ventricle, and then into the **aorta**, the largest artery in the body. Major arteries such as the coronary, common carotid, and renal arteries divide the blood flow from the aorta toward the different peripheral tissues. Arteries branch into **arterioles** and these ultimately lead to **capillaries**, which perfuse the tissues. On the venous side of a capillary network, the capillaries join together into **venules** that join into **veins**. The deoxygenated blood travels through the veins into the inferior and superior **vena cavae** (IVC and SVC), the largest veins in the body, which carry the blood to the right atrium. Blood then moves into the right ventricle, which pumps the blood to the lungs via the pulmonary arteries for gas exchange. Finally, blood leaves the lungs through the pulmonary veins and goes to the left atrium, where we started. Written out in shorthand, the pathway appears like this:

Left atrium → left ventricle → aorta → arteries → arterioles → capillaries → venules → veins → IVC and SVC → right atrium → right ventricle → pulmonary arteries → lungs → pulmonary veins → left atrium

In some cases, blood actually passes through two capillary beds, which are connected by venules, before being returned to the heart. Each of these networks has a special purpose and is referred to as a **portal system**. There is a hepatic portal system (see Chapter 7) connecting the vasculatures of the intestines and the liver, and a hypophyseal portal system in the brain, connecting the vasculatures of the hypothalamus and the pituitary gland (see Chapter 12). Both are test-worthy topics that you should review and understand.

Bridge

The heart and blood vessels are analogous to a pair of batteries that are linked in series. The right heart is a low-pressure system (like a low-voltage battery) that sends blood to the lungs, whereas the left heart is a high-pressure system (like a high-voltage battery) that sends blood to the body.

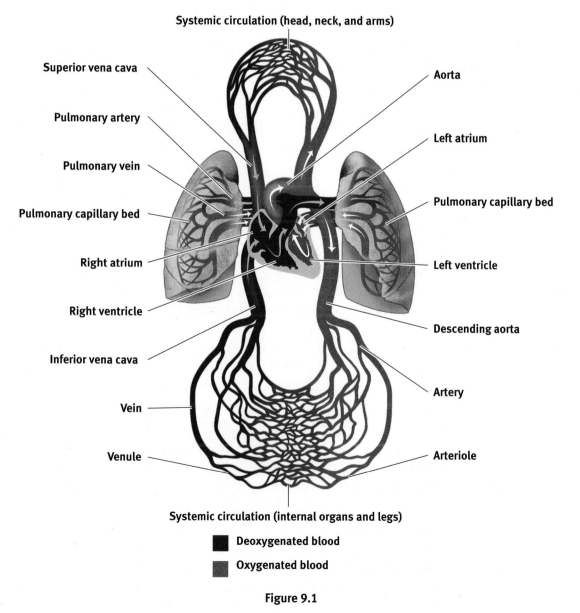

Figure 9.1

Real World

Oxygen and nutrients are supplied to the heart muscle by the coronary arteries. A delicate balance exists between the supply of oxygen to the heart (coronary blood flow) and the myocardial oxygen demand. Deprivation of oxygen and nutrients to the heart is called myocardial ischemia. The most common clinical manifestation of this condition is a type of chest pain called *angina*. If this ischemia goes on unchecked, parts of the heart muscle may become irreversibly damaged. This is called myocardial infarction (heart attack). Although there are many possible causes for decreased coronary blood flow, the most common by far is atherosclerosis of the coronary arteries (the formation of a plaque composed primarily of cholesterol).

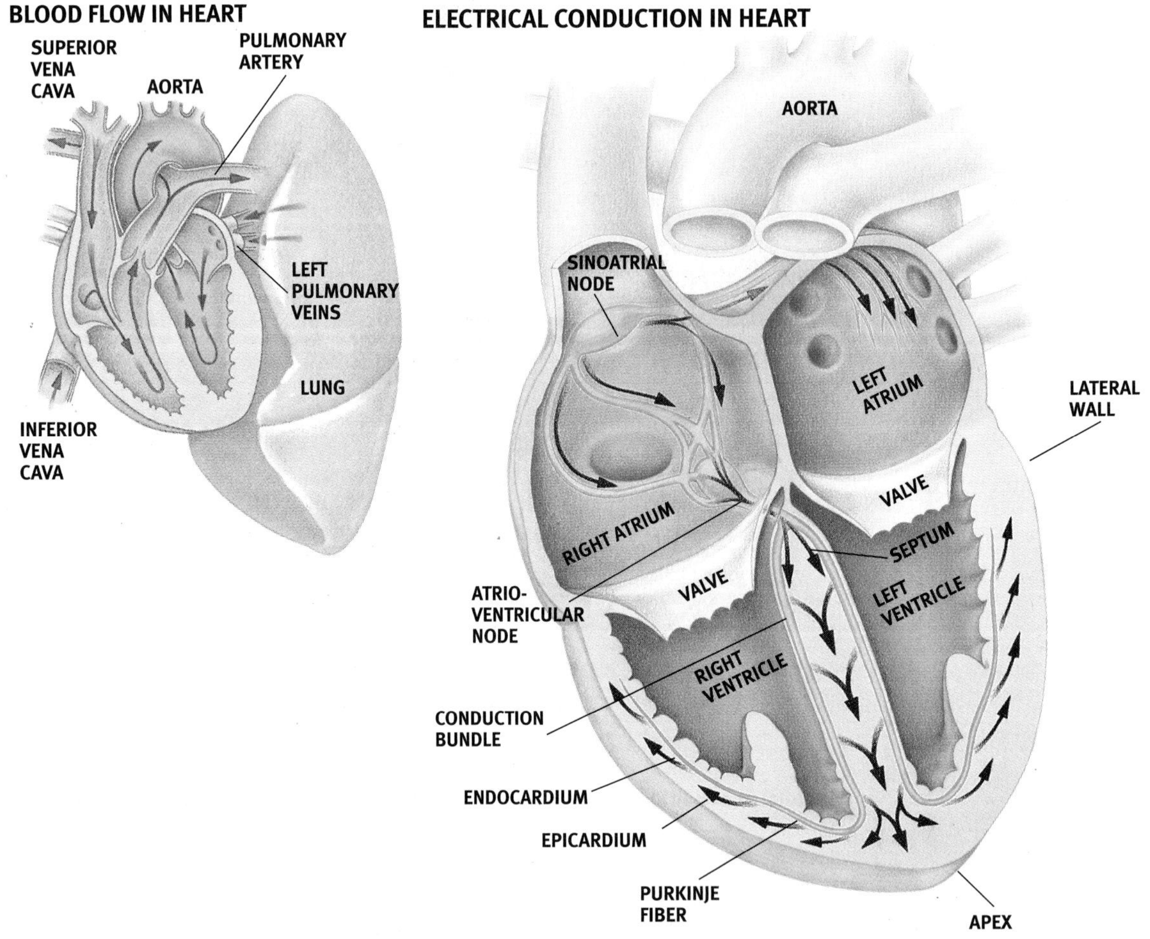

THE HEART

Alas, the human heart is not the lacy pink object associated with Valentine's Day. (Can you imagine the utter shock of the cardiothoracic surgeon who finds, upon opening up a patient's chest cavity, a heart-shaped box of chocolates?) Nor is the human heart merely a square four-room apartment with two entrances, two exits, and two sets of French doors connecting the anterior and posterior room—although for simplicity and clarity, the heart is usually drawn like the floor plan of said apartment: a box divided into four square chambers. The heart is a muscular organ a little larger than your fist, weighing between 7 and 15 ounces. Located between the lungs, it lies behind and a little to the left of the sternum, and it is tilted ever so slightly so that the exterior wall of the right ventricle forms the base of the heart. The walls of the heart are composed of cardiac muscle of varying thickness. It may seem to be an obvious point, but we've known students to make this mistake, so let's be as clear as possible: Cardiac muscle is found only in the heart, and no other muscle type composes the muscle tissue of the heart.

Figure 9.2

Can we make an MCAT-worthy prediction concerning whether the left or right heart will be more muscular? Let's think about which side works at higher pressures and has to pump the blood farther. The left heart is responsible for pumping blood to all the tissues of the body by way of the systemic circulation. In order to do so, it must be able to generate high pressures. The right heart, on the other hand, is responsible for pumping blood to the lungs via the pulmonary circulation. It can do so at lower pressures (because there's little resistance to the blood flow through the pulmonary circulation). Therefore, the left heart must be more muscular, since it has to generate higher pressures to pump the blood over greater distances. In fact, the wall of the left ventricle is the thickest in the heart, at about half an inch. You may have heard that there is a difference in the volumes of arterial blood and venous blood (see below); indeed, that is true. Nevertheless, because the right and left sides of the heart are in series with each other, the total volumes of blood passing through the two sides (about 5 liters per minute) are the same.

Valves

As we discussed, the heart moves blood through the systemic and pulmonary vasculatures by generating pressures through contraction. It is critical for blood to move in a single direction (forward) in the system. Different valves in the heart and in veins ensure that the blood will flow only in one direction. The heart contains four valves. Between each of the atria and ventricles are the aptly named **atrioventricular (AV) valves**. These valves also have colloquial names, which you should know for Test Day. The right AV valve is also called the **tricuspid** valve because it has three leaflets; the left AV valve has only two leaflets and is also known as the **bicuspid** or **mitral** valve. When the heart beats by ventricular contraction, the blood must move forward into the pulmonary arteries and aorta. These two valves prevent backflow into the right and left atria, respectively.

There are also valves that prevent backflow into the ventricles. Each ventricle is protected by a **semilunar valve** with three cusps. The right semilunar valve is called the **pulmonary** valve, because it sits between the right ventricle and pulmonary arteries; the one on the left is the **aortic** valve, as it separates the left ventricle from the aorta. They prevent backflow of blood from the pulmonary arteries and aorta into the ventricles during ventricular relaxation (**diastole**), whereas the AV valves prevent backflow from ventricles into atria during contraction (**systole**).

Contraction

Phases

The heart is a muscle that must contract in order to move blood. Each heartbeat is composed of two phases known as systole and diastole. During systole, ventricular contraction and closure of the AV valves occur and blood is pumped

Key Concept

Because the right heart pumps blood only to the lungs, which are close by and whose vasculature offers lower resistance, it can operate at lower pressures. Consequently, the walls of the right heart are not as thick as those of the left. In the left heart, which is responsible for systemic circulation, the walls are thicker and more muscular because they must generate stronger contractions to maintain higher pressures, to move blood over a longer distance and against higher resistance.

Real World

The rhythmic impulses ("*lub dub*") we hear when we listen to someone's heart with a stethoscope are referred to as the heart sounds. The first heart sound, S1, is produced when the two atrioventricular valves close at the start of systole to prevent blood from flowing back into the atria. The second heart sound, S2, is produced when the two semilunar valves close at the conclusion of systole to prevent blood from flowing back into the ventricles. Heart murmurs, which may be so loud as to be audible without a stethoscope, arise when the valves malfunction and become either narrow and stiff or wide and floppy, resulting in abnormal flow patterns across the valve.

Real World

There is a limit to how fast the heart can beat and still pump blood effectively. Since the heart fills with blood when it is relaxing (diastole), the faster it beats, the less time there is for blood to enter the heart during relaxation. Thus, a faster heartbeat means diminishing returns in terms of the amount of blood supplied to the body. A dangerous condition called ventricular tachycardia (often abbreviated *v tach*) describes rates upward of 200 beats per minute. The heart in v tach cannot properly fill with blood and, paradoxically, stops pumping blood. Systemic pressures drop precipitously. Death will result unless the heart is forced out of this abnormal rhythm.

Key Concept

Recall from Chapter 6 that cardiac muscle is functionally a hybrid of smooth muscle and striated muscle. Cardiac muscle can beat without descending (neural) input due to the automaticity of its internal contraction system; however, as with smooth muscle, this rate can be modulated by the descending input.

out of the ventricles. During diastole, the heart is relaxed, semilunar valves are closed, and blood from the atria is filling the ventricles. Contraction of the ventricular muscles generates the higher pressures of systole, whereas their relaxation during diastole causes the pressure to decrease. The elasticity of the walls of the large arteries, which stretch out to receive the volume of blood from the heart, allows the vessels to maintain sufficient pressure while the ventricular muscles are relaxed. In fact, if it weren't for the elasticity of the large arteries, your diastolic blood pressure (which is a gauge pressure; see below) would plummet to zero and you wouldn't survive for very long: *die*-astolic indeed!

A measure we should be aware of is the **cardiac output,** the total blood volume pumped by the ventricle in a minute. Does it matter which ventricle we choose? No. The two pumps are connected in series, so the volumes of blood passing through each side are the same. This sort of critical thinking is exactly what we need on Test Day. Cardiac output is the product of **heart rate** (beats per minute) and **stroke volume** (volume of blood pumped per beat). For humans, cardiac output is about 5 L/min. Incidentally, the average total volume of blood in a human is about 5 liters. Cardiac output will depend on size and age of person, as well as cardiovascular and systemic health of the individual. During periods of rest or exercise, the autonomic nervous system will decrease (parasympathetic) or increase (sympathetic) cardiac output, respectively.

Mechanism and Control

The autonomic nervous system will regulate cardiac output by increasing or decreasing the heart rate, similar to the way in which it regulates breathing (see Chapter 8). However, cardiac muscle, like smooth muscle, demonstrates myogenic activity (see Chapter 6). In other words, neural signals can modulate the rate at which the heart beats, but the heart will continue to function even without input from the nervous system. We might even say that the heart marches to the beat of its own drummer.

The coordinated, rhythmic contraction of cardiac muscle originates in an electrical impulse generated by and traveling through a pathway formed by four electrically excitable structures. This commonly tested pathway consists of, in order, the **sinoatrial (SA) node**, the **atrioventricular (AV) node**, the **bundle of His (AV bundle)**, and the **Purkinje fibers**. **Impulse** initiation occurs at the SA node, which generates 60–100 signals per minute without any neural input. This small collection of cells is located in the wall of the right atrium. As the depolarization wave spreads from the SA node, it causes the two atria to contract simultaneously. Atrial systole (contraction) results in an increase in atrial pressure and more blood pumped into the ventricles. This additional volume of blood forced from the atria into the ventricles is called the atrial kick and accounts for about 5–30% of the cardiac output. Next, the signal reaches the AV node, which sits at the junction of the atria and ventricles. The signal may be delayed here to allow for the ventricles to fill completely before they contract. It then travels down the bundle of His, embedded in the interventricular septum (wall), and to the Purkinje fibers, which distribute the electrical signal through the ventricular muscle, causing ventricular contraction.

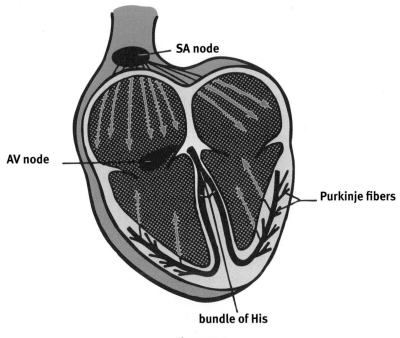

Figure 9.3

The SA node has an intrinsic rhythm of 60–100 signals per minute, so the normal human heart rate is 60–100 beats per minute. Highly conditioned athletes (most famously, triathletes) may have heart rates significantly lower than 60, in the range of 40–50 beats per minute. Stress, exercise, excitement, surprise, or danger can cause the heart rate to rise significantly above 100. We wouldn't advise doing so, but you could test this by suddenly clapping and yelling very loudly in the middle of the MCAT testing session and then immediately measuring the heart rate of the other test takers. We guarantee that you would observe tachycardia (elevated heart rate) in every person. Granted, you might not survive the violent anger directed toward you long enough to collect the data for your little Test Day experiment.

So what part of the nervous system influences cardiac contractions? The auto-nomic division, which consists of **parasympathetic** ("rest and digest") and **sym-pathetic** ("fight or flight") branches, controls the heart. Parasympathetic neu-rotransmitters slow the heart via the **vagus nerve** (more on this in Chapter 12), whereas sympathetic neurotransmitters speed it up. Quick review: Which system

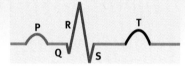
would jump into action when we're in the woods, running away from an angry bear? The sympathetic branch of the autonomic division. We exploit this autonomic control of heart rate in medicine all the time. For example, after suffering a heart attack, a patient will often be given a drug called a β-blocker, which blocks sympathetic β-receptors. The β-blocker reduces the heart rate and blood pressure, thereby reducing the cardiac workload and reducing the heart's need for oxygen. It is thought that by preventing the heart from overworking after a heart attack, the risk of death and of future heart attacks can be reduced.

Blood Vessels

We have considered how the heart acts as a pump to move blood through systemic and pulmonary circulation, and we have even compared the two sides of the heart to low- and high-voltage batteries connected in series. Now let's consider the conductive pathway of this vascular circuit, by examining the vessels through which the blood flows. The three major types of vessels are arteries, veins, and capillaries. Arteries are strong, thick-walled structures that always carry blood *away* from the heart (*ar*teries = *a*way) to the lungs and all other parts of the body, like our brain (which will need a lot of nourishment for critical thinking on Test Day!). Most arteries contain oxygenated blood. Only the pulmonary arteries and (fetal) umbilical arteries carry deoxygenated blood. Veins are thin-walled and inelastic vessels that transport blood *to* the heart (*v*eins con*v*erge near the heart). Except for the pulmonary and umbilical vessels, all veins carry deoxygenated blood. Take a look at Figure 9.4. Notice that arteries and veins share the same components, simply in different proportions. Don't worry about the names of all the different layers. Simply be able to recognize that the same types of cells comprise both types of vessels, and that arteries have much more smooth muscle than veins.

Due to their high elasticity, arteries offer high resistance to the flow of blood, which is why the left ventricle must generate the higher pressures. After they are filled with blood, the elastic recoil from their walls maintains a high pressure and forces blood forward. Conversely, veins are capacitive and can carry large amounts of blood owing to their thin, inelastic walls, which stretch out easily and do not recoil. Indeed, three-fourths of our total blood volume may be in venous circulation at any given moment.

Given that the heart is located in the chest, the blood flow in most veins is upward from the lower body back to the heart, against gravity. In the inferior vena cava, this translates into a lot of blood in a large column. As you might imagine, the pressure at the bottom of this venous column in, say, the large veins of the legs, can be quite high. In fact, it can exceed systolic pressure (120 mmHg) going as high as 200 mmHg or more. In light of this, two questions must be answered: How do veins prevent backflow in the venous circulation? And, how do veins move blood forward

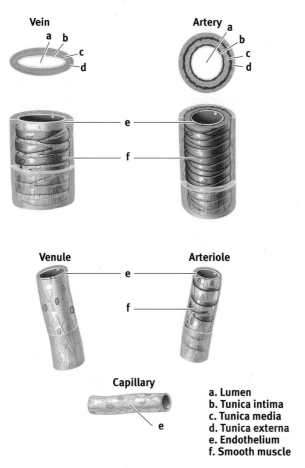

Vein

a b
c
d

Artery a
b
c
d

e
f

Venule   **Arteriole**

e
f

Capillary

e

a. Lumen
b. Tunica intima
c. Tunica media
d. Tunica externa
e. Endothelium
f. Smooth muscle

Figure 9.4

toward the heart, given the inelasticity and the thinner or absent layer of smooth muscle in their walls? First, the larger veins have one-way valves to prevent backflow. Blood flowing forward pushes the valves open, but if blood begins to move backward, the valves are pushed shut. Failure of the venous valves results in the formation of varicose veins, which are distended where the blood has pooled. Pregnant women are especially susceptible to the formation of varicose veins because the total blood volume increases dramatically during pregnancy resulting in increased venous pressure, especially in the lower body due to the fetus compressing the IVC.

The second question is answered by considering the relationship between the large veins and skeletal muscles. Most large veins are surrounded by skeletal muscle, which squeezes the veins as muscles contract, forcing the blood up against gravity, in much the same way that squeezing the bottom of a tube of toothpaste causes the contents to be expelled onto your toothbrush. This is why sitting motionless for long periods of time, such as in a cramped middle seat on a long transatlantic flight, can increase the risk of pulmonary embolism. Blood pools in the lower extremities; sluggish blood coagulates more easily. If a blood clot forms in the vein and becomes dislodged, it may be carried through the heart into the pulmonary vasculature, where it may get stuck in a small vessel.

The third and final type of blood vessel is the capillary. Capillaries are vessels with a single endothelial cell layer that allows for exchange of nutrients and gases. Capillaries can be quite delicate. The punch that you so rudely received from your sibling in Chapter 6 probably left a bruise, an area in which broken capillaries allowed erythrocytes to escape into the interstitial space. Capillaries are usually so small that blood cells must traverse them single file.

BLOOD PRESSURE

The voltage or potential difference between two points in a circuit is analogous to blood pressure: The pressure gradient from left to right is the fundamental determinant of the movement of blood through the closed vascular circuit, just as the electric potential difference between two points causes charge to move between them. Blood pressure is a measure of the force per unit area that is exerted on the wall of the blood vessels. This is exactly how we define pressure when discussing any fluid or solid: force per unit area. The device used to measure blood pressure is called a **sphygmomanometer** (and is quite a mouthful!). Sphygmomanometers measure the gauge pressure in the systemic circulation, which is the pressure above atmospheric pressure (760 mmHg at sea level). Blood pressure is expressed as a ratio of the systolic (ventricular contraction) to diastolic (ventricular relaxation) pressures. Pressure gradually drops from the arterial to venous circulation, although the largest drop is across the arterioles.

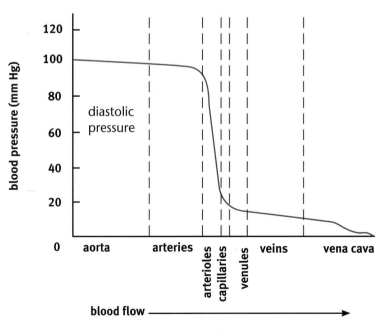

Figure 9.5

Blood

Now that we have examined the pump and the pipes, let's talk about the fluid that travels through them.

COMPOSITION

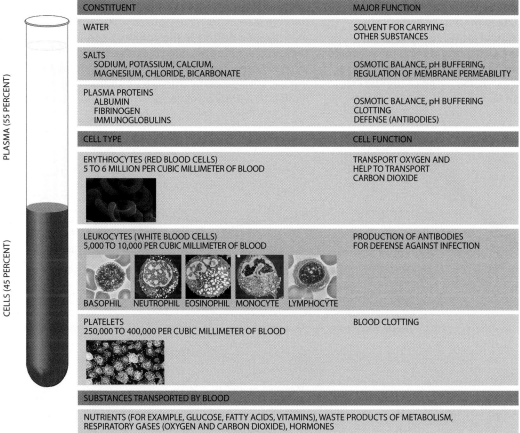

THE COMPOSITION OF BLOOD

CONSTITUENT	MAJOR FUNCTION
WATER	SOLVENT FOR CARRYING OTHER SUBSTANCES
SALTS SODIUM, POTASSIUM, CALCIUM, MAGNESIUM, CHLORIDE, BICARBONATE	OSMOTIC BALANCE, pH BUFFERING, REGULATION OF MEMBRANE PERMEABILITY
PLASMA PROTEINS ALBUMIN FIBRINOGEN IMMUNOGLOBULINS	OSMOTIC BALANCE, pH BUFFERING CLOTTING DEFENSE (ANTIBODIES)

CELL TYPE	CELL FUNCTION
ERYTHROCYTES (RED BLOOD CELLS) 5 TO 6 MILLION PER CUBIC MILLIMETER OF BLOOD	TRANSPORT OXYGEN AND HELP TO TRANSPORT CARBON DIOXIDE
LEUKOCYTES (WHITE BLOOD CELLS) 5,000 TO 10,000 PER CUBIC MILLIMETER OF BLOOD BASOPHIL NEUTROPHIL EOSINOPHIL MONOCYTE LYMPHOCYTE	PRODUCTION OF ANTIBODIES FOR DEFENSE AGAINST INFECTION
PLATELETS 250,000 TO 400,000 PER CUBIC MILLIMETER OF BLOOD	BLOOD CLOTTING

SUBSTANCES TRANSPORTED BY BLOOD
NUTRIENTS (FOR EXAMPLE, GLUCOSE, FATTY ACIDS, VITAMINS), WASTE PRODUCTS OF METABOLISM, RESPIRATORY GASES (OXYGEN AND CARBON DIOXIDE), HORMONES

PLASMA (55 PERCENT)

CELLS (45 PERCENT)

Figure 9.6

We learn from those pesky paper cuts that blood is a bright red substance and that it's never a good idea to run the edge of paper over your skin, even on a dare. To learn more about blood, we'll need some help from our MCAT biologist's toolbox. First, using a centrifuge, we can spin blood down to separate its components by density. Doing so separates the blood into two compartments: by volume, blood is 55% liquid and 45% cells, as seen above in Figure 9.6. **Plasma** is the liquid portion of blood, an aqueous mixture of nutrients, salts, respiratory gases, hormones, and blood proteins. Finally, if we pull out our handy-dandy microscope, we can examine the components of the cell compartment, which fall into three major categories: **erythrocytes**, **leukocytes**, and **platelets**. All blood cells are formed from the same hematopoietic stem cells, which originate in the bone marrow. See Figure 9.7 for a schematic of how blood cells are all ancestrally related.

HIERARCHY IN BLOOD-FORMING CELLS

Stem cells in the blood-forming, or hematopoietic, system illustrate principles governing the activity of stem cells in other tissues as well. A small population of hematopoietic stem cells (HSC) in the bone marrow is the source of most of the different blood and immune cell types that circulate in the human body. HSCs reside in an environmental niche, surrounded by stromal cells that provide important regulatory signals to the stem cell. When new blood or immune cells are needed, an HSC divides to produce one daughter cell that remains in the niche and retains the long-term

HSC identity and another short-lived daughter termed a multipotent progenitor cell (MPP). The MPP, in turn, divides to produce progenitors committed to generating cells in the myeloid (blood) or lymphoid (immune) lineages. As the descendants of progenitors become increasingly specialized they experience a programmed decline in their ability to proliferate until they stop dividing and are said to be terminally differentiated. Only the stem cell retains unlimited proliferative potential through its ability to renew itself indefinitely by dividing without differentiating.

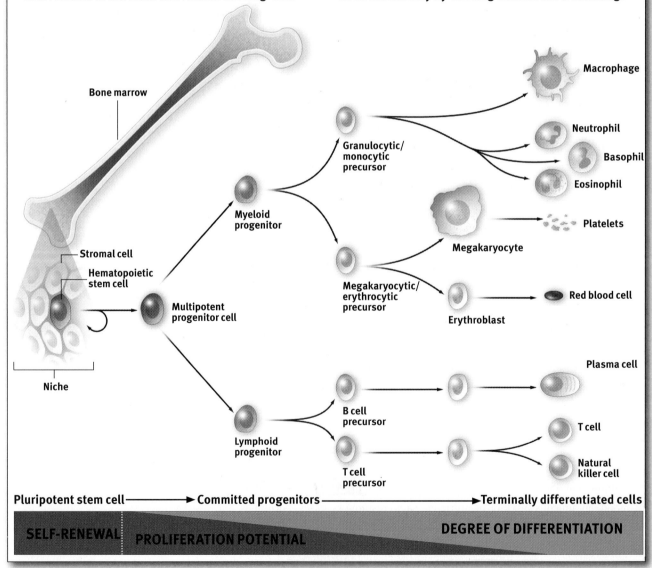

Figure 9.7

Erythrocytes (Red Blood Cells)

In the body, oxygen and nutrients are delivered to the peripheral tissues, and carbon dioxide and other wastes (e.g., hydrogen ions, ammonia) are picked up from the peripheral tissues and delivered to the organs of waste management—the lungs, liver, and kidneys. The erythrocyte is a specialized cell designed for oxygen transport. Red blood cells are like couriers who travel up and down elevators all day, delivering goods and picking up packages. Oxygen is not simply dissolved in the cytoplasm of the red blood cell. (Remember, molecular oxygen is nonpolar and therefore has low solubility in aqueous environments.) Rather, each erythrocyte contains about 250 million molecules of **hemoglobin** protein, and each hemoglobin can bind four molecules of oxygen. That's one billion molecules of oxygen per cell! Red blood cells are unique in other ways, as well, and the modifications reflect their special role in the human body. On the surface, they look different from other cells: They have a biconcave disk shape that serves a dual purpose. First, this shape assists them in traveling through tiny capillaries. Second, it increases the cell's surface area, which allows for greater gas exchange.

However, beauty isn't only skin deep; when we peer beneath the cell membrane of the erythrocyte, we discover many more fascinating characteristics—fascinating more for what is not there than what is. As red blood cells mature, they lose their nuclei, mitochondria, and other membranous organelles. (You'll recall from our discussion in Chapter 6 that red blood cells form and mature in the bone marrow before they are released into the circulation.) The loss of membrane-bound organelles is a dramatic modification, to say the least. What purpose does this serve? It essentially clears some room, which allows the cell to carry a maximal amount of hemoglobin for gas exchange. Additionally, since no mitochondria are present to enable aerobic respiration, none of the transported oxygen will be used up for cellular respiration. Of course, this means that red blood cells must rely on fermentation (lactic acid, not ethanol—human cells are not microbreweries!) for ATP production. Furthermore, without nuclei, erythrocytes cannot divide. They live for about 120 days in the bloodstream, getting knocked about, dented, and dinged, before cells in the spleen and liver phagocytize them for recycled parts. There are about 5 million erythrocytes per milliliter of blood. This translates into a total of about 25 billion red blood cells that can carry up to 100 billion oxygen molecules in the total blood volume!

Leukocytes (White Blood Cells)

Like erythrocytes, leukocytes, or white blood cells, form in the bone marrow. Leukocytes usually comprise less than 1% of total blood volume. This translates into about 500–1,000 leukocytes per milliliter of blood, which is a small number relative to the erythrocyte concentration. This number can massively increase under certain conditions when we need supplemental white blood cells, most notably during infection. White blood cells are a crucial part of the immune system, acting as our defenders against pathogens, foreign cells, and other materials not recognized as self. Let's briefly discuss five basic types of leukocytes, which are all categorized as **granulocytes** or **agranulocytes**.

The granular leukocytes (**neutrophils, eosinophils**, and **basophils**) are so named because cytoplasmic granules are visible under microscopy. These granules are like miniature bombs containing a variety of compounds that are toxic to invading microbes. (Remember how we mentioned viral and bacterial infections as invaders and spies in Chapter 1.) Granular lymphocytes are involved in inflammatory reactions, allergies, pus formation, and destruction of bacteria and parasites.

The agranulocytes, which do not contain granules, consist of **lymphocytes** and **monocytes**. Lymphocytes are important in the **specific immune response**, the body's targeted fight against particular pathogens such as viruses and bacteria. Some lymphocytes are involved in the immediate fight against an infection, while others function to maintain a long-term memory bank of pathogen recognition. These cells, in a very real sense, help our body learn from experience and are prepared to mount a lightning-fast response to repeated exposure to familiar pathogens. For example, most children in the United States receive different vaccines to help build their immune systems. One such vaccine is the chickenpox vaccine, which includes a live but weaker strain of the virus (varicella) that causes chickenpox. When the vaccine is administered, the virus is recognized as foreign and an immune response is activated. In the process, certain immune cells develop that maintain a memory of the virus; our body learns what it looks like and prepares itself to ward off the virus later in life.

Lymphocyte maturation takes place in one of three locations. Those lymphocytes that mature in the spleen or lymph nodes are referred to as B-cells, and those that mature in the thymus are called T-cells. B-cells are responsible for antibody generation, whereas T-cells kill virally infected cells and activate other immune cells.

The other agranulocytes are monocytes, which phagocytize foreign matter such as bacteria. They are renamed to **"macrophages"** once they leave the marrow, travel through the bloodstream, and move into tissue outside the vascular system. In the brain, they are called **microglia**.

Platelets

Platelets are actually cell fragments derived from the breakup of cells known as **megakaryocytes** in the marrow. Their function is to clot blood. They are present in concentrations of 200,000–500,000 per milliliter. The enzymatic reactions involved in the formation of a clot (the clotting cascade) will be discussed shortly.

Real World

Human immunodeficiency virus (HIV) causes a loss of a certain subset of T-cells known as helper T-cells (CD4⁺). Although the loss of helper T-cells alone is not fatal, the destruction of these lymphocytes prevents the generation of immune responses against opportunistic infections. This is why people infected with HIV (often referred to as *immunocompromised*) are more susceptible to a variety of diseases against which an intact immune system would normally be able to defend.

BLOOD ANTIGENS

How do we know who we are? Existential questions of self, identity, being, and purpose are beyond the scope of the MCAT. (But we would certainly encourage you to think about these questions when you're not studying for the MCAT!) In part, we each define ourselves based on an outward projection, an image or representation of an interior sense of self. Our mannerisms, speech patterns, style of dress, and political or religious activities, to name but a few outward expressions of interior processes, help us recognize ourselves as self and distinguish ourselves from others. Cells operate in similar ways to identify themselves and recognize each other. Cells put on a style of dress or a manner of acting reflective of the processes going on deep inside the cell. For example, a direct way of identifying cell type is to examine the proteins expressed on the extracellular surface of the cell membrane. Since surface proteins expressed by a cell may initiate an organism's immune system, we call these proteins *antigens*. The two major antigen families that we need to discuss relative to blood groups are the **ABO antigens** and the **Rh factor** protein.

ABO Group

First up is the ABO classification. Take a look at Table 9.1, and we will discuss it below.

Table 9.1

Blood Type	Antigen in Red Blood Cell	Antibodies Produced
A	A	anti-B
B	B	anti-A
AB (universal recipient)	A and B	none
O (universal donor)	none	anti-A and anti-B

Now that we know what we are looking at, let's fill in the details. The ABO system is based on the existence of three alleles for blood type. But, as we will discuss in Chapter 13 (and we may already know), the human genome is diploid and for each gene there will be two alleles, one of maternal and the other of paternal origin. For this particular class of erythrocyte cell-surface protein, the A and B alleles are codominant. This is to say, if the allele for A is present (I^A), it will be expressed; if the allele for B is present (I^B), it will be expressed; and if we have an allele for each, both will be expressed. O is recessive to both. People with type O blood don't express either variant of this protein (antigen). For the type O blood phenotype, the genotype is ii. The naming system of blood types based on the presence or absence of these protein variants doesn't refer to the alleles themselves, but to the proteins, and the four blood types are: A, B, AB, and O. Be aware that there are two possible

MCAT Expertise

You are almost guaranteed to see at least one question on blood groups on Test Day. It is critical that you learn how the system works (A/B codominant).

genotypes each for type A and type B blood. The possible genotypes for type A blood are I^AI^A or I^Ai; and for type B blood, the possible genotypes are I^BI^B or I^Bi.

Why are we making such a big deal about this? Because the MCAT makes a big deal about this. "And why is that?" you might be asking. Because the ABO classification has such important implications for medical practice. For example, it is critical to match blood types for transfusions. It's no exaggeration to say that blood type matching is a life and death matter, given the severe hemolysis that can result if the donor blood antigen is recognized as foreign by the recipient's immune system. The foreign antigens are recognized by antibodies. For example, a person with type A blood will recognize the type A protein variant as self but the type B variant protein as foreign, and will make antibodies to type B. Since type O blood cells express neither antigen variant, they will not initiate any immune response, regardless of the recipient's actual blood type. However, a recipient who is type O, and whose immune system does not recognize either protein variant as self, will produce both anti-A *and* anti-B antibodies. This leads to our recognition of **universal recipients and donors**. People with type AB blood (universal recipients) can receive from all blood types. No blood antigen is foreign to AB blood group members, so no adverse reactions will occur upon transfusion. People with type O blood can donate to all groups (universal donor) as their blood cells have no ABO antigens on the surface for anti-A or anti-B antibodies to recognize.

Rh Factor

The Rh factor (so named because it was first described in Rhesus monkeys) is also a surface protein expressed on red blood cells. Although at one time it was thought to be a single antigen, it has since been found to exist as several variants. However, there is one predominant variant whose presence or absence is indicated by a plus or minus superscript on the ABO blood type (e.g. O⁺, AB⁻). Rh⁺ individuals express the Rh protein on their erythrocytes and Rh⁻ individuals do not. The presence of the Rh factor is a dominant condition; one positive allele is enough for the protein to be expressed.

The Rh factor status is particularly important in maternal-fetal medicine. During childbirth, women are often exposed to fetal blood. If a woman is Rh⁻ and her fetus is Rh⁺, she will become sensitized to the Rh factor and her immune system will begin making antibodies against it. This is not a problem during first pregnancies because sensitization and antibody production begin only at the time of delivery. However, any subsequent pregnancy in which the fetus is Rh⁺ will present a problem because maternal anti-Rh antibodies can cross the placenta and attack the fetal blood cells, resulting in hemolysis of the fetal cells. This condition is known as **erythroblastosis fetalis**, which can be fatal to the fetus. Today, we can use medicine to prevent this condition (see the sidebar). There is less concern with ABO mismatching between mother and fetus, because these maternal antibodies do not readily cross the placenta (they are a different subclass of antibody). ABO and Rh typing often appear as discrete MCAT questions.

Functions of the Cardiovascular System ★★★★☆

We have fully discussed the anatomical components of the cardiovascular system—the heart, blood vessels, and blood—and we are now ready to discuss the overarching purpose of the system. The cardiovascular system transports many compounds including gases, nutrients, and waste products to and from the body's tissues, through the red blood cells and plasma. Furthermore, it serves an important role in immunity through the production of the different types of leukocytes and delivery of those immune cells to fight against localized or systemic pathogens. Finally, through the activity of platelets and clot formation, the system has a built-in mechanism for repairing damaged vessels. Let's start with gas transport.

TRANSPORT OF GASES

Two major gases are transported in the blood: oxygen and carbon dioxide. Oxygen is delivered from the lungs to the tissues and carbon dioxide is removed from the tissues for transport to the lungs. We will investigate each one separately.

Oxygen is primarily carried by hemoglobin in the blood. We should recall that hemoglobin is a protein made up of four separate but interacting chains, each of which has a prosthetic heme group to bind an oxygen molecule. The actual binding of oxygen is accomplished by the heme group's central iron atom, which can undergo changes in its oxidation state. The binding or releasing of oxygen to or from the iron atom in the heme group is a redox reaction.

As the first oxygen binds to a heme group, it induces a conformational shift in the shape of hemoglobin from taut to relaxed. This shift results in an increase in hemoglobin's affinity for oxygen, making it easier for subsequent molecules of oxygen to bind to the other unoccupied heme groups. Once hemoglobin is full, the removal of one molecule of oxygen also results in a conformational shift. This shift results in a decrease in hemoglobin's affinity for oxygen, making it easier for the other molecules of oxygen to leave the heme groups. This phenomenon is referred to as cooperative binding and results in the classic sigmoidal (S-shaped) hemoglobin-binding curve. From our discussion of enzymes in Chapter 2, you should recognize this pattern of binding as an allosteric effect (due to the quaternary structure of the hemoglobin protein).

Key Concept

Remember that hemoglobin is composed of four subunits (i.e., hemoglobin protein has quaternary structure). The interaction among the four subunits (allosteric effect) results in a change in hemoglobin's binding affinity for oxygen and gives the classic sigmoidal binding curve. Myoglobin, the globular protein responsible for transferring oxygen from hemoglobin to the muscle cells, is composed of only one subunit and lacks quaternary structure. Its curve is not sigmoidal, but shows rapid saturation at low P_{O_2}.

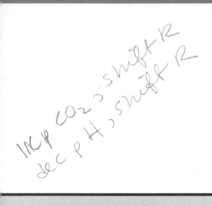

To make sure that we fully understand this important concept, let's draw a second curve to the right of the normal one in Figure 9.8. Notice that at the same partial pressure of O_2 (e.g., 60 mmHg), the O_2 saturation level will be lower on the right curve than on the normal one. The oxygen saturation is lower because the hemoglobin is more readily giving up its oxygen.

MCAT Expertise

The hemoglobin–oxygen dissociation curve is not static—it can shift to the right or left depending on the circumstances. A shift to the right means that for a given partial pressure of O_2, less O_2 will be bound to hemoglobin (more oxygen has been unloaded and the hemoglobin has a lower percent saturation) due to a decrease in affinity. Several conditions produce a right shift, including an increase in the partial pressure of CO_2, a decrease in pH, and an increase in temperature. These seemingly disparate conditions are associated with periods of increased metabolic rate and signal a need for more oxygen, such as during exercise. For example, we would predict that rapidly and repeatedly contracting muscles would have higher pCO_2 (increased metabolism), lower pH (because of increased pCO_2 and lactic acid build up), and higher temperature (increased thermal energy release). Conversely, a shift to the left means that for a given partial pressure of O_2, more O_2 will be bound to hemoglobin (the hemoglobin has a higher percent saturation) due to an increase in affinity. Fetal hemoglobin, which has a higher affinity for O_2 than adult hemoglobin, has a left-shifted curve.

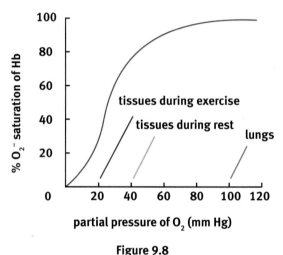

Figure 9.8

Delivering oxygen to tissues is only part of the job of transporting respiratory gases; removing CO_2 (the primary waste product of cellular respiration) is also important. Carbon dioxide gas, like oxygen gas, is essentially nonpolar and therefore has low solubility in the aqueous plasma; only a small percentage of the total CO_2 being transported in the blood to the lungs is dissolved in the plasma. Carbon dioxide can be directly carried by hemoglobin, but hemoglobin has a much lower affinity for carbon dioxide than for oxygen. The vast majority of CO_2 exists in the blood in a disguised form, as the bicarbonate ion (HCO_3^-). How does that happen? When CO_2 enters a red blood cell, it encounters the enzyme carbonic anhydrase, which catalyzes the combination reaction between CO_2 and H_2O to form carbonic acid (H_2CO_3). Carbonic acid, as a weak acid, will then dissociate into a proton and the bicarbonate anion. The hydrogen ion (proton) and bicarbonate ion both have high solubilities in water, and thus provide a much more effective means of transporting cellular respiration's waste product to the lungs for excretion. We hear your silent protest, "But we breathe out CO_2 gas, not hydrogen ions and bicarbonate ions!" And you are absolutely correct: the same reactions that led to the formation of the ions can be reversed once the blood reaches the alveolar capillaries in the lungs. Carbon dioxide gas is rapidly reformed by the reverse action of carbonic anhydrase in the lungs and is breathed out.

$$CO_2\,(g) + H_2O\,(l) \xrightleftharpoons[\text{carbonic anhydrase}]{} H_2CO_3\,(aq) \leftrightarrow H^+\,(aq) + HCO_3^-\,(aq)$$

This chemical reaction is important not only because it provides an effective means of ridding the body's tissues of carbon dioxide gas, but also because the concentration of free protons in the blood affects pH, and the pH can have allosteric effects on the hemoglobin–oxygen dissociation curve. Increased proton concentration (lowered pH) shifts the curve to the right; this is known as the **Bohr Effect**. When will a right shift occur? When we have high energy demands (such as running a race) which require an increased rate of cellular respiration and a concomitant increase in oxygen supply. Higher rates of cellular metabolism will yield greater P_{CO_2} and accumulation of lactic acid, both of which will decrease the pH, signaling to the hemoglobin that the tissue needs more oxygen. Consequently, hemoglobin will experience a reduced affinity for oxygen (the allosteric effect of the hydrogen ion) and will be able to give off (or dump) more oxygen to the metabolically active tissue. If we believe that it is a *downright* shame to not have enough oxygen to finish the race, then we'll remember which way the curve shifts.

Equally important is the link between blood pH homeostasis and the respiratory and renal systems. You'll recall from general chemistry that a solution containing a weak acid and its conjugate base in roughly equal concentrations is called a buffer. The presence of the weak acid–conjugate base pair in solution helps to minimize dramatic shifts in pH. We might characterize a buffer as an acid–base sponge, soaking up excess hydrogen ions or hydroxide ions, to keep the solution's pH relatively steady. The carbonic acid–bicarbonate ion pair is the most important buffer system for the blood. The pH of blood must be maintained within a narrow range around 7.4, slightly alkaline. Metabolic or respiratory disturbances can cause the pH to shift down (acidosis) or up (alkalosis), giving rise to potentially dangerous and life-threatening conditions in which other systems malfunction and proteins become denatured. In response to changing blood pH, the respiratory rate may rise or fall to increase or decrease the amount of carbon dioxide gas excreted and the kidneys can increase or decrease the amount of bicarbonate ion secreted into the nephron filtrate. For example, in response to a metabolic acidosis (decreased pH), the respiratory rate will increase to reduce the systemic P_{CO_2} so as to shift the reversible system to the left, resulting in a decrease in hydrogen ion concentration (and an increase in the pH).

TRANSPORT OF NUTRIENTS AND WASTES

The blood serves as a way to mobilize nutrients, vitamins, minerals, and other compounds necessary for proper cell and tissue functions. Let's quickly review how each of our major nutrients enters the blood:

Carbohydrates and amino acids: absorbed in the small intestine capillaries, enter systemic circulation via hepatic portal system.

Key Concept

Only a small percentage of carbon dioxide is actually bound directly to hemoglobin (as carboxyhemoglobin); most of the CO_2 is dissolved in plasma and lives as HCO_3^-.

Fats: absorbed into lacteals in the small intestine; bypass the hepatic portal circulation and enter systemic circulation via the thoracic duct. Once in the bloodstream, fats are packaged in lipoproteins, which are water-soluble.

Wastes such as carbon dioxide (see previous discussion), ammonia and urea enter the bloodstream throughout the body as they travel down their concentration gradients from the tissues into the capillaries. The blood eventually passes through the excretory organs, where these waste products are filtered or secreted for removal from the body (see Chapter 10), just as the building maintenance staff might remove waste products from the office building.

An essential concept that has come up again and again is the movement of compounds and molecules along the gradients, which may be electrical, chemical, pressure, or a combination of these. This should indicate how important understanding the roles of gradients is to your performance on the MCAT, in both the Physical Sciences and the Biological Sciences sections. In the bloodstream, two pressure gradients are essential for maintaining a proper balance of fluid volume and solute concentrations in the interstitium. These are the opposing but related **hydrostatic** and **oncotic (osmotic) pressures**. Let's take a look at Figure 9.9 and figure out why.

At the arteriole end of the capillary, hydrostatic pressure (generated by the contraction of the heart and the elasticity of the arteries; measured upstream in the large arteries

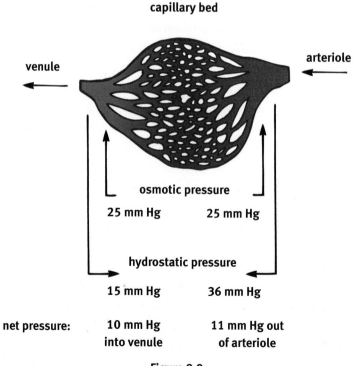

capillary bed

venule

arteriole

osmotic pressure

25 mm Hg   25 mm Hg

hydrostatic pressure

15 mm Hg   36 mm Hg

net pressure: 10 mm Hg   11 mm Hg out
                 into venule   of arteriole

Figure 9.9

as blood pressure) is relatively high. Hydrostatic pressure is the force per unit area that the blood exerts against the vessel walls. Capillaries are leaky by design, so fluid will be forced out of the bloodstream into the interstitial space of the tissues, carrying with it some of the nutrients. As fluid moves out of the vessels, the hydrostatic pressure drops significantly. At the venule end of the capillary bed, the hydrostatic pressure has dropped below the oncotic pressure, which is the osmotic pressure generated by the concentration of particles in the plasma compartment. Because the primary determinant of plasma osmotic pressure is the concentration of plasma proteins, it is called oncotic pressure. The osmotic/oncotic pressure is essentially constant along the capillary as nutrients filter out and wastes filter in at a relatively equal rate. Unlike hydrostatic pressure, oncotic pressure exerts an inward force and draws fluid, nutrients, and wastes out of the tissues into the bloodstream.

The balance of these opposing pressures, which are also called the Starling forces, is essential for maintaining the proper fluid volumes and solute concentrations inside and outside the vasculature. Imbalance of these pressures can result in too much or too little fluid in the tissues. For example, accumulation of excess fluid in the interstitium results in a condition called edema. We should note that some interstitial fluid is also taken up by the lymphatic system, which is another venous circulatory system that runs parallel to the venous central circulatory system. Lymphatic fluid (lymph) returns to the central circulatory system by way of a channel called the thoracic duct. Blockage of lymph nodes by infection or surgical invasion can also result in edema. Although you do not need to learn or memorize the Starling equation, which quantifies the net filtration rate between two fluid compartments, you should understand that the movement of solutes and fluid at the capillary level is governed by pressure differentials, just like the movement of carbon dioxide and oxygen in the lungs.

CLOTTING

We have now covered most of the functions of red blood cells and the plasma. Let's turn to platelets. As we have already discussed, platelets protect the vascular system in the event of damage to a vessel, by forming a clot, which prevents (or at least minimizes) the pathological loss of blood through the vascular damage or injury. Recall from Chapter 6 that connective tissue underlies most of our other tissues and is partly composed of collagen. When platelets come into contact with exposed collagen, they sense this as evidence of injury. In response, they release their contents and begin to aggregate, or clump together. One of the important chemicals they release is a clotting factor known as **thromboplastin**. Thromboplastin converts **prothrombin** into **thrombin** with some help from its enzymatic cofactors, calcium and Vitamin K. Thrombin then converts **fibrinogen** into **fibrin**. Fibrin is a protein that functions just as its name suggests. It makes little fibers that aggregate into a woven structure, like a net, which captures red blood cells and other platelets, forming a

Key Concept

Note how much lower hydrostatic pressure is in the capillaries than in the arteries (normal arterial pressure is 120 mmHg during systole and 80 mmHg during diastole). Recall that this pressure drop occurs across the arterioles and is necessary because the delicate capillaries cannot handle such high pressure. Capillary walls are only a single cell thick so that water flow and nutrient and waste exchanges can occur quickly and efficiently.

clot (a plug) over the area of damage. If the clot forms on a surface vessel that has been cut (e.g., a paper cut), we call the clot a scab.

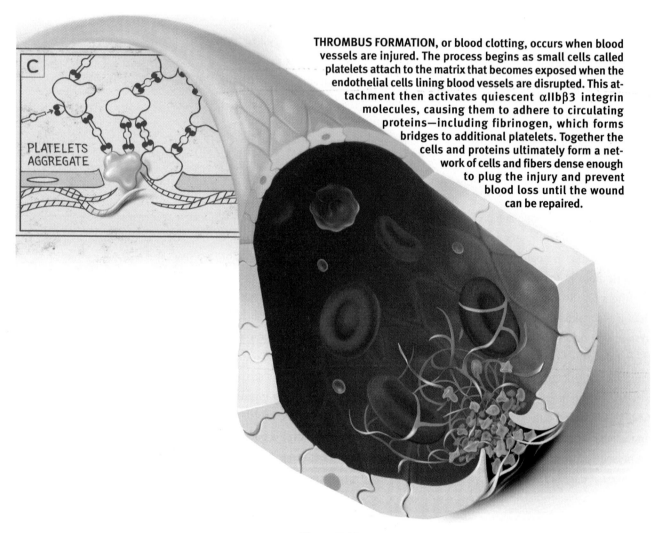

THROMBUS FORMATION, or blood clotting, occurs when blood vessels are injured. The process begins as small cells called platelets attach to the matrix that becomes exposed when the endothelial cells lining blood vessels are disrupted. This attachment then activates quiescent $\alpha IIb\beta 3$ integrin molecules, causing them to adhere to circulating proteins—including fibrinogen, which forms bridges to additional platelets. Together the cells and proteins ultimately form a network of cells and fibers dense enough to plug the injury and prevent blood loss until the wound can be repaired.

PLATELETS AGGREGATE

C

Figure 9.10

Certain genetic diseases, such as hemophilia, cause malfunctions in the cascade of clotting reactions and increase the risk of life-threatening blood loss from even relatively minor injuries. Hemophilia, which is a recessive disorder, has run surprisingly commonly through some branches of European royal families, leading to all sorts of scandalous court gossip and innuendos. We will take a closer look at the inheritance patterns of these diseases and other traits in Chapter 14.

IMMUNOLOGICAL REACTIONS

As we discussed before, the body has the ability to differentiate between self and foreign by identifying cell-surface antigens. The development of immunity and the roles and activities of the different cell types in the immune system are discussed in more detail in Chapter 10.

Conclusion

The cardiovascular system is one of the most commonly tested MCAT topics. You should be familiar with its basic structure: a system with two pumps in series, which we have compared with two batteries in series in a circuit. We discussed the basic anatomy of the heart and its connection to the systemic and pulmonary circulations. We discussed the myogenic activity of cardiac muscle and the pathway that electricity follows in the heart through the SA node, AV node, bundle of His, and Purkinje fibers. The movement of blood through the vascular system is a function of the heart pumping to generate pressure. Blood pressure is a measure of the blood's force per unit area on the vessel walls, and is recorded as a gauge pressure (pressure above atmospheric pressure). We discussed the differences among arteries, veins, and capillaries and how these anatomical differences are reflective of the different functions. We then took a look at the composition of blood and discussed the three major cell types. Red blood cells and platelets were discussed in detail. We examined the ABO and Rh antigen systems, which commonly appear on the MCAT due to their widespread clinical relevance. Hemoglobin's ability to carry oxygen and carbon dioxide was also described; recall that carbon dioxide is primarily carried as bicarbonate ion in the blood. The conversion of carbon dioxide to and from this ion is accomplished by the enzyme carbonic anhydrase. We will revisit white blood cells when we discuss the immune system.

CONCEPTS TO REMEMBER

☐ The electrical signal travels from the SA node to the AV node to the bundle of His and down the Purkinje fibers. Thus, the heart can fire without descending input from the nervous system. This is known as myogenic activity.

☐ During the contraction phase (systole), blood is pumped from the heart and through the vasculature. During the relaxation phase (diastole), the heart fills with blood.

☐ The pipes of the circulatory system are the arteries, veins, and capillaries. Whereas arteries have intrinsic smooth musculature that is used to regulate capacity, veins rely on adjacent skeletal muscles to squeeze venous blood progressively back to the heart.

☐ Capillaries are a single cell-layer thick to allow for efficient gas and nutrient exchange.

☐ Blood pressure is a gauge pressure. It is highest in the arterial side of the circulation.

☐ Leukocytes have two classes: granulocytes and agranulocytes. Each of these cell types is involved in different parts of the immune response.

☐ Blood can be classified by the set of surface antigens that are expressed on RBCs. The ABO classification is based on the codominant expression patterns of the I^A and I^B alleles. Blood can also be Rh^+ or Rh^-.

☐ Oxygen (and carbon dioxide, to a lesser degree) is carried by hemoglobin. The relative affinity of oxygen for hemoglobin is depicted by a sigmoidal curve and may be affected by temperature, pH, altitude, and CO_2.

☐ Carbon dioxide is primarily carried as bicarbonate ion. The formation of the ion is catalyzed by carbonic anhydrase.

☐ Platelets are involved in forming clots. Deficiency will result in bleeding disorders.

Practice Questions

1. Which of the following is a FALSE statement regarding erythrocytes? *red blood cells.*

   A. They contain hemoglobin.
   B. They are anaerobic.
   C. Their nuclei are located in the middle of the cells' disk-like depression.
   D. They are phagocytized in the spleen and liver after a certain period of time.

2. Which is the correct sequence of a cardiac impulse?

   A. SA node → AV node → Purkinje fibers → bundle of His → ventricles
   B. AV node → bundle of His → Purkinje fibers → SA node → ventricles → atria
   C. SA node → atria → AV node → bundle of His → Purkinje fibers → ventricles
   D. SA node → AV node → atria → bundle of His → Purkinje fibers → ventricles

3. Hemoglobin's affinity for O_2

   A. increases in exercising muscle tissue.
   B. decreases as blood pH increases.
   C. decreases as blood pH decreases.
   D. is higher in maternal blood than in fetal blood.

4. Which of the following correctly traces the circulatory pathway?

   A. Superior vena cava → right atrium → right ventricle → pulmonary artery → lungs → pulmonary veins → left atrium → left ventricle → aorta
   B. Superior vena cava → left atrium → left ventricle → pulmonary artery → lungs → pulmonary veins right atrium → right ventricle → aorta
   C. Aorta → right atrium → right ventricle → pulmonary artery → lungs → pulmonary veins → left atrium → left ventricle → superior vena cava
   D. Superior vena cava → right atrium → right ventricle → pulmonary veins → lungs → pulmonary artery → left atrium → left ventricle → aorta

5. The tricuspid valve prevents backflow of blood from the

   A. left ventricle into the left atrium.
   B. aorta into the left ventricle.
   C. pulmonary artery into the right ventricle.
   D. right ventricle into the right atrium.

6. At the venous end of a capillary bed, the osmotic pressure

   A. is greater than the hydrostatic pressure.
   B. results in a net outflow of fluid.
   C. results in a net reabsorption of fluid into the blood.
   D. both A and C.

7. A patient's chart reveals that he has a cardiac output of 7,500 mL/min and a stroke volume of 50 mL. What is his pulse (in beats per minute)?

A. 50 beats/min

B. 100 beats/min

C. 150 beats/min

D. 400 beats/min

8. An unconscious patient is rushed into the emergency room and needs a fast blood transfusion. Because there is no time to check his medical history or determine his blood type, which type of blood should you, as his doctor, give him?

A. A⁻

B. AB⁺

C. O⁺

D. O⁻

9. Which of the following is TRUE regarding arteries and veins?

A. Arteries are thin-walled, muscular, and elastic, whereas veins are thick-walled and inelastic.

B. Arteries always conduct oxygenated blood, whereas veins always carry deoxygenated blood.

C. The blood pressure in the aorta is always higher than the pressure in the superior vena cava.

D. Arteries facilitate blood transport by using skeletal muscle contractions, whereas veins make use of the pumping of the heart to push blood.

10. At any given time, there is more blood in the venous system than the arterial system. Which of the following features of a vein allows this?

A. Relative lack of smooth muscle in the wall

B. Presence of valves

C. Proximity of veins to lymphatic vessels

D. Thin endothelial lining

11. Which of the following is involved in the body's primary blood-buffering mechanism?

A. Fluid intake

B. Absorption of nutrients in the gastrointestinal system

C. Carbon dioxide produced from metabolism

D. Reabsorption in the kidney

Small Group Questions

1. Why does O⁻ blood not elicit an immune response when transferred to an individual with AB blood?

2. In which direction does the dissociation curve for fetal hemoglobin shift compared with adult hemoglobin? Explain.

3. How does the pH of arterial blood affect the rate of ventilation?

4. Erthryocytes are anaerobic. Why is this advantageous for the organism?

Explanations to Practice Questions

1. C

Erythrocytes, or red blood cells, are produced in the red bone marrow and circulate in the blood for about 120 days, after which they are phagocytized in the spleen and the liver. Red blood cells have a disk-like shape and lose their membranous organelles (like mitochondria and nuclei) during maturation. Erythrocytes thus cannot multiply on their own, and are anaerobic. Their main role is the transport of oxygen to the tissues and of the carbon dioxide to the lungs; this task is accomplished through the use of hemoglobin, which carries oxygen and a limited amount of carbon dioxide. From the given statements, (C) is false and, therefore, the correct answer to this question.

2. C

An ordinary cardiac contraction originates in, and is regulated by, the sinoatrial (SA) node. The impulses travel through both atria, stimulating them to contract simultaneously. The impulse then arrives at the atrioventricular (AV) node, which momentarily slows conduction, allowing for completion of atrial contraction and ventricular filling. The impulse is then carried by the bundle of His, which branches into the right and left bundle branches and through the Purkinje fibers in the walls of both ventricles, generating a strong contraction. The only choice that correctly depicts this sequence is (C).

3. C

Let's quickly review how hemoglobin's affinity for O_2 changes. According to the Bohr effect, decreasing the pH in the blood decreases hemoglobin's affinity for O_2. A decrease in the pH of the blood generally occurs during heavy exercise, when the muscles produce a lot of lactic acid. This decreased affinity for O_2 facilitates the unloading of O_2 to tissues in need. Based on this, (C) is the correct

answer. (A) and (B) state the opposite. (D) is incorrect, because hemoglobin's affinity for O_2 is higher in the fetal blood than in adult blood.

4. A

Blood drains from the superior vena cava into the right atrium. It passes through the tricuspid valve and into the right ventricle, and then through the pulmonary valve into the pulmonary artery, which leads to the lungs. Oxygenated blood returns to the left atrium via the pulmonary veins. It flows through the mitral valve into the left ventricle. From the left ventricle, it is pumped through the aortic valve into the aorta for distribution throughout the body. The only choice that correctly illustrates this path is (A).

5. D

The atrioventricular valves are located between the atria and the ventricles on both sides of the heart. Their role is to prevent backflow of blood into the atria. The valve on the right side of the heart has three cusps and is called the tricuspid valve. As such, it prevents backflow of blood from the right ventricle into the right atrium, making (D) the correct answer. The valve on the left side of the heart has two cusps and is called the bicuspid or mitral valve (early anatomists thought this valve looked like a miter, the hat traditionally worn by bishops). The mitral valve prevents backflow from the left ventricle into the left atrium.

6. D

The exchange of materials is greatly influenced by the relative balance between the hydrostatic and osmotic pressures of blood and tissue fluids. The osmotic pressure of the surrounding tissue remains constant; however, the hydrostatic pressure at the arterial end is greater than the hydrostatic pressure at the venous end. As a result, fluid moves out of the capillaries at the arterial end, and back in at the venous end. To answer this question, fluid is reabsorbed at the venous end because the osmotic pressure exceeds the hydrostatic pressure. (D) is thus the correct answer.

7. C

The first step in solving this problem is to define cardiac output:

cardiac output = heart rate × stroke volume

We are given the stroke volume and the cardiac output, so we can calculate the heart rate, or pulse, according to the following equation:

heart rate = cardiac output/stroke volume
heart rate = (7500 mL/min)/(50 mL)
heart rate = 150 beats/min

The patient thus has a pulse of 150 beats/min; (C) is the correct answer.

8. D

Without knowing a patient's blood type, the only type of transfusion that we can safely give is O^-. People with O^- blood are considered universal donors because their blood cells contain no surface antigens. Therefore, O^- blood can be given to anyone without causing potentially life-threatening consequences. (D) is therefore the correct answer.

9. C

The only answer choice that correctly describes arteries and veins is (C); the pressure in the aorta is usually about 120 or 80 mmHg, depending on whether the heart is in systole or diastole, whereas the pressure in the superior vena cava is extremely low. (A) is wrong because arteries are thick-walled and veins are thin-walled. (B) is also incorrect; this relationship is reversed in pulmonary circulation. (D) is an opposite answer choice. Arteries make use of the pumping of the heart and the "snapping back" of their elastic walls to transport blood, whereas venous blood is "pumped" by skeletal muscle contractions.

10. A

The relative lack of smooth muscle in venous walls allows stretching, to store most of the blood in the body. Valves in the veins allow for one-way flow of blood toward the heart. Both arteries and veins are close to lymphatic vessels, which has no bearing on their relative difference in volume. Both arteries and veins have a thin endothelial lining.

11. C

Carbon dioxide is a by-product of metabolism in cells, which later combines with water to form bicarbonate in a reaction catalyzed by carbonic anhydrase. This system is blood plasma's most important buffer system. Food and fluid absorption are not significant sources of buffering.

The Immune System

Within the past decade or so, the public's imagination has been captured by alarming reports of "flesh-eating" bacteria and diseases. Descriptions and images that seem to have been lifted directly from the neural synapses of Wes Craven suggest a bacterial entity, large and ravenous, capable of consuming a person in one pustulant gulp. In fact, flesh-eating bacteria do not actually eat flesh, but that doesn't make them any less dangerous. The pathological and life-threatening impact of necrotizing fasciitis, caused by many different types of bacteria, including group A streptococcus, *Clostridium perfringens*, and methicillin-resistant *Staphylococcus aureus* (MRSA), is a massive destruction of skin, muscle, and connective tissue by the release of bacterial toxins called superantigens. These proteins cause the immune system to become nonspecifically overactivated, resulting in the overproduction of cytokines, a set of chemical messengers that are important for activation and regulation of the immune system. Overproduction of cytokines, sometimes called a cytokine storm, consists of a positive feedback loop between cytokines and immune cells, and results in destruction of host tissues and organs as well as a systemic inflammatory response, which can severely impact cardiovascular and respiratory functions. Necrotizing fasciitis is a serious disease that requires aggressive medical and surgical treatment including intravenous antibiotics and surgical debridement (removal) of the necrotic tissue, and sometimes even amputation. Mortality rates have been recorded as high as 73%.

In Chapter 1, we introduced bacteria and viruses as invaders and spies. Our immune system is the counterespionage force (think Homeland Security) that attempts to neutralize these threats. We will consider both specific and nonspecific defenses. Nonspecific defenses, such as the skin, are the initial barriers against infection. If microbes breach them, we then rely on the activities of specific defense, which are mediated by the leukocytes that we introduced in Chapter 9. We will also discuss advances in medical techniques, which allow us to manipulate and control the immune system to our advantage, such as immunizations, which can prevent us from ever having to suffer a debilitating disease (e.g., hepatitis vaccination). By examining each of these topics, we will be ready to search and destroy any questions related to the immune system on Test Day.

Anatomy ★★★☆☆

The immune system is not housed in a single organ. The structures and components that serve as nonspecific defenses (discussed next) often serve functions in other organ systems. Leukocytes, which are vital for specific immunity, are born in the bone marrow and may contribute to either **innate immunity** or **adaptive immunity**. We introduced the three major classes of leukocytes in Chapter 9. **Granulocytes** include neutrophils, eosinophils, and basophils. **Agranulocytes** include the **lymphocytes**, which are responsible for antibody production, immune system modulation, and

targeted killing of infected cells. Finally, **monocytes** (primarily macrophages) are also agranulocytes and serve as nonspecific sanitation workers that travel the body picking up debris, both foreign (invaders) and domestic (our own). The lymphocytes that contribute to adaptive immunity are B-cells and T-cells, so named because of their site of maturation: T-cells mature in the thymus and B-cells mature in the spleen (in birds, the B-cells mature in an organ called the bursa of Fabricius, from which these leukocytes originally derived their moniker).

THE DIVISIONS OF THE IMMUNE SYSTEM

The mammalian immune system has two overarching divisions. The innate part (*left side*) acts near entry points into the body and is always at the ready. If it fails to contain a pathogen, the adaptive division (*right side*) kicks in, mounting a later but highly targeted attack against the specific invader.

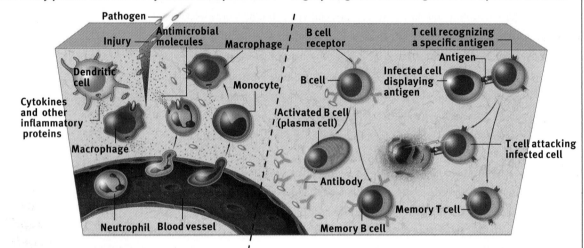

INNATE IMMUNE SYSTEM

This system includes, among other components, antimicrobial molecules and various phagocytes (cells that ingest and destroy pathogens). These cells, such as dendritic cells and macrophages, also activate an inflammatory response, secreting proteins called cytokines that trigger an influx of defensive cells from the blood. Among the recruits are more phagocytes—notably monocytes (which can mature into macrophages) and neutrophils.

ADAPTIVE IMMUNE SYSTEM

This system "stars" B cells and T cells. Activated B cells secrete antibody molecules that bind to antigens—specific components unique to a given invader—and destroy the invader directly or mark it for attack by others. T cells recognize antigens displayed on cells. Some T cells help to activate B cells and other T cells (*not shown*); other T cells directly attack infected cells. T and B cells spawn "memory" cells that promptly eliminate invaders encountered before.

Figure 10.1

Innate immunity refers to the responses cells can carry out without learning; for this reason, it is also known as the **nonspecific immune response**. Conversely, adaptive immunity is developed as immune cells learn to recognize and respond to particular antigens, and is often aptly referred to as the **specific immune response**. We can also parse the specific immune system into **humoral immunity** (driven by B-cells and antibodies) and **cell-mediated immunity** (provided by T-cells).

How do these defense mechanisms know to destroy microbial targets and not attack our own cells? Remember that antigens are proteins and carbohydrates present on the outer membranes of most cells. They allow our immune systems to distinguish between self and nonself (or foreign) and to recognize our self-antigens and antigen-presenting cells as nonthreatening. Antigens that the immune cells learn to recognize as foreign will cause activation of the immune response. When the immune system fails to learn the distinction between self and foreign, it may attack self-antigens as if they were foreign, a condition termed **autoimmunity**. Note that autoimmunity is only one potential problem with immune functioning; another problem arises when the immune system misidentifies a foreign antigen as dangerous, when, in fact, it is not. Pet dander, pollen, and peanuts are not inherently threatening to human life, and yet some people's immune systems are hypersensitive to these antigens and become overactivated (to varying degrees) when these antigens are encountered. **Allergies** and autoimmunity are part of a family of immune disorders classified as hypersensitivity reactions.

Nonspecific Defense Mechanisms

★★★★☆☆

Our first line of defense is the skin (integument). In the next chapter, we will discuss its homeostatic functions, but for now, let's focus on how it keeps us protected. By providing a physical barrier between the outside world and our internal organs, the skin keeps microbes at bay. Additionally, sweat contains an enzyme that attacks bacterial cell walls, and therefore serves an antibacterial purpose in addition to its better-known role in thermoregulation. A cut or abrasion on the skin provides an entry point for pathogens into the body, and the deeper the wound is, the deeper the pathogens can gain initial entry. This is why painful puncture wounds from nails or playful bites from kittens can lead to serious infections.

We outlined another mechanism of defense in the respiratory chapter. The respiratory passages, which are mucous membranes, are lined with cilia to trap particulate matter and push it up toward the oropharynx where it is swallowed. We definitely don't want to breathe in smoke and dirt, but we *really* want to prevent the bacteria and viruses that may be hitching a ride on the particulate matter suspended in the air from reaching deep lung tissue where they may set up serious infection. Several other mucous membranes, including around the eye and in the oral cavity, produce a nonspecific bactericidal enzyme (lysozyme), which is secreted in the tears and saliva, respectively.

If foreign particles do make it past the skin, macrophages will phagocytize them. Macrophages may be called to a site of **inflammation** by chemicals such as

THE PLAYERS

The immune system consists of innate cells, which form a first line of defense against pathogens, and members of the adaptive system, which targets invaders with greater specificity.

INNATE

MACROPHAGE
This immune defender engulfs and consumes pathogen invaders.

MAST CELL
This cell releases histamine and other chemicals that promote inflammation.

GRANULOCYTE
Three cell types with tiny granules in their interior—the neutrophil, eosinophil and basophil—participate in the inflammatory response.

DENDRITIC CELL
It presents antigens—fragments of protein or other molecules from pathogens or cancer cells—to adaptive immune cells, inducing the cells to attack bearers of the displayed antigens.

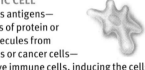

NATURAL KILLER CELL
This cell destroys the body's own cells that have become infected with pathogens; it also goes after cancer cells.

ADAPTIVE

B CELL
Antigens stimulate this cell to divide and produce antibodies that neutralize invaders or tag them for killing.

T CELL
A killer T cell destroys an infected cell in which it detects the presence of antigens. Other T cells—such as helper and regulatory types—coordinate the immune response.

histamine, which causes vasodilation and allows macrophages to move out of the bloodstream and into the tissue. The granulocytes, especially neutrophils, may be called out in a similar manner. This process works well against pathogens that are extracellular, like bacteria. But how do we contain viruses, which are obligate intracellular pathogens? Immune cells and cells that have been infected with viral particles may produce **interferon**, a protein that prevents viral replication and dispersion. Note that interferon is directed against viruses but not against specific viruses, so it is considered a nonspecific defense.

Each of these mechanisms is a part of the innate immune system. Interferon, for example, doesn't have to be previously exposed to virus to know how to defeat it. The protein is produced upon infection and is immediately effective against the viral particle. Innate immunity is useful because it can begin to fight disease immediately. However, its major drawback is that, as a defense mechanism, it is not adaptive. Organisms cannot make their innate defense mechanisms more effective over time. This is of particular interest when dealing with quickly mutating viruses that evolve the ability to overcome interferon. Whereas the innate, nonspecific immune defenses form an important first barrier system, this system has its limitations. As a more sophisticated defense mechanism, the adaptive immune system works by forming **immunological memory**, which improves the effectiveness and alacrity of the immune response.

Humoral Immunity

When we are exposed to a pathogen, it may take a few days for the physical symptoms to be relieved. This occurs because the adaptive immune response takes time to get geared up. **Humoral immunity**, which involves the production of antibodies, may take as long as a week to become fully effective. These antibodies are specific to the antigens of the invading microbe. Antibodies are produced by B-cells, which are lymphocytes that originated in the bone marrow and matured in the spleen and lymph nodes.

Antibodies (also called **immunoglobulins [Ig]**) can carry out many different jobs in the body. Once they bind to their specific antigens, they may attract other leukocytes to phagocytize those antigens immediately, or they may clump together (agglutinate) with the antigens to form large insoluble complexes that can be phagocytized. Antibodies are *Y*-shaped molecules (see Figures 10.2 and 10.3) that are made up of two identical **heavy chains** and two identical **light chains**. Disulfide linkages and noncovalent interactions hold the heavy and light chains together. Each antibody has an **antigen-binding region** at the two top tips of the *Y*. Within this region, there are specific polypeptide sequences that will bind one, and only one, specific antigenic sequence. Each B-cell makes one antibody, but we have many B-cells so that our immune system can recognize many antigens. The remaining part of the antibody molecule is known as the **constant region**, which is involved in recruitment and binding of other immune modulators (e.g., macrophages).

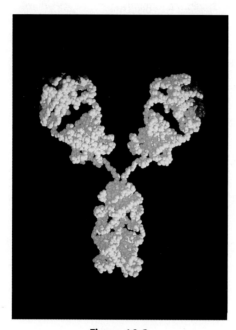

Figure 10.2

Not all B-cells that are generated actively or constantly produce antibodies. Why wouldn't we want all of our B-cells to be active? Antibody production is an energetically expensive process; there is no reason to expend energy producing antibodies we don't need. Instead, B-cells wait in the lymph nodes for their particular antigens to come along. Upon exposure to the correct antigen, a B-cell will proliferate and produce two types of daughter cells. **Plasma cells** produce large amounts of antibody, whereas **memory cells** stay in the lymph nodes for use upon being re-exposed to the same antigen. This initial activation takes approximately seven to ten days and is known as the **primary response**. The plasma cells will eventually die, but the memory cells may last the lifetime of the organism. If the same microbe is ever encountered again, the memory cells jump into action and produce the antibodies specific to that pathogen. This immune response, called the **secondary response**, will be more rapid and robust. The development of these lasting memory cells is the basis for the efficacy of **vaccinations**.

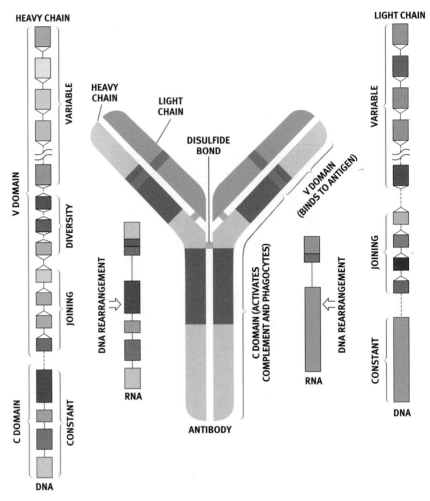

Figure 10.3

Cell-mediated Immunity ★★★★☆☆

Whereas humoral immunity is based on the activity of B-lymphocytes, cell-mediated immunity involves the T-lymphocytes. Although both B-cells and T-cells originate from the same set of stem cells in the bone marrow, T-cells mature in the thymus, unlike the B-cells, which mature in the spleen and lymph nodes. There are three major types of T-cells: **helper T-cells**, **suppressor T-cells**, and **killer (cytotoxic) T-cells**. Helper T-cells, also called T4 cells because they express the CD4 cell-surface protein, coordinate the immune response by secreting chemicals known as **lymphokines**. These molecules are capable of recruiting other immune cells (e.g., plasma cells, cytotoxic T-cells, macrophages) and increasing their activity. The loss of these cells prevents the immune system from mounting an adequate response to infection. HIV destroys T4 cells, essentially immobilizing the host immune system and paving the way for opportunistic infections. Cytotoxic T-cells, also called T8 cells because of their expression of the CD8 surface protein, are capable of directly killing virally infected cells by secreting toxic chemicals. Suppressor T-cells, another group of T8 cells, help to tone down the immune response once infection has been adequately contained. T-cells may also form memory cells, so that the next exposure to the same antigen will result in a more robust response.

helper T cells — CD4
suppressor T cells ⎫
killer T cells ⎬ CD8

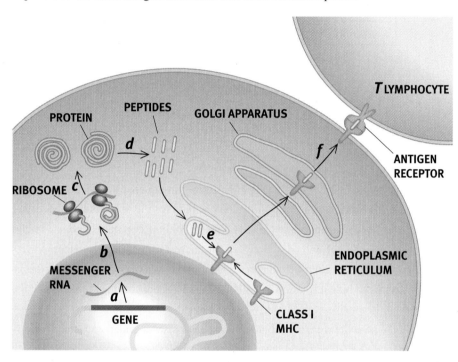

Figure 10.4

A sidebar in a previous chapter referred to the transplantation of a liver from a donor to a patient in need. However, the donated liver would have antigens native to the donor, that would be recognized as foreign in the recipient. Rejection will occur as the cytotoxic T-cells, having identified the transplanted liver cells as foreign, try to destroy it. Organ transplantation requires the use of **immunosuppressants**, which are drugs that can prevent activation of the immune system. Autoimmunity, mentioned before, can be treated in a similar manner.

Refer to the following figure for an overview of lymphocyte differentiation and the cell types involved in each branch of specific immunity.

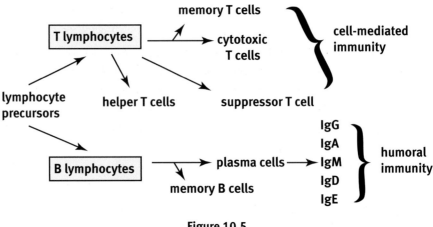

Figure 10.5

Immunization

Often, diseases can have significant, long-term consequences. Infection with the poliovirus, for example, can leave a person disabled for the remainder of his or her life. The former President of the United States, Franklin Roosevelt, contracted polio in the summer of 1921 and was paralyzed for the rest of his life. So concerned was he that the paralysis would be interpreted as political weakness, he went to extraordinary lengths to hide it. In fact, he commissioned a special train car into which the presidential limousine could be driven and carried from Washington, DC, to New York City, where the train would stop in a special station underneath the Waldorf-Astoria Hotel so that he would never have to leave his car and expose his malady to the public eye. Polio used to be a widespread illness; however, today we hardly hear about it as a result of a highly effective **vaccinization** program that led to the virtual eradication of polio in this country.

Immunization can be achieved in an active or passive fashion. In active immunity, the immune system is stimulated to produce antibodies against a specific pathogen. The means by which we are exposed to this pathogen may either be natural or artificial. Through natural exposure, antibodies are generated by B-cells once an individual becomes infected. Artificial vaccination also results in the production of antibodies; however, the individual never experiences true infection. Instead, he receives an injection containing an antigen that will activate B-cells to produce antibodies to fight the specific infection. The antigen may be a weakened or killed form of the microbe, or it may be a part of the microbe's protein structure. A recent example is the vaccination against chicken pox, which became available in 1995 in the United States. Once exposed to chicken pox, people usually are immune to it and do not become infected again. Prior to 1995, immunity was achieved by natural means; individuals became infected and were protected from future bouts of the disease. In fact, some parents were known to intentionally expose their children to the virus to ensure infection at a young age (when the virus resulted in a milder form of illness). After 1995, inoculation began with a live but weakened (attenuated) form of the virus (artificial active immunization). This allowed for B-cells and antibodies to be generated, but did not result in the normal course of infection.

Immunization may also be achieved passively. Passive immunity results from the transfer of antibodies to an individual. The immunity is transient as only the antibodies, and not the B-cells that produce them, are given to the immunized individual. A natural example is the transfer of antibodies across the placenta during pregnancy to protect the fetus, or the transfer of antibodies from a mother to her nursing infant through breast milk. An artificial example is the administration of RhoGAM to an Rh⁰ woman (see Chapter 9) to prevent sensitization to her Rh⁺ fetus's blood.

See Figure 10.6 to see how DNA vaccines incite an immune response. You'll notice that the primary response to the vaccine is no different than a primary response to any other antigen.

Real World

Sometimes the organisms that cause different diseases are so alike in structure that the immune system can be fooled—even for our benefit. When Edward Jenner was trying to find a treatment for smallpox, he inoculated his son with infectious particles from a different, but related disease, cowpox. His experience with cowpox immunized him to smallpox, thanks to the similarity of the two diseases!

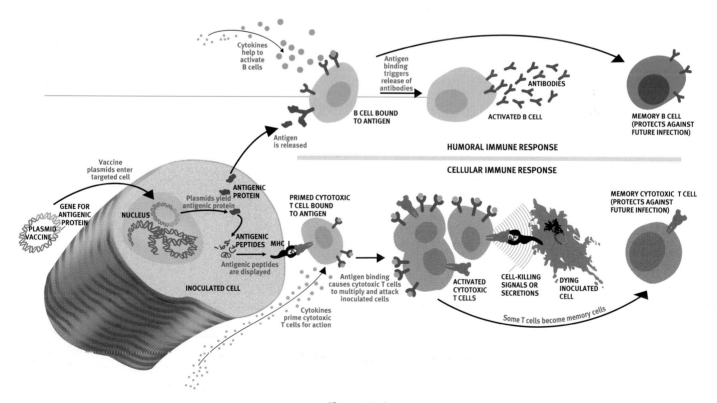

Figure 10.6

Lymphatic System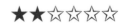

The lymphatic system, along with the cardiovascular system, is a type of circulatory system. It is made up of one-way vessels that become larger as they move toward the center of the body (toward the heart). Hence, the lymphatic system is a venous system. These vessels carry lymphatic fluid and join to comprise a large thoracic duct in the chest, which then delivers the fluid into the left subclavian vein (near the heart).

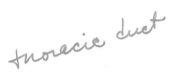

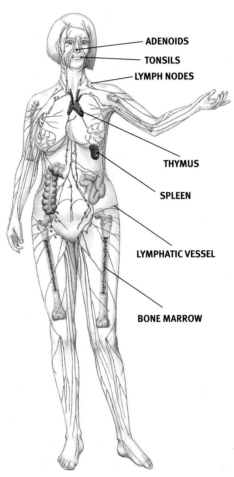

Figure 10.7

We mentioned in Chapter 9 that at the capillary level, not all the fluid is reabsorbed from the interstitial space; the excess fluid is collected by the lymphatic vessels and then returned to cardiovascular circulation. We also saw in Chapter 7 that the smallest lymphatic vessels (**lacteals**) collect fats in the form of chylomicrons from the villi in the small intestine and deliver them into the bloodstream, bypassing the liver. Along the lymphatic vessels are swellings (**lymph nodes**) that contain immune cells (primarily B-cells). These areas provide a place for antigens from microbes to first interact with the adaptive immune system and allow its activation. You can think of lymph nodes as security checkpoints for fluid that is being returned from the peripheral tissues to the central circulation. It makes sense that this fluid should be checked for pathogens only before being returned to the systemic highway system. In fact, physicians often discover underlying disease by the presence of enlarged or hardened lymph nodes during a physical exam.

Conclusion

The ability to fend off microbial invasion is critical to our survival. The immune system is housed in many locations in the body and involves many different organs and cell types. Nonspecific mechanisms, such as intact skin, mucous membranes, interferon, and lysozyme, constitute a first line of defense; these mechanisms also make up part of the innate immune system, which is capable of an immediate response but cannot learn from experience. The adaptive immune system, comprised of T- and B-lymphocytes, allows for our immune system to learn from past exposure. Thus, once we are infected with a certain strain of virus, activation of specific immunity confers long-term protection against that particular virus. Immunization is a type of adaptive immunity. In active immunization, our immune cells are stimulated in response, resulting in long-term immunity. Passive immunization results from the transfer of antibodies alone; therefore the protection it provides is transient.

CONCEPTS TO REMEMBER

☐ Leukocytes are the functional cells of the immune system. They consist of granulocytes, lymphocytes, and monocytes.

☐ Nonspecific defenses are activated immediately upon infection; however, they cannot learn from past exposure.

☐ Humoral immunity is mediated by B-cells. B-cells proliferate to make plasma cells and memory cells. Antibodies are made by the plasma cells.

☐ Humoral immunity is more effective at combating bacterial infections, whereas cell-mediated immunity fights viral and fungal infections.

☐ Antibodies fight infection by binding to foreign antigens, thereby allowing other immune cells (e.g., macrophages) to phagocytize them.

☐ Cell-mediated immunity requires T-cells. The three major classes are helper T-cells, suppressor T-cells, and killer (cytotoxic) T-cells.

☐ Immunizations may be active or passive. Active immunization results in a sustained immune response mediated by B-cells, whereas the effects of passive immunization are short-lived.

☐ Immunizations may also be natural or artificial. Natural immunization is the result of exposure to the antigen in nature or transfer of antibodies from mother to fetus. Artificial active immunization uses weakened or dead forms of microbes to generate an immune response without causing active infection.

☐ The lymphatic system is a secondary circulation system that removes excess fluid from the interstitial space. It also transports fat molecules from the intestinal epithelial cells to the bloodstream and serves as a conduit for the movement of immune cells.

Practice Questions

1. If a virus, such as HIV, destroys the body's T lymphocytes, to which type of diseases would the patient be most susceptible?

   A. Viral infections
   B. Bacterial infections
   C. Autoimmune diseases
   D. Immunoglobulin deficiencies

2. Which of the following is NOT involved in cell-mediated immunity?

   A. Memory cells
   B. Plasma cells
   C. Cytotoxic cells
   D. Suppressor cells

3. The lymphatic system

   A. transports hormones throughout the body.
   B. transports absorbed chylomicrons to the circulatory system.
   C. filters the blood.
   D. both A and B.

4. Which of the following is involved in antibody production?

   A. Plasma cells
   B. Memory cells
   C. Helper cells
   D. Cytotoxic cells

5. Which of the following is TRUE regarding passive and active immunity?

   A. Active immunity requires weeks to build, whereas passive immunity is acquired immediately.
   B. Active immunity is short-lived, whereas passive immunity is long-lived. *opposite*
   C. Active immunity may be acquired during pregnancy through the placenta.
   D. Passive immunity may be acquired through vaccination.

6. Which of the following is NOT an example of a nonspecific defense mechanism?

   A. Skin provides a physical barrier against invasion.
   B. Macrophages engulf and destroy foreign particles.
   C. An inflammatory response is initiated in response to physical damage.
   D. Cytotoxic T cells destroy foreign antigens.

Small Group Questions

1. Explain the basis of autoimmunity.

2. Under what conditions is there a risk for erythroblastosis fetalis? Explain why subsequent pregnancies are at greater risk than the first.

Explanations to Practice Questions

1. A

T lymphocytes act primarily against the body's own cells that are infected by a fungus or virus. Therefore, if the patient lacks T cells, he would be prone to viral and fungal infections, as choice (A) indicates.

2. B

The lymphocytes involved in cell-mediated immunity are the T lymphocytes, or T cells. There are four different types of T cells, each playing a different role in cell-mediated immunity: cytotoxic T cells, helper T cells, memory T cells, and suppressor T cells. Thus, from the answer choices, the only cells not involved in cell-mediated immunity are the plasma cells, which are differentiated immunoglobulin-secreting B lymphocytes involved in humoral immunity. Choice (B) is therefore the correct answer.

3. B

The main function of the lymphatic system is to collect excess interstitial fluid and return it to the circulatory system, maintaining the balance of body fluids. However, this is not one of the answer choices. In addition, the lymphatic system absorbs chylomicrons from the small intestine and delivers them to the cardiovascular circulation. Transport of hormones and filtration of blood are not functions of the lymphatic system, so (A), (C), and (D) are incorrect. Thus, (B) is the correct answer.

4. A

Humoral immunity is involved in the production of antibodies following exposure to an antigen. Antibodies are produced by plasma cells derived from B lymphocytes. Antibodies recognize and bind to specific antigens, marking them so they can be recognized by specific cells called phagocytes. Antibodies may also cause the antigens to agglutinate and form insoluble complexes, facilitating their removal. (A) is therefore the correct answer.

5. A

Active immunity refers to the production of antibodies during an immune response. Active immunity may be conferred by vaccination, such as an individual injected with a weakened, inactive, or related form of a particular antigen, which stimulates the immune system to produce antibodies. Active immunity may require weeks to build. Passive immunity, on the other hand, involves the transfer of antibodies either passively or by injection. An example would be during pregnancy when some maternal antibodies cross the placenta and enter fetal circulation, conferring passive immunity upon the fetus. Although passive immunity is acquired immediately, it is very short-lived, lasting only as long as the antibodies circulate in blood. (A) is therefore the correct answer.

6. D

The body employs a number of nonspecific defense mechanisms against foreign invasion. The epithelium provides a physical barrier against bacterial invasion. In addition, sweat contains an enzyme that attacks bacterial cell walls. Certain passages, such as the respiratory tract, are lined with ciliated mucous-coated epithelia, which filter and trap foreign particles. Macrophages engulf and destroy foreign particles. The inflammatory response is initiated in response to physical damage. The only choice not mentioned is (D), the correct answer. Cytotoxic T cells are involved in cell-mediated immunity.

Homeostasis

Have a headache? Pop an ibuprofen. Backache? Works for that, too. Swollen foot? Sure, why not? It's easy enough. Ibuprofen, which has been around for over 40 years, is an inexpensive, over-the-counter, nonsteroidal anti-inflammatory drug (NSAID). Because of its ability to relieve pain, it's also known as an analgesic. It's often said to be safer than aspirin, and usually proves successful with minimal side effects. Many people use it as a cure-all for aches and pains throughout the body; and when used in moderation, that seems to work just fine.

The problem arises when people take multiple doses every day for several years. Usually the drug is taken orally, which means that it circulates to the affected location and all other organs, too. These other organs include the kidneys, which are sensitive to overuse of analgesics. They are especially sensitive to combination analgesics, (e.g., acetaminophen + codeine). Years of analgesic use (usually self-therapy) can lead to kidney failure, known as analgesic nephropathy. If untreated, kidney failure is fatal. If caught, however, dialysis and perhaps a kidney transplant can save the patient's life. All over-the-counter painkillers will have to be discontinued and other methods, such as counseling or behavior modifications, will need to be employed to control pain.

This isn't an issue for people who have a headache once a week. This is an issue for people who suffer from chronic pain due to injury, lifestyle (job demands, etc.), or simply as a side effect from another condition. Chronic pain afflicts millions of Americans each year. The subset of this group that suffers from analgesic nephropathy is primarily composed of females over 30 years of age, who have some sort of chronic pain (head or backaches, severe menstrual pain), often emotional or behavioral changes, and sometimes a history of tobacco or alcohol use. Luckily, the painkiller most associated with analgesic nephropathy (phenacetin) is no longer on the market, and combination analgesics usually need to be prescribed by a clinician. It is currently estimated that analgesic nephropathy affects 0.004% of the population.

How does dialysis save an analgesic nephropathy patient experiencing kidney failure? Dialyzing fluid has many of the same solutes as blood (in strategic concentrations), and it is separated from blood by a semipermeable membrane. As blood is filtered through the dialysis machine, fluid and solutes diffuse down their concentration gradients, limited only by size. The dialysis machine therefore performs filtration, a crucial first step in which healthy kidneys would participate to purify the blood and excrete wastes. In this chapter, we'll learn more about filtration and the major processes that accompany it, reabsorption and secretion. These processes are collectively involved in osmoregulation. Osmoregulation is just one mechanism that the body uses to stabilize its fluids and tissues. In this chapter, we'll also discuss other organs such as the liver, large intestine, and skin, all of which play a role in upholding a constant internal environment. Together, these processes contribute to a necessary stable state known as homeostasis.

Key Concept

Maintenance of an internal environment wouldn't really be that hard if the external environment were static. However, we know that in the real world it does change; thus, homeostasis becomes an absolutely critical adaptation to life.

The Kidneys

The kidneys are located behind the abdomen at the level of the bottom rib. Cleverly enough, they are shaped like kidney beans. The functional unit of the kidney is the **nephron**, of which each kidney has approximately 1 million.

STRUCTURE

Each kidney is subdivided into the **cortex** and the **medulla**, as shown in Figure 11.1. The definitions for these areas hold constant for all organs to which they apply. The kidney's cortex is the outermost layer, much like the brain's. Also like the brain, the medulla of the kidney sits beneath the cortex (see Chapter 13). Each kidney also has a renal pelvis, which is its deepest layer. Although our brain certainly doesn't have a pelvis, the renal pelvis is so named because its shape appears similar to the pelvic bone structure. The **renal artery**, **renal vein**, and **ureter** enter and exit the kidneys through the renal pelvis.

> ### Mnemonic
>
> The brain and kidney both refer to their outer layer as the cortex, and have their medullas underneath (we'll see in Chapter 11 that the adrenal glands follow this scheme, too). The renal pelvis acts much like the bony pelvis in that it serves as a passageway for key structures.

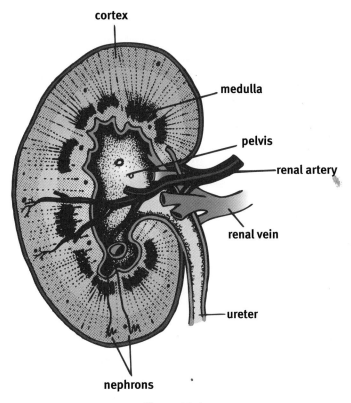

Figure 11.1

As we mentioned in Chapter 9, the kidney has one of the few **portal systems** in the body. Remember that a portal system consists of two sets of capillaries in series through which blood must travel before returning to the heart. The renal artery branches out much like the limbs of a tree and travels through the medulla and into the cortex as **afferent arterioles**. The capillaries that are derived from these afferent arterioles are known as **glomeruli** (sing: **glomerulus**) and together form a highly convoluted structure. After blood passes through the glomerulus, the **efferent arterioles** lead blood away from it.

As is the case in portal systems, the glomerular capillaries lead to a second set of arterioles (the efferents), rather than venules. Like most arterioles, the efferent arterioles also lead to a set of capillaries. This second set of capillaries is known as the **vasa recta**.

Nephrons are the functional units of the kidney. Figure 11.2 will help us understand their microanatomy.

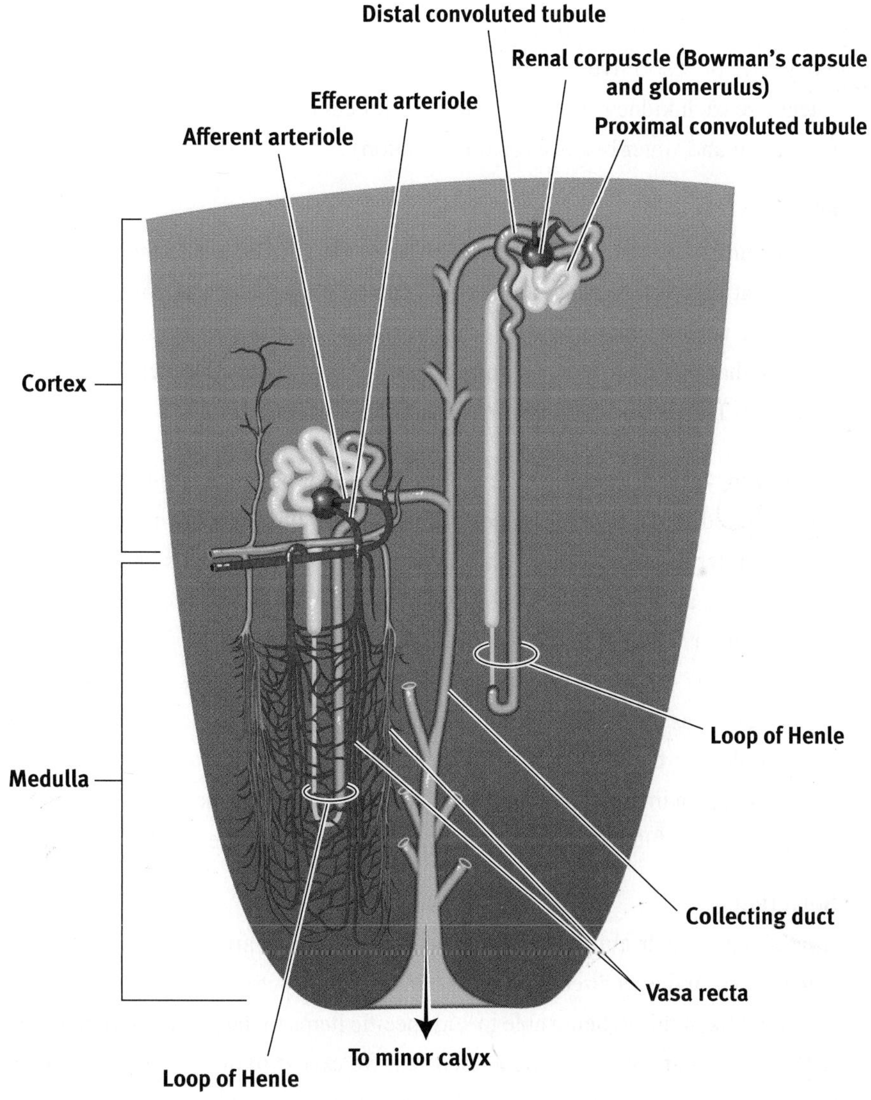
Distal convoluted tubule
Renal corpuscle (Bowman's capsule and glomerulus)
Efferent arteriole
Afferent arteriole
Proximal convoluted tubule
Cortex
Medulla
Loop of Henle
Collecting duct
Vasa recta
To minor calyx
Loop of Henle

Figure 11.2

Key Concept

The kidneys have two sets of arterioles: afferent and efferent. The afferent arterioles lead into capillaries and the efferent arterioles branch out from them. How can we remember this distinction on Test Day? *A* comes before *E* in the alphabet, with *C* in between, just as the *A*fferent arterioles come before the *E*fferent ones, with the *C*apillaries in between.

Bridge

Our discussion of nerves (Chapter 13) uses some of the same terms as do the blood vessels when we describe their organization. Afferent nerves carry sensory information toward the brain much as afferent arterioles carry blood toward the glomeruli. Efferent nerves relay signals away from the brain toward muscle just as efferent arterioles carry blood away from the glomerulus.

We will begin with the glomerulus. Our complex net of capillaries will be surrounded by a cuplike structure known as **Bowman's capsule**. Bowman's capsule leads to a long tubule with many distinct areas; in order, they are the **proximal convoluted tubule**, **descending** and **ascending limbs of the loop of Henle**, the **distal convoluted tubule**, and the **collecting duct**. Although we may think of these distinctions as trivial, the kidney's ability to excrete waste is intricately tied to the proper order and placement of these structures. When building a skyscraper, for instance, it is important that the plumbing be properly installed. We want the restrooms and water fountains and tap water to be connected in the right fashion. This requires the coordinated integration of many pipes, just as in our kidneys.

OSMOREGULATION BASICS

Now that we are experts on kidney structure (both macroscopic and microscopic), we can analyze function. Similar to the way we divided parts of the digestive system into digestive or absorptive roles, we can use **filtration**, **secretion**, and **reabsorption** to categorize each kidney structure. The three processes work together to ensure appropriate salt and water balance (osmoregulation) .

Filtration

The nephron's first step is filtration. Many of the offices inside that skyscraper filter what they throw away. Some items can be reused (such as paper), whereas others are useless and can only be discarded (the banana peel from lunch). Now, imagine that this filtering goes on in a special room right off the elevators in the basement. This is basically how the glomerulus is set up.

In the kidneys, approximately 20% of the blood that passes through the glomerulus is filtered into Bowman's space. The collected fluid is known as the filtrate, and is similar in composition to blood but does not contain cells or proteins due to the filter's ability to select based on size. In other words, molecules or cells that are larger than glomerular pores will remain in the blood. Where does that blood go next? On to the efferent arterioles and then through a second capillary network, the vasa recta. The filtrate is isotonic (Chapter 1) to blood so that neither the capsule nor the capillaries swell. Our kidneys filter about 180 liters a day, which is approximately 36 times our blood volume. This means that our entire blood volume is filtered about 36 times per day—truly impressive!

Secretion

In addition to their ability to filter blood, the nephrons are able to secrete salts, acids, bases, and urea directly into the tubule by both active and passive transport. We might liken this to being able to add specific items to the pile in our trash room in the skyscraper basement due to their relative excess in the building (e.g., if we received a duplicate shipment of light bulbs and had no room to store them, we might choose to discard the excess). Similarly, our kidneys can get rid of ions or other substances when they are present in relative excess in the blood. Secretion is also a mechanism for excreting wastes that are simply too large to pass through glomerular pores.

Reabsorption

The kidneys are firm believers in "Waste not, want not." Some compounds that are filtered and/or secreted may be taken back up for use. Certain substances are always reabsorbed, like glucose and amino acids. Imagine realizing that you threw away a lot of paper that could actually be reused in the copy machines. Sorting through the trash to find that paper would be similar to reabsorption in the kidney (without the *ick* factor, of course!).

NEPHRON FUNCTION

If our last few paragraphs had you wondering how the kidney could possibly stay on top of its to-do list, don't worry. The kidneys make use of selective permeability and osmolarity gradients to support all of their tasks. They allow the kidney to reabsorb water, salt, and nutrients from the filtrate while selectively excreting waste products. As we have probably noticed by now, a solid understanding of gradients will help us make the grade on Test Day!

Selective Permeability

In the same way that molecules must be able to cross the cell membrane to enter a cell, compounds that we want to reabsorb and keep must be able to leave the filtrate (by crossing the plasma membranes of the cells lining the tubule). Remember that failure to leave the tubule will result in excretion from the body. Where does reabsorption occur? The proximal and distal tubules are capable of reabsorbing most substances (including water). The ascending and descending limbs of the loop of Henle and the collecting duct are a bit more selective. The descending limb is permeable to water but not salt, whereas the ascending limb is permeable to salt but not water. The collecting duct almost always reabsorbs water, but the amount is variable. When the body is very well hydrated, the collecting duct will be fairly impermeable to salt and water. When in conservation mode (imagine walking on a hot day with no water bottle), antidiuretic hormone and aldosterone will each act to increase the permeability of the collecting duct, allowing for greater water reabsorption and more concentrated urine output. We will discuss these hormones shortly.

Osmolarity Gradient

The kidney is capable of altering the osmolarity of the interstitium (the tissue surrounding the tubule). This creates a gradient that, coupled with the selective permeability mentioned above, will allow us to reabsorb and excrete compounds as we need. Together, they work together as a **countercurrent multiplier system**. In the normal physiological state, the osmolarity in the cortex is approximately

Real World

In certain conditions (e.g., congestive heart failure), the body tends to accumulate excess water as fluid in the lungs or peripheral tissues (edema). The judicious use of a diuretic drug can help the body get rid of excess fluids. Diuretics typically inhibit the reabsorption of sodium in one or more regions of the nephron, thereby increasing sodium excretion. Sodium, as an osmotically active particle, will pull water with it, thereby relieving the body of some of its excess fluid.

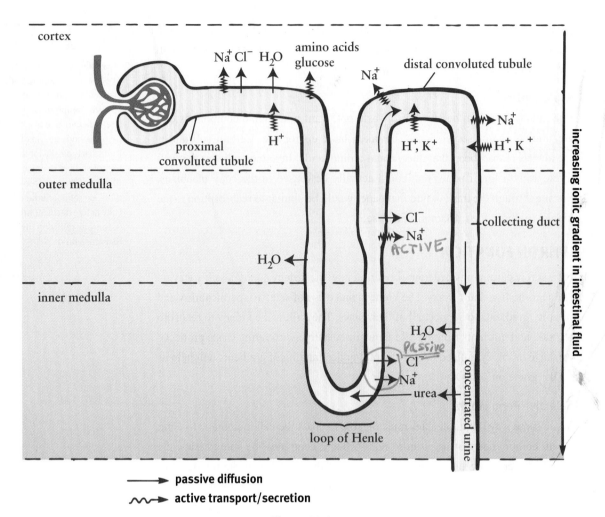

Figure 11.3

the same as that in the blood and remains at that level. As we descend deeper into the medulla, the osmolarity in the interstitium can range from isotonic with blood (when trying to excrete water) to four times as concentrated (when trying to conserve water). Water will move out of the tubule, into the interstitium, and eventually back into the blood if the concentration of solute is very high in the surrounding tissue, thereby conserving the water. If the concentration is the same in the tubule and in the interstitium, there is no driving force (gradient), and the water will be lost in urine. The solute movements that set up the countercurrent gradients are going to be major concepts for us to learn in medical school; however, for the MCAT, we just want to know that altering the osmolarity of the interstitium and selective permeability of the tubule are what allow this system to work.

Flow of Filtrate

Following the anatomical path we described before and integrating the two characteristics we just discussed, let's follow the filtrate through the nephron. In the proximal convoluted tubule, glucose, amino acids, soluble vitamins, and the majority of salts

Bridge

The entire system under which the kidney operates is based on membrane transport and gradients (Chapter 1). Both active and passive transport are used and the extent of each depends on the specific section of the nephron in question. The takeaway is that membrane permeability is absolutely necessary for the kidneys to work.

are reabsorbed, along with water. Almost 70% of filtered sodium will be reabsorbed here, but the filtrate remains isotonic to the interstitium. The descending limb of the loop of Henle is only permeable to water. As we travel down it, the concentration of the surrounding tissue will increase (we could also say it's hypertonic), which will drive water out of the tubule. Water loss increases the filtrate's osmolarity to roughly the same level as the interstitium's. The ascending limb is permeable only to salt. As the filtrate moves back up the loop toward the cortex, the concentration in the area surrounding the tubule drops and salt will be actively pumped out. Again, the filtrate is isotonic to the interstitium. The distal convoluted tubule maintains the same concentration as the cortex by reabsorbing salt and water in roughly equal proportions. The final concentration of urine will depend on the permeability of the collecting duct. As permeability increases, so does water removal, which concentrates the urine. Ultimately, the duct itself works under the directions of antidiuretic hormone (ADH) and aldosterone. Let's examine these hormones in a bit more detail.

HORMONAL REGULATION

We've mentioned ADH and aldosterone several times now because of their influence on renal function, but haven't yet discussed how they exert their effects. Both are hormones (Chapter 12) that alter the permeability of the collecting duct in different ways. We will look at each in turn briefly and discuss their regulation by the endocrine system in the next chapter.

Aldosterone

Aldosterone is a steroid hormone that is secreted by the adrenal cortex in response to decreased blood volume. A decreased blood volume means we have less fluid in our "pipes," which would lead to low blood pressure (hypotension). Aldosterone is released from the adrenal glands in response to an increase in angiotensin, which itself is positively regulated by renin (see Chapter 12).

Aldosterone works by altering the ability of the collecting duct to reabsorb sodium. Remember that water doesn't move on its own; it travels down the osmolarity gradient. If we reabsorb more sodium, water will follow it. This has the net effect of increasing blood volume and therefore blood pressure. Aldosterone will also increase potassium excretion. We exploit this often in medicine for people with high blood pressure (hypertension). By giving a drug that blocks aldosterone's receptor, we can prevent its activity. If aldosterone doesn't bind its receptor because of the drug, less sodium (and therefore less water) are reabsorbed. Less water means less blood volume and a lower blood pressure!

ADH

Antidiuretic hormone (also known as vasopressin) is a peptide hormone that directly alters the permeability of the collecting duct. It allows more water to be reabsorbed by making the cell junctions of the duct leaky. Increased concentration

Key Concept

Water is not reabsorbed alone. In fact, water is not usually pumped at all. The kidney moves ions (primarily Na^+ and Cl^-) to create gradients that water will follow by osmosis.

Bridge

As a quick flashback to Chapter 5, we can quiz ourselves on which embryonic germ layer the adrenal cortex arises from (...the mesoderm). Also recall that the adrenal medulla is generated from the ectodermal cell layer.

in the interstitium (i.e., hypertonic to the filtrate) will then cause the reuptake of water from the tubule. ADH is made in the hypothalamus, stored in the posterior pituitary, and secreted when blood osmolarity is high. Alcohol and caffeine both inhibit ADH, and lead to the frequent excretion of dilute urine.

EXCRETION

Anything that doesn't leave the tubule will be excreted. The collecting duct is essentially the point of no return. After that, there are no further transporters for reuptake. As the filtrate leaves the tubule, it collects in the renal pelvis. The fluid, which carries mostly urea, uric acid, and excess ions (e.g., sodium, potassium, magnesium, calcium), flows through the ureter to the bladder, where it is stored until voiding. Urine is excreted through the urethra.

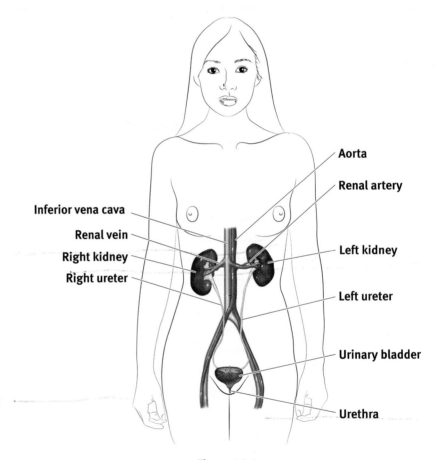

Figure 11.4

Three compounds that should always be absent from healthy urine are blood, protein, and glucose. Their presence indicates kidney pathology. Erythrocytes are too large to filter, so their appearance in urine usually indicates a problem with the glomerulus; glucose, amino acids, and small proteins are freely filtered but should be fully reabsorbed.

The Liver

We have already discussed the function of the liver in digestion. It produces bile, which aids in the absorption of fats by solubilizing them. The liver is also responsible for assisting with blood glucose regulation and the elimination of nitrogen waste through urea. We previously learned that the nutrients absorbed during digestion are delivered to the liver through the **hepatic portal vein** (Chapter 7).

In times of plenty (like just after a meal), the liver will combine circulating glucose molecules into glycogen, a polymerized storage form. During times of famine (the early morning hours before we wake up and also the later morning if we skip breakfast) this glycogen can be broken back down into glucose and released into the bloodstream. Additionally, the liver can make new glucose from a variety of precursors through **gluconeogenesis**.

The liver simply serves as a storage depot for glucose; we will see how this process is controlled in the next chapter.

In addition to glucose regulation, the liver also has the responsibility of dealing with nitrogenous waste products. Proteins are composed of amino acids, which contain amino groups. When there is a shortage of glucose, amino acids are used for vital processes such as cellular respiration. They must first undergo deamination (removal of the amino group), which would normally result in the formation of toxic ammonia. In order to prevent an ammonia buildup, the liver combines it with carbon dioxide to create urea—which we already learned can be excreted by the kidneys. The liver has several other functions, including:

- Detoxification
- Storage of vitamins and cofactors (iron and B$_{12}$)
- Destruction of old erythrocytes
- Synthesis of bile
- Synthesis of various blood proteins
- Defense against antigens
- Beta-oxidation of fatty acids to ketones
- Interconversion of carbohydrates, fats, and amino acids

The Large Intestine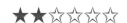

Although we already saw in Chapter 7 that the large intestine is capable of reabsorbing salt and water (but not directing overall fluid balance), this organ can also excrete certain salts such as calcium and iron.

Mnemonic

We have seen several word roots in previous chapters that can help us on Test Day. The liver is no different. *Hepato-* refers to the liver and its processes. In fact, we can remember this on the MCAT by thinking of hepatitis, which is an inflammation of the liver resulting from bacterial or viral infection.

Mnemonic

The name says it all: *gluco–* for *glucose*, *neo–* for *new*, and *genesis* for *creation*; thus gluconeogenesis creates new glucose.

Key Concept

When we discussed eukaryotic cells, organelle compartmentalization helped cells carry out fairly dangerous reactions without damaging themselves. Here again in the liver, we see the compartmentalization of a damaging molecule (ammonia) and its conversion to a nontoxic intermediate (urea) that can be safely excreted.

The Skin

STRUCTURE

By both weight and size, the skin (integument) is the largest organ in our bodies. It makes up about 16% of total body weight, on average. Just as we might cover our building in panels to keep heat in and soot-filled air out, skin protects us from the elements and disease (as we saw in Chapter 10). In fact, our skyscraper may have multiple layers of exterior paneling, and the same goes for the skin. Starting from the outside and working in, these layers are the **epidermis**, **dermis**, and **hypodermis**. Remember that the skin is derived from the ectodermal germ layer.

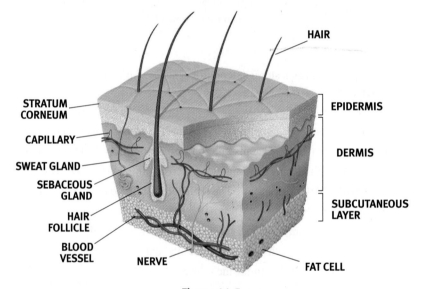

Figure 11.5

The epidermis is also subdivided into layers (strata). From the skin surface inward, these are the **stratum corneum, stratum lucidum, stratum granulosum, stratum spinosum, and stratum basalis**. The deepest layer is responsible for further proliferation. The outer layers are formed from cells that have pushed up from the stratum basalis. As these cells reach the outermost layer, they die and lose their nuclei, forming the scales (squames) of keratin that we mentioned way back in Chapter 1. The tight packing of these cells serves an immune function (as we discussed in the previous chapter) and helps to prevent loss of fluids and salt. Hair projects above the skin, and there are openings for sweat glands.

The dermis also consists of multiple layers. The upper layer (right below the epidermis) is the **papillary layer**, which consists of loose connective tissue. Below the papillary layer is the denser **reticular layer**. In addition to the three major layers of

Mnemonic

Squamata is the name of the order of scaly reptiles that includes snakes and lizards.

skin in Figure 11.5, we can also see the sweat glands, sense organs for touch and temperature, blood vessels, and hair follicles in the dermis.

Finally, we reach the hypodermis, which is the layer of connective tissue that connects our skin to our bodies. Imagine the walls in a house. The deepest layer is the drywall; this is analogous to the hypodermis. We then add paint and wallpaper, and hang pictures from the drywall, the same way that the dermis and epidermis are layered on top of the hypodermis. We can't get attachment for our dermis and epidermis (paint, wallpaper, and pictures) without the hypodermis (drywall) connecting the skin to the body.

FUNCTION

We have already mentioned that skin is capable of protecting us from the elements and microbes. It also has other functions, including ultraviolet protection, thermoregulation in **endotherms**, and transduction of sensory information from the outside world. When we go to celebrate our excellent MCAT scores on the beach, we will need full use of our **melanocytes**. These epidermal cells secrete the pigment **melanin**, which helps keep us safe from ultraviolet light and its consequent DNA damage.

The skin can also serve as a receptor for touch and temperature. Thermoregulation is achieved by vasodilation, vasoconstriction, and sweating. Sweating, while it may seem unsightly, is actually an excellent cooling mechanism. By using the heat of our bodies as the heat of vaporization (a significant energy barrier), sweat helps us keep cool.

Heat loss is prevented in a variety of ways. Pads of subcutaneous fat provide insulation. Hair also contributes by trapping heat close to the skin's surface. Shivering in the cold is a result of involuntary muscle contraction and relaxation, a byproduct of which is heat. Fat, as we mentioned in Chapter 3, also serves as a storage depot for excess energy, generating close to 100 ATP per molecule of triacylglycerol. We will see in the next chapter how epinephrine can alter the metabolic rate, affecting how rapidly this fat is stored and utilized.

Although we are all mammals, dogs rid themselves of excess heat a bit differently than we do: they pant. The basic concept is the same: evaporation of warmth results in a cooling effect, but they evaporate warm air from the respiratory passages rather than warm water from skin. Moreover, all mammals, by definition, have hair. In some (especially our canine friends), it is quite thick and is called **fur**. Their fur serves the same function as the hair we already discussed, but does so much more effectively. Animals that maintain a constant temperature are known as **endotherms** or homeotherms, whereas those whose temperature depends on the external

Real World

People who have albinism suffer from a genetic metabolic disorder characterized by the inability to synthesize melanin. Typically, albinism is inherited in an autosomal recessive fashion. As would be expected, patients with albinism are exquisitely sensitive to the harmful effects of the sun. A more common pigmentation disorder is vitiligo. Vitiligo is caused by the loss of epidermal melanocytes. Vitiligo is easily diagnosed, as there are usually well-defined zones of pigment loss. It is now believed that vitiligo is primarily an autoimmune disorder (homemade antibodies against self-melanocytes cause the depigmentation).

Bridge

The skin is also involved in the production of vitamin D with the aid of sunlight. Recall that vitamin D is critical in bone maintenance.

[handwritten margin note: • Vasoconstriction is a response to cold that inc. body temp • Vasodilation is a response to heat that dec body temp]

environment (e.g., snakes) are called **ectotherms** (previously, we may have heard these animals called cold-blooded or poikilotherms).

Finally, some animals may choose to enter a state of decreased arousal (**torpor**) during periods of excessive heat or cold. During the warm months, some desert animals may choose to **aestivate** (*aestas* is Latin for *summer*). During the winter months, the analogous process is called **hibernation**. In both cases, metabolic rate, heart rate, and respiration are far below normal. The benefit of these modes is the minimal expenditure of energy in an inhospitable environment.

Conclusion

This chapter introduced us to a new organ system (renal) and shed a different light on some organs we've already discussed (liver, large intestine, and skin). Each of these plays an integral role in maintaining a constant internal environment. For their small size, the kidneys have the immense task of filtering the blood and regulating water balance. The liver is a jack-of-all-trades; it acts a storage depot, waste handler, and detoxifier, in addition to several other roles. We've seen the skin play a role in immunity, and now we've also seen it serve in the regulation of temperature and sense perception. Now that we know how these systems work, let's move on to Chapter 12 to discuss how they are controlled.

Bridge

Homeostatic mechanisms are largely maintained involuntarily by the autonomic nervous system. The endocrine system plays a significant role, which we'll review in the next chapter.

CONCEPTS TO REMEMBER

- ☐ Homeostasis is the ability to maintain a constant internal environment despite a changing external environment.

- ☐ The kidneys use selective permeability and osmolarity gradients to maintain the body's water and salt balance.

- ☐ The functional unit of the kidney is the nephron, which has five basic sections: glomerulus, proximal convoluted tubule, distal convoluted tubule, loop of Henle (ascending and descending), and the collecting duct.

- ☐ Aldosterone is a steroid hormone that increases the amount of reabsorbed salt (directly) and thereby water (indirectly). It is secreted as part of a hormone cascade in response to low blood pressure.

- ☐ ADH is a peptide hormone that increases the ability of water to flow out of the collecting duct. It is secreted in response to an increase in blood osmolarity.

- ☐ The liver allows for excretion of excess nitrogenous waste by coupling ammonia to carbon dioxide, thereby creating the relatively nontoxic compound urea.

- ☐ The large intestine is capable of directly secreting ions and metals into solid waste.

- ☐ Thermoregulation in the skin is accomplished by vasodilation and vasoconstriction of surface blood vessels. Vasodilation of surface vessels allows more blood to run close to the skin's surface. Heat will be carried away by convection. Vasoconstriction of these same vessels prevents convection by minimizing the amount of blood at the skin's surface.

- ☐ Melanocytes in the epidermis secrete melanin, giving skin its pigmentation and protecting it from ultraviolet damage.

- ☐ Hibernation and aestivation are states of decreased metabolic activity and awareness. They serve to conserve resources in a time of scarcity.

Practice Questions

1. Which of the following would most likely be filtered through the glomerulus into Bowman's capsule?

   A. Erythrocytes
   B. Monosaccharides
   C. Platelets
   D. Proteins

2. In which of the following segments is sodium NOT actively transported out of the nephron?

   A. Proximal convoluted tubule
   B. Loop of Henle
   C. Distal convoluted tubule
   D. Sodium is always actively transported out of the nephron.

3. Which region of the kidney has the lowest solute concentration?

   A. Nephron
   B. Cortex
   C. Medulla
   D. Pelvis

4. Which of the following sequences correctly shows the passage of blood flow through the vessels of the kidney?

   A. Renal artery → afferent arterioles → glomerulus → efferent arterioles → vasa recta → renal vein
   B. Afferent arterioles → renal artery → glomerulus → vasa recta → renal vein → efferent arterioles
   C. Glomerulus → renal artery → afferent arterioles → efferent arterioles → renal vein → vasa recta
   D. Renal vein → efferent arterioles → glomerulus → afferent arterioles → vasa recta → renal artery

5. Which of the following statements is FALSE?

   A. ADH increases water reabsorption in the kidney.
   B. Aldosterone indirectly increases water reabsorption in the kidney.
   C. ADH acts directly on the proximal convoluted tubule.
   D. Aldosterone stimulates reabsorption of sodium from the collecting duct.

6. In the nephron, amino acids enter the vasa recta via the process of

   A. filtration.
   B. secretion.
   C. excretion.
   D. reabsorption.

7. On a very cold day, a man waits for over an hour at the bus stop. Which of the following structures helps his body set and maintain a normal body temperature?

   A. Hypothalamus
   B. Kidneys
   C. Heart
   D. Brain stem

8. Glucose reabsorption in the nephron occurs in the

   A. loop of Henle.
   B. distal convoluted tubule.
   C. proximal convoluted tubule.
   D. collecting duct.

9. All of the following are functions of the liver EXCEPT

    A. destruction of erythrocytes.
    B. storage of bile.
    C. detoxification of toxins.
    D. β-oxidation of fatty acids.

10. The primary function of the nephron is to create urine that is

    A. hypertonic to the blood.
    B. hypotonic to the blood.
    C. hypertonic to the filtrate.
    D. hypotonic to the vasa recta.

11. The liver

    A. decreases blood glucose levels.
    B. increases blood glucose levels.
    C. synthesizes glucose.
    D. All of the above are functions of the liver.

Small Group Questions

1. The kidneys of desert animals have modified nephrons, which help them survive long periods without water. What modifications would you expect to see in such a desert animal?

2. The glomeruli filter out a tremendous amount of water and molecules needed by the body, which must later be reabsorbed by an energy-requiring process. The Malpighian tubules of insects might seem to function more logically, secreting molecules and ions that need to be excreted. What advantages might a filtration–reabsorption process provide over a strictly secretion method of elimination?

3. You are planning to travel to a hot and arid desert region where little water is available. What kind of modifications to your epithelium would you expect to occur?

Explanations to Practice Questions

1. B

The glomerulus functions like a sieve; small molecules dissolved in the fluid will pass through the glomerulus (e.g., glucose, which is later reabsorbed), whereas large molecules such as proteins and blood cells will not. Some proteins can be filtered if they are small enough, but (B), monosaccharides, is always true and therefore the correct answer.

2. B

Sodium is actively transported out of the nephron in the proximal and distal convoluted tubules, where the concentration of sodium outside of the nephron is higher than inside; thus, energy is required to transport the sodium molecules against their concentration gradient. In the inner medulla, however, sodium and other ions (such as chloride) diffuse passively down their concentration gradient. The loop of Henle is the only structure that dips into the medulla, making (B) the correct answer.

3. B

The region of the kidney that has the lowest solute concentration is the cortex, where the proximal convoluted tubule and a part of the distal convoluted tubule are found. (B) is thus the correct answer.

4. A

Blood enters the kidney through the renal artery, which divides into many afferent arterioles that run through the medulla and into the cortex. Each afferent arteriole branches into a convoluted network of capillaries called a glomerulus. Rather than converging directly into a vein, the capillaries converge into an efferent arteriole, which divides into a fine capillary network known as the vasa recta. The vasa recta capillaries enmesh the nephron tubule where they reabsorb various ions, and then converge into the renal vein. This arrangement of tandem capillary beds is known as a portal system. (A) correctly describes the passage of blood through the kidney.

5. C

Glancing at the answer choices, we notice right away that they all test us on our knowledge about ADH and aldosterone. These two hormones ultimately act to increase water reabsorption in the kidney; their respective mechanisms of action, however, are different. ADH increases water reabsorption by increasing the permeability of the collecting duct to water, whereas aldosterone stimulates reabsorption of sodium from the DCT. Using this knowledge, we can now attack the answer choices. (A), (B), and (D) are all true statements, while (C) is false; ADH does not act on the proximal convoluted tubule. (C) is thus the correct answer.

6. D

Essential substances such as glucose, salts, amino acids, and water are reabsorbed from the filtrate and returned to the blood in the vasa recta. This results in the formation of concentrated urine, which is hypertonic to the blood. (D) correctly identifies the process through which amino acids enter the vasa recta. By knowing that the body does not want to lose any proteins, and thus amino acids, we could eliminate (A), (B), and (C).

7. A

The hypothalamus functions as a thermostat that regulates body temperature. When it's cold outside, nervous stimulation to the blood vessels in the skin is increased, causing the vessels to constrict. This constriction diminishes blood flow to the skin surface and prevents heat loss. Sweat glands are turned off to prevent heat loss through evaporation.

Skeletal muscles are stimulated to shiver (rapidly contract), which increases the metabolic rate and produces heat. Furthermore, the cerebrum stimulates warmth-seeking behaviors, such as foot stamping. If the cold stress becomes severe, the hypothalamus will stimulate the secretion of thyroid and adrenal hormones, which will provide additional heat by further increasing the metabolic rate. Since the hypothalamus is the main structure involved in maintaining body temperature, (A) is therefore correct.

8. C

The filtrate enters Bowman's capsule and then flows into the proximal convoluted tubule, where virtually all glucose, amino acids and other important organic molecules are reabsorbed via active transport. (C) is thus the correct answer.

9. B

The liver is a complex organ and plays many crucial roles in the maintenance of homeostasis. Among the main functions, we can enumerate the conversion of glucose into glycogen, the destruction of erythrocytes, the detoxification of toxins, and the β-oxidation of fatty acids. From the given choices, the only function that cannot be attributed to the liver is (B). Although bile is produced in the liver, it is stored in the gallbladder. (B) is therefore the correct answer.

10. A

The kidneys function to eliminate wastes such as urea, while reabsorbing various important substances such as glucose and amino acids for reuse by the body. Generation of a solute concentration gradient from the cortex to medulla allows a considerable amount of water to be reabsorbed. Excretion of concentrated urine serves to limit water losses from the body and helps to preserve blood volume. Thus, the primary function of the nephron is to create urine that is hypertonic to the blood, making (A) the correct answer.

11. D

The liver helps regulate blood glucose levels through three main mechanisms: conversion of glucose to glycogen, conversion of glycogen to glucose, and gluconeogenesis (synthesis of glucose from noncarbohydrate precursors). Thus, (A), (B), and (C) all identify functions of the liver, making (D) the correct answer to this question.

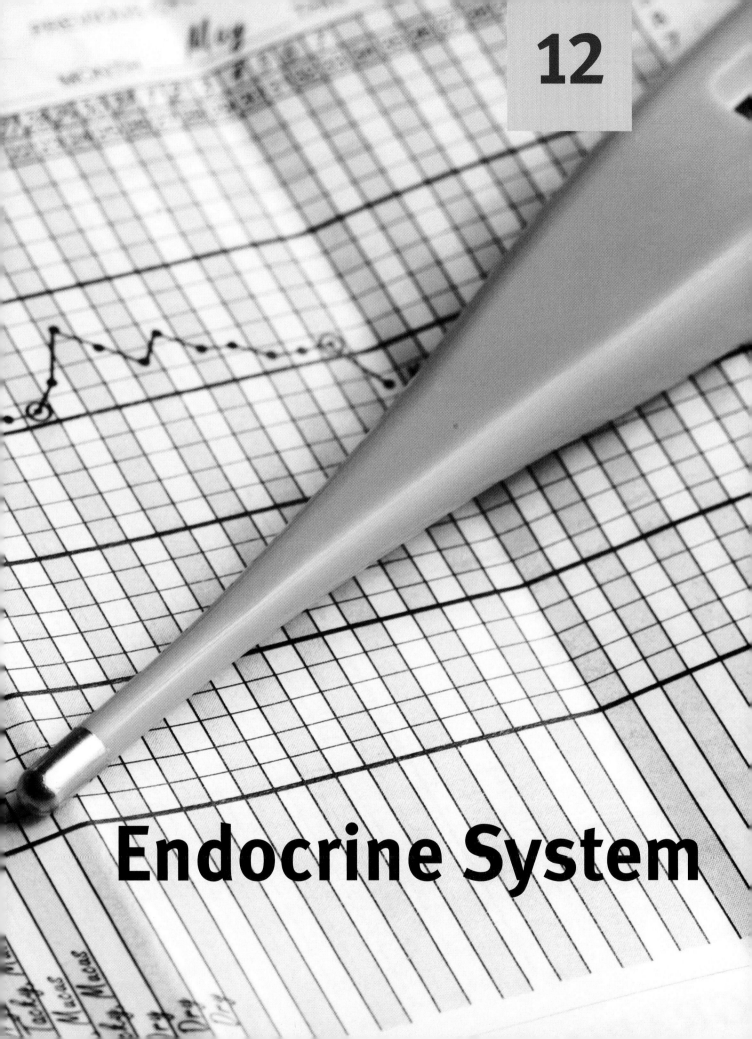

12

Endocrine System

In medicine, there are certain terms used that have onomatopoeic qualities: the *lub dub* of the heart sounds, the *rhonchi* of respiratory illnesses. Although ovulation, the rupture of the follicle and release of the oocyte from the surface of the ovary, is a silent event, the pain that some women experience in the hours around ovulation is described by a term that possesses the sensory equivalent of onomatopoeia: *mittelschmerz*. It just *sounds* unpleasant, doesn't it? German for *middle pain, mittelschmerz* is experienced by about 20 percent of ovulating women. Ranging from dull to sharp, typically located in the lower abdomen and pelvis, the pain may last anywhere from a few hours to a couple of days. In some women, the pain is so localized that they can tell from which ovary the egg was released, and because ovulation occurs randomly from each ovary every month, the pain may switch sides month to month. Analgesics (pain relievers) may be used in cases of moderate to severe discomfort. The source of the pain may be related to irritation of the abdominal cavity wall by the fluid and blood released from the ruptured ovarian follicle.

Ovulation is a key event in the cycle of female fertility. Highly controlled by a complex system of positive and negative feedback loops involving chemical messengers called hormones, the menstrual cycle is the example par excellence of endocrine system activity. The MCAT will test your general understanding of the endocrine system, which is a complex association of many different organs and tissues working together to control the activity of other organs and maintain homeostasis. Although the menstrual cycle is a primary focus for the MCAT, you must also be sure to understand endocrine regulation of blood glucose concentration, renal function and osmoregulation, and thyroid function as it relates to thermoregulation, to name but a few aspects of the overall concept of homeostasis.

Although the hypothalamus is one of the major regulators of the endocrine system, there is no single control center. Glands throughout the organism contribute to endocrine effects. We will briefly examine the anatomy of the endocrine glands and then jump into the functional products, hormones. The hypothalamus and pituitary will get special attention because they are involved in many disparate functions, including menstrual regulation, the stress response, and tissue growth and development. Hormones can appear in antagonistic pairs, in a way analogous to the antagonistic pairing of muscles. We will see examples of hormone antagonist pairs that control blood glucose and calcium concentrations. The effects of hormones are mediated through their receptors, so we will close with a discussion of the chemical classes of hormones. Table 12.1 at the end of the chapter will be an important study resource for you. As we discuss each hormone, we will draw your attention to the source of each hormone, its general structure, receptor location, and effect on the target cell.

Key Concept

Unlike the other organ systems that we have discussed thus far, the basis of the endocrine system is *action at a distance*. Each organ has a local effect that can then be passed though the blood stream to affect the entire organism.

[handwritten margin notes:]
endocrine system — system of glands, each of which secretes a type of hormone to regulate the body.

hypothalamus — portion of the brain; links the nervous system to the endocrine system via the pituitary gland

Anatomy

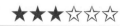

Endocrine organs exert their influence, sometimes over long distances, upon other areas in the body to provide both feedback and stimulation. Depending on the distance between the endocrine organ and the intended site of action of its hormone, signaling may be described as **autocrine**, **paracrine**, or **endocrine**. In autocrine signaling, the same cell is stimulated. For example, some T-cells (see Chapter 10) will release interleukin-2. This cytokine can then bind to the same T-cells to increase their immune functionality. Paracrine signaling occurs between cells that are placed close to one another. Here, we can use two neurons signaling between the hypothalamus and pituitary as an example. Finally, endocrine signaling involves our classic action at a distance. We can think of follicle-stimulating hormone (FSH), which is released by the anterior pituitary, but exerts its effects at the level of the gonads. We need to be mindful of the involvement of the different hormones in the various types of signaling (autocrine, paracrine, and endocrine). Table 12.1 at the end of the chapter will help guide us.

Endocrine Glands

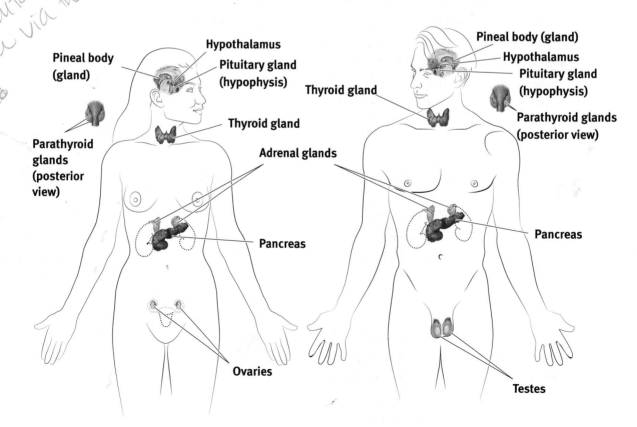

Figure 12.1

Many organs in the body have endocrine capabilities, and we have mentioned several of them already! This group includes the **hypothalamus**, the **pituitary**, the **testes** and **ovaries**, the **pineal gland**, the **kidneys**, the **gastrointestinal glands**, the **heart**, and the **thymus**. Each of these organs is capable of synthesizing and secreting one or more hormones. Furthermore, we may identify collections of cells within organs that serve important endocrine roles. Perhaps the most well-known collection of cells having endocrine activity are the pancreatic Islets of Langerhans, which are primarily responsible for glucose homeostasis. Hormones come in two varieties: **peptide** and **steroid**. We will discuss the physiological consequences of this shortly, but in either case, hormones must bind to their receptors to be effective. Thus, we can say that hormone activity is not only controlled by the release of hormone, but also by the presence of receptors on target organs.

HYPOTHALAMUS

We will start with the hypothalamus, the master control gland in the brain. If the endocrine system was a complex political organization, we might characterize the hypothalamus as the president. By regulating the pituitary (see below), the hypothalamus is capable of having organism-wide effects. The hypothalamus is located in the forebrain (see Chapter 13), directly above the pituitary gland and below the thalamus (hence, *hypo*thalamus). Since the hypothalamus and the pituitary are close to each other, the hypothalamic control of the pituitary is by paracrine release of

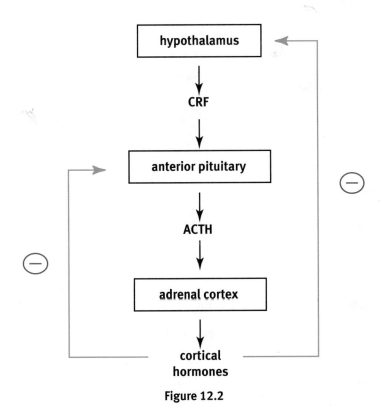

Figure 12.2

> **Bridge**
>
> Enzymes are also often regulated via feedback inhibition. The endocrine system is regulated in a similar manner. As concentrations of the final effector molecule rise (e.g., cortisol), negative feedback to the hypothalamus and pituitary decreases their release of the upstream signaling molecules (e.g., CRF and ACTH, respectively).

pituitary gland — located @ bottom of hypothalamus, secretes hormones regulating homeostasis, also trophic hormones that stimulate other endocrine glands.

hormones into a portal system that directly connects the two organs. The hypothalamus receives input from a wide variety of neural sources; for example, a part of the hypothalamus called the suprachiasmatic nucleus (which we don't need to remember for Test Day) receives some of the light input from the retinas and helps control sleep–wake cycles. The release of hormones by the hypothalamus is also regulated by negative feedback (recall Chapter 2 and control of enzymatic activity). As part of our discussion of the hypothalamus, we should note that the pituitary has an **anterior** and **posterior** component. The different roles of each will be examined shortly. The hypothalamus controls both parts, but in different ways.

Interactions with the Anterior Pituitary

The hypothalamus secretes compounds into the **hypophyseal portal system** (see Chapters 7 and 9), which is shown in Figure 12.3. Although the name may sound funny, **hypophysis** is just the medical name for the pituitary (remember, *hypo*– means *below*; the pituitary is below the hypothalamus). Hormones are released from the hypothalamus into this portal bloodstream, then travel down the pituitary stalk and bind to receptors in the anterior pituitary, where they stimulate the release of other hormones.

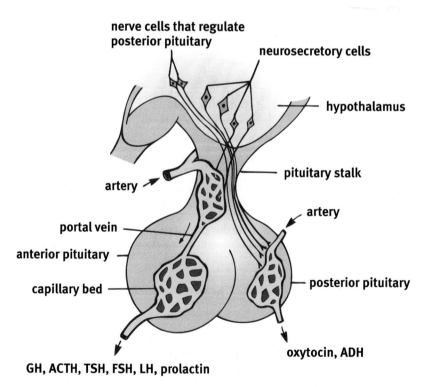

nerve cells that regulate posterior pituitary

neurosecretory cells

hypothalamus

pituitary stalk

artery

portal vein

artery

anterior pituitary

capillary bed

posterior pituitary

GH, ACTH, TSH, FSH, LH, prolactin

oxytocin, ADH

Figure 12.3

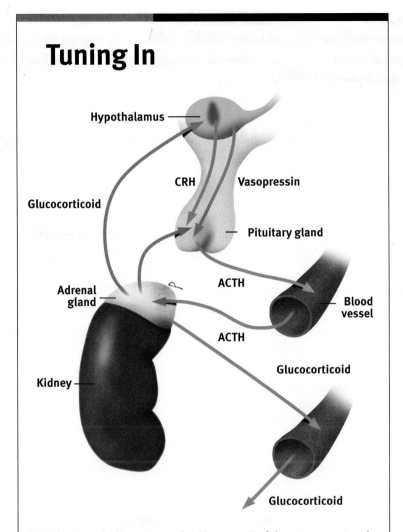

Tuning In

The hypothalamus runs the "long arm" of the stress system by secreting the hormone CRH. CRH flows through veins (*green arrow*) to the pituitary, which in turn releases the hormone ACTH into the blood. ACTH stimulates the adrenal glands to produce glucocorticoid hormones, which put the body on alert. In acute stress, the hypothalamus secretes vasopressin as well, to further activate the adrenals. The system regulates itself down after a threat is over via a negative feedback loop (*blue arrows*), in which gluco-corticoids bathe both the hypothalamus to suppress CRH secretion and the pituitary to suppress ACTH. But daily stress may endlessly activate the system.

Figure 12.4

For each of the next pairs of hormones, the first is the hypothalamic hormone whose binding in the anterior pituitary causes the release of the second hormone: **gonadotropin-releasing hormone (GnRH)** with **follicle-stimulating hormone (FSH)** and **luteinizing hormone (LH); growth hormone-releasing hormone**

Mnemonic

To remember the seven products of the anterior pituitary, think FLAT PEG:

FSH

LH

ACTH

TSH

Prolactin

Endorphins

GH

(GHRH) with growth hormone (GH); prolactin inhibitory factor (PIF) with prolactin; thyroid-releasing hormone (TRH) with thyroid-stimulating hormone (TSH); and corticotropin-releasing factor (CRF) with adrenocorticotropic hormone (ACTH). Each of the hypothalamic–anterior pituitary hormone pairs, with one exception, operates in the same manner: Increased release from the hypothalamus will cause increased release of the corresponding hormone from the anterior pituitary. The oddball in the bunch is PIF/prolactin. Prolactin is constitutively released from the anterior pituitary and is *inhibited* by prolactin inhibitory factor.

Excessive levels of hormones can be detrimental. To keep the amounts within a healthy range, the hypothalamus and pituitary are both subject to feedback inhibition. Let's take a look at an example of this, diagrammed back in Figure 12.2.

Release of CRF (also known as CRH, cortisol-releasing hormone) from the hypothalamus will stimulate the anterior pituitary to generate ACTH. ACTH will then cause the adrenals to increase the level of cortisol being secreted into the blood. However, we wouldn't want cortisol levels to rise too high (we will see why shortly). To prevent excess cortisol secretion, cortisol can inhibit the hypothalamus and anterior pituitary from releasing CRF and ACTH, respectively. This makes sense as CRF and ACTH have now had their desired effect: namely, getting more cortisol into the blood. What does this mean in terms of receptors in the hypothalamus and pituitary? They must contain receptors for cortisol; otherwise, they wouldn't be able to recognize that cortisol levels had increased.

Interactions with the Posterior Pituitary

Connection between the hypothalamus and the posterior lobe of the pituitary is not by way of the hypophyseal portal system. Rather, neurons in the hypothalamus send their axons (see Chapter 13) down the pituitary stalk and into the posterior pituitary, where they can release oxytocin and anti-diuretic hormone (ADH). ADH, also called vasopressin, is a hormone we have discussed already in the context of renal function; oxytocin is new to us, but will be described in detail in the next section.

PITUITARY

We have already introduced the anatomical divisions in the pituitary, the anterior and posterior lobes, which are also functionally distinct. We will consider each in turn.

Anterior Pituitary

One distinction that can help us organize the anterior pituitary hormones is categorizing them into direct or tropic roles. Direct hormones will bind to receptors on their target organs and have a direct effect (i.e., no intermediate is needed). Tropic hormones also bind to receptors on organs, but rather than resulting in immediate changes, they cause the release of effector hormones (i.e., they act as an intermediate). Both are important mechanisms. The FLAT PEG mnemonic helps us not only to remember the hormones, but also to separate them according to their direct versus tropic effects.

Direct Hormones

Growth hormone is named for what it does: It promotes the growth of bone and muscle. This sort of growth is energetically expensive (think of how much hungrier you were and how much you ate during puberty). Growth hormone prevents glucose uptake in certain tissues (nongrowing ones) and stimulates the breakdown of fatty acids. We can see that this will increase the availability of glucose overall, allowing the muscle and bone to use it. If we think back to the hypothalamus, we know that the release of GH is tied to GHRH stimulation.

We mentioned in Chapter 6 that growth occurs at the epiphyseal plates of the long bones; these plates seal during puberty. An excess of GH released in childhood (before this closure) can cause **gigantism**. A deficit results in **dwarfism**. In adults, the situation is slightly different. Because the long bones are sealed, GH still has an effect but it is in the smaller bones. Bone remodeling occurs throughout life, and an excess of GH in adulthood will affect smaller bones disproportionately. The medical condition is known as **acromegaly**. The bones most commonly affected are those in the hands, feet, and head. Patients will present because they have had to buy larger shoes, they cannot wear their rings, and they can no longer fit into their hats.

The other two direct hormones are prolactin and the endorphins. Prolactin is more important in females than in males, where it stimulates milk production in the **mammary glands**. Milk production in the male is pathologic, as stated previously.

Finally, endorphins have a direct effect on pain modulation, by decreasing the perception of pain. Many pharmaceutical agents, such as morphine, mimic the effect of these naturally occurring painkillers. A real-life example of this occurs in runners. After completing a marathon, many people will say they are on an endorphin "high" or "rush." Endorphins mask the pain from just having run 26.2 miles and induce a sense of euphoria. People who eat very spicy food claim a similar sensation in response to capsaicin, the compound found in peppers.

Tropic Hormones

We are going to mention the tropic hormones only briefly here. They work by causing the release of another hormone at the organ level. We will discuss those effector hormones with each organ system. ACTH is regulated by CRF. It induces the adrenal cortex to release glucocorticoids. As we might expect with a root like *gluco–*, glucocorticoids can affect sugar balance in the body. TSH is released in response to TRH stimulation. TSH is appropriately named, as it stimulates the thyroid to take up iodine and release **thyroid hormone**. Both LH and FSH are secreted when GnRH levels rise. They affect the ovaries and testes. The specific effects of each hormone with which we want to be familiar for the MCAT will be discussed later.

Posterior Pituitary

The posterior pituitary contains the nerve terminals of neurons whose bodies are in the hypothalamus. The posterior pituitary receives and stores two hormones produced by the hypothalamus, ADH and oxytocin. These hormones are released into the bloodstream by the posterior pituitary. Oxytocin is secreted during childbirth and allows for coordinated contraction of uterine smooth muscle. Its secretion may also be stimulated by suckling, which in turn will lead to increased milk production.

We already examined the details of ADH in Chapter 11, but as a quick review, we will highlight key points. ADH is secreted in response to increased blood osmolarity (sensed by **osmoreceptors**) or low blood volume (sensed by **baroreceptors**). Its action is at the level of the collecting duct, where it increases the permeability of the duct to water. The net effect is a greater reabsorbtion of water from the nephron filtrate, resulting in greater retention of water and expansion (and dilution) of the vascular compartment.

THYROID GLAND

The thyroid is controlled by the pituitary (TSH) and the hypothalamus (TRH). The human thyroid is on the front surface of the trachea; if you put your fingers gently on the front of your windpipe, you can feel it as the organ that moves up and down with swallowing. The thyroid has two major functions: setting basal metabolic rate and calcium homeostasis. It mediates the first effect by releasing **thyroxine** and **triiodothyronine (the thyroid hormones)**, whereas calcium levels are controlled by **calcitonin**.

Thyroid Hormones (Thyroxine and Triiodothyronine)

Thyroxine (T_4) and triiodothyronine (T_3) are both produced by the iodination of the amino acid tyrosine in the follicular cells of the thyroid. The numbers 3 and 4 refer to the number of iodine atoms attached. Thyroid hormones are capable of resetting the basal metabolic rate of the body by making energy production more or less efficient, as well as altering the utilization of glucose and fatty acids. Increased amounts of T_3 and T_4 will lead to increased cellular respiration. They will also cause a greater amount of protein and fatty acid turnover by speeding up both synthesis and degradation of these compounds. High plasma levels of thyroid hormones will lead to decreased TSH and TRH synthesis; we expect this negative feedback so that T_3 and T_4 levels don't become excessive.

Key Concept

The posterior pituitary is controlled differently from the anterior. The posterior pituitary simply serves as a jumping-off point for the hormones ADH and oxytocin (made in the hypothalamus). It serves no synthetic functions of its own.

Real World

Iodine is absolutely required for the thyroid to carry out its function. In the Western world, shortage of iodine is rare as most table salt is now iodized.

A deficiency of iodine or an inflammation of the thyroid may result in **hypothyroidism**, in which thyroid hormones are secreted in insufficient amounts or not at all. The condition is characterized by lethargy, decreased body temperature, slowed respiratory and heart rate, cold intolerance, and weight gain. Thyroid hormones are required for appropriate neurological and physical development in children. Most children are tested at birth for appropriate levels because a deficiency will result in mental retardation and developmental delay (**cretinism**). An excess of thyroid hormones, which may result from a tumor or thyroid over-stimulation, may lead to **hyperthyroidism**. We can predict its clinical course by considering the opposite of each of the effects seen in hypothyroidism: heightened activity level, increased body temperature, increased respiratory and heart rate, heat intolerance, and weight loss.

In both hyperthyroidism and hypothyroidism, the organ itself may enlarge and become visible by external examination. This is known as a **goiter.**

Calcitonin

If we were to examine thyroid tissue under a light microscope, we would see two distinct cell populations within the gland. Follicular cells produce thyroid hormones and C-cells produce **calcitonin**. Calcitonin acts to decrease plasma calcium levels in three ways: increase excretion from the kidneys, decrease absorption from the gut, and increase storage in the bone. High levels of calcium in the blood stimulate secretion of calcitonin from the C-cells.

PARATHYROID GLANDS

The hormone produced by the parathyroid glands is aptly, if unimaginatively, named **parathyroid hormone (PTH)**. The parathyroids are four small pea-shaped structures that sit on the surface of the thyroid. PTH serves as an antagonistic hormone to calcitonin. It functions to increase plasma levels of calcium by reversing the effects of calcitonin; namely, it decreases excretion of calcium through the kidneys, increases absorption of calcium in the gut, and increases bone resorption, thereby freeing up calcium. PTH also activates vitamin D to its active form, which is required for the absorption of calcium in the gut. Like the hormones we have already seen, PTH is also subject to feedback inhibition. As levels of plasma calcium rise, PTH secretion is decreased.

ADRENAL GLANDS

The adrenal glands are the next endocrine organ we will examine as we continue our whirlwind journey through the body. The adrenals are located on top of the kidneys, one on each side (*adrenal*, meaning near or next to the kidney). As we discussed in Chapter 5, they consist of a cortex and a medulla. The distinction is more than anatomical; each part of the gland is responsible for secretion of a different hormone. Let's take a look.

Adrenal Cortex

The adrenal cortex secretes a set of hormones called the **corticosteroids**. These compounds are secreted in response to ACTH stimulation from the anterior pituitary, which itself responds to CRF from the hypothalamus. All of the corticosteroids are steroid hormones (derived from cholesterol); they may be divided into three functional classes: **glucocorticoids**, **mineralocorticoids**, and **cortical sex hormones**. One way to remember the corticosteroids is to think of the three *s*'s of the adrenal cortex: sugar, salt, and sex. A medical school professor once said that we should no longer have any problem remembering these, given how much of our waking (and dreaming) hours are spent fantasizing about or actually pursuing each one of them.

Glucocorticoids

The name of this class of hormones gives us an insight to their function. The prefix *gluco–* gives us the clue that they help regulate glucose levels. In addition, they affect protein metabolism. Two glucocorticoids we should be familiar with for Test Day are **cortisol** and **cortisone**. How might these compounds raise blood glucose? They increase gluconeogenesis (see Chapter 11) and decrease protein synthesis. Cortisol and cortisone can also decrease inflammation and immunological responses. When we see football players receiving steroid shots to cut down on inflammation in their knee joints, glucocorticoids are being used. Cortisol is often known as the stress hormone, as it is released in response to physical or emotional stress. As we can see in the next figure, stress affects several parts of the body, so it should make sense that it stimulates an endocrine release.

Mineralocorticoids

Considering the name of this class of hormones, we can predict that mineralocorticoids will help us to keep a healthy mineral balance. And they do, in fact, control salt balance in coordination with the kidneys. You should recall the mineralocorticoid that we discussed in Chapter 11. **Aldosterone** causes increased reabsorption of sodium, and thereby water. The increased sodium and water will lead to expansion of the blood volume and a higher blood pressure. Aldosterone can also affect the levels of potassium and hydrogen ions. It enhances the secretion of these two atoms into the tubule. What will be the net result of this movement? Potassium and hydrogen will be excreted from the body in the urine.

The secretion of aldosterone is under the control of the **renin–angiotensin–aldosterone** system. Decreased blood volume causes the juxtaglomerular cells of the kidney to secrete renin, which cleaves an inactive plasma protein **angiotensinogen** to its active form, **angiotensin I.** Angiotensin I is then

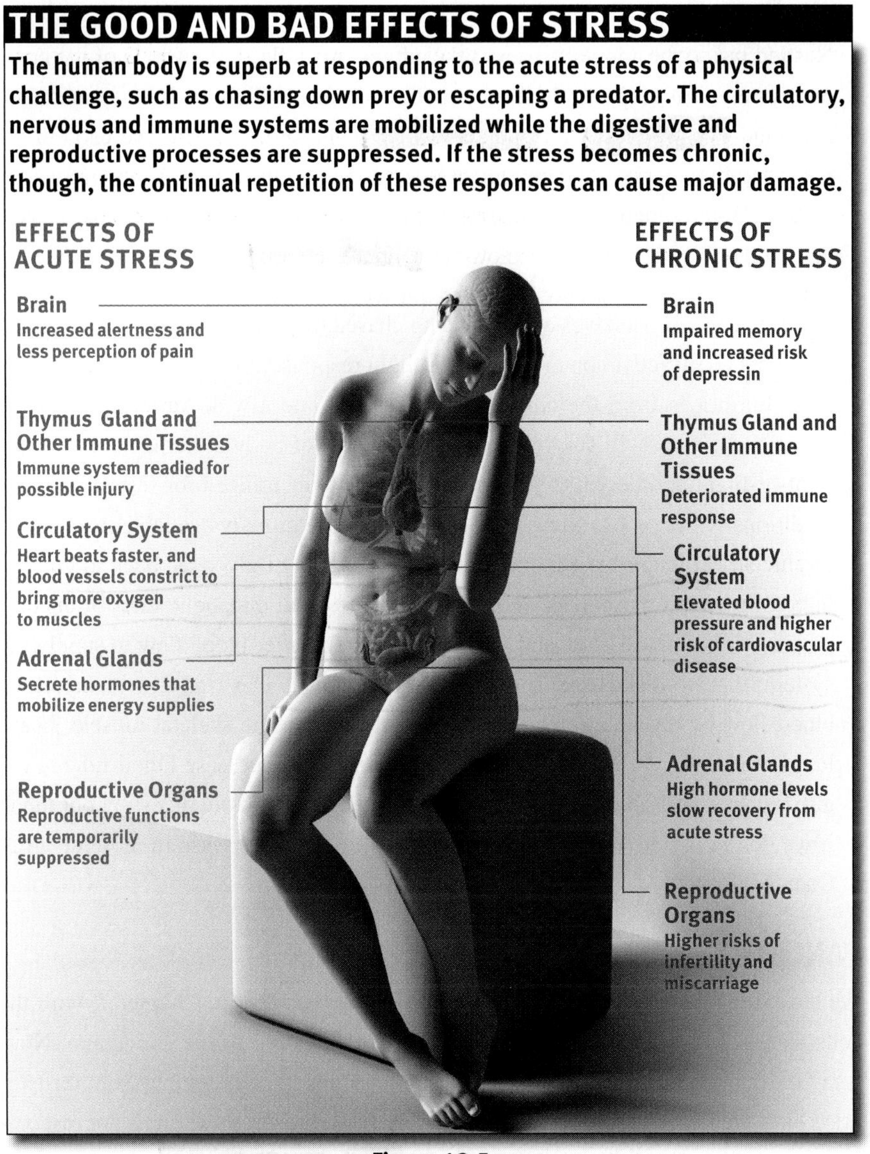

THE GOOD AND BAD EFFECTS OF STRESS

The human body is superb at responding to the acute stress of a physical challenge, such as chasing down prey or escaping a predator. The circulatory, nervous and immune systems are mobilized while the digestive and reproductive processes are suppressed. If the stress becomes chronic, though, the continual repetition of these responses can cause major damage.

EFFECTS OF ACUTE STRESS

Brain
Increased alertness and less perception of pain

Thymus Gland and Other Immune Tissues
Immune system readied for possible injury

Circulatory System
Heart beats faster, and blood vessels constrict to bring more oxygen to muscles

Adrenal Glands
Secrete hormones that mobilize energy supplies

Reproductive Organs
Reproductive functions are temporarily suppressed

EFFECTS OF CHRONIC STRESS

Brain
Impaired memory and increased risk of depressin

Thymus Gland and Other Immune Tissues
Deteriorated immune response

Circulatory System
Elevated blood pressure and higher risk of cardiovascular disease

Adrenal Glands
High hormone levels slow recovery from acute stress

Reproductive Organs
Higher risks of infertility and miscarriage

Figure 12.5

converted to **angiotensin II** (see the sidebar), which will stimulate the adrenal cortex to secrete aldosterone. Once fluid volume is restored, there is a decreased drive to stimulate renin release, thus serving as the negative feedback mechanism for this system.

Cortical Sex Hormones

The adrenals are also capable of making male sex hormones (**androgens**). Because normal males make much larger amounts of androgens in the testes, the hormones secreted from the adrenals are relatively unimportant. In females, however, the lower baseline of androgens is subject to greater perturbation. An increase in adrenal sex hormones may have masculinizing effects such as excess hair growth and an increase in other male secondary sex characteristics.

Real World

In addition to stimulating the secretion of aldosterone, which increases blood volume and hence blood pressure, angiotensin II also increases blood pressure directly by a powerful vasoconstrictive effect. Angiotensin converting enzyme (ACE) inhibitors block the conversion of angiotensin I to angiotensin II, inhibiting vasoconstriction and actually producing vasodilation. Therefore, ACE inhibitors frequently are prescribed for the treatment of high blood pressure and congestive heart failure. (In the latter case, vasodilation helps reduce the resistance against which the failing heart must pump.)

Adrenal Medulla

Nestled inside the adrenal cortex is the adrenal medulla. A derivative of the nervous system, it is responsible for the production of the flight-or-fight sympathetic hormones **epinephrine** and **norepinephrine**. The specialized nerve cells in the medulla are capable of secreting these compounds directly into the circulatory system. Both epinephrine and norepinephrine are peptide hormones that belong to a larger class of molecules known as **catecholamines**.

If we ever found ourselves actually being chased by a bear, our survival would, in part, depend on activation of the fight or flight response. As a part of this response, these hormones from the adrenal medulla modulate a wide variety of systems in the body. They will act to increase the activity of body systems necessary for fight-or-flight and decrease activity to those systems utilized for rest-and-digest. Additionally, we would want to make energy more directly available in the form of glucose. Epinephrine can increase the conversion of glycogen back to glucose in both liver and muscle, as well as increase the basal metabolic rate. Both compounds will increase heart and respiratory rate and alter blood flow to supply the systems that would be used in a sympathetic response. This would mean increased blood flow by vasodilation of the arteries leading to the skeletal muscle, heart, lungs, and brain. In addition, vasoconstriction would decrease blood flow to the gut, kidneys, and skin. After all, we won't need to worry about digesting our lunch if we don't escape! We will discuss the fight-or-flight response in more detail in Chapter 12.

PANCREAS

We have already seen the exocrine function of the pancreas in Chapter 7, with the cells that secrete digestive enzymes into the ducts leading to the duodenum. Now, we will examine the *endocrine* function. Small groups of cells distinct from the exocrine ones are known as **islets of Langerhans**. If we look at these areas microscopically, we will see three distinct types of cells: **alpha**, **beta**, and **delta** cells. The alpha cells secrete **glucagon**, whereas the beta cells are responsible for the production of **insulin**. Delta cells make **somatostatin**.

Glucagon

Glucagon is a hormone whose actions are antagonistic to those of insulin. It is secreted during times of famine (the word "famine" might sound a bit harsh, so perhaps we'll imagine the hunger we feel before breakfast!). When glucose levels run low, it stimulates degradation of protein and fat, conversion of glycogen to glucose, and production of new glucose via gluconeogenesis. In addition to being secreted by low blood glucose, certain gastrointestinal hormones (e.g., CCK and gastrin; see Chapter 7) will increase glucagon release from the alpha cells. In times of feast, or high glucose levels, secretion will be inhibited.

> ## Bridge
>
> The secretions of the exocrine pancreas are components of the pancreatic juice that enters into the duodenum:
>
> - Amylase (carbohydrate digestion)
> - Lipase (lipid digestion)
> - Trypsin, chymotrypsin, and carboxypeptidase (protein digestion)

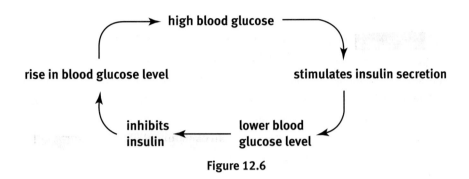

Figure 12.6

Mnemonic

We can remember when glucagon levels are high because it is secreted when glucose is *gone*.

Insulin

If insulin is antagonistic to glucagon, when would we expect it to be secreted? Insulin levels in plasma rise in conjunction with blood glucose levels. Insulin induces muscle and liver cells to take up glucose and store it as glycogen for later use. In addition, since it is active when glucose levels are high, insulin stimulates anabolic processes such as fat and protein synthesis.

In excess, insulin will cause **hypoglycemia**, which is characterized by low blood glucose. Underproduction, insufficient secretion, or insensitivity to insulin all can result in **diabetes mellitus**, which is clinically characterized by **hyperglycemia**, excess glucose in the blood. As we saw in Chapter 10, excessive glucose in the filtrate will result in its presence in the urine. Since it is an osmotically active particle, its (abnormal) presence in the filtrate leads to excess excretion of water and expansion, sometimes dramatic, of the urine volume. Diabetics often report **polyuria**, increased frequency of urination, and **polydipsia**, increased thirst. There are two types of diabetes. **Type I** (insulin-dependent diabetes mellitus) is caused by autoimmune destruction of the beta cells of the pancreas; these individuals produce little to no insulin, as the majority of beta cells have been destroyed. Type I diabetics require regular injections of insulin to prevent hyperglycemia. **Type II** (non–insulin dependent diabetes mellitus) is a result of the body resisting the effects of insulin at its receptor. It is partially inherited and partially due to high-sugar diets. Certain pharmaceutical agents can be taken orally to help the body more effectively use the insulin it produces. These individuals require insulin only when their body cannot naturally control glucose levels, even when aided by these other medications.

Somatostatin

Somatostatin is an inhibitor of both insulin and glucagon. High blood glucose and amino acid concentrations stimulate its secretion.

TESTES

The testes, present only in the male, are the site of spermatogenesis (Chapter 4). To carry out this function properly, there is a delicate interplay of FSH and LH stimulation on two structures in the testes. FSH stimulates the Sertoli cells and is

Key Concept

Insulin decreases plasma glucose. Glucagon increases plasma glucose. Don't forget that growth hormone, the glucocorticoids, and epinephrine are also capable of increasing plasma glucose.

necessary for sperm maturation, whereas LH causes the interstitial cells to produce **testosterone**, the major androgen in the male. In addition to being important for spermatogenesis, testosterone is necessary for male embryonic differentiation, male sexual development at puberty, and maintenance of secondary sex characteristics (e.g., axillary and pubic hair). It provides negative feedback to FSH, LH, and GnRH. If the receptors for testosterone are absent from an individual, it cannot exert its effects. The result is a condition called **androgen insensitivity syndrome**, in which a genetic male (XY) has secondary female sexual characteristics.

OVARIES

The ovaries, which are derived from the same embryonic structure as the testes, are found only in females. They are also under the control of FSH and LH secreted from the anterior pituitary, which itself is directed by GnRH release from the hypothalamus. The ovaries produce both **estrogens** and **progesterone**.

Hormones

Estrogens

Estrogens, which are secreted in response to elevated FSH and LH, are responsible for the development and maintenance of secondary female sexual characteristics. They also lead to thickening of the **endometrium** each month in preparation for implantation of a zygote. In the embryo, they stimulate development of the female reproductive tract. Estrogens are secreted by the ovarian follicles and the **corpus luteum**.

Progesterone

Progesterone is secreted in response to LH stimulation from the anterior pituitary. It is released from the corpus luteum (the remnant follicle on the ovary surface) and is responsible for the development and maintenance (but not generation) of the endometrium. By the end of the first trimester of a pregnancy, progesterone is supplied by the placenta and the corpus luteum ceases functioning.

The Menstrual Cycle

Each month after the onset of puberty and until menopause, the endometrial lining will grow and shed in a cyclical manner. This is known as the **menstrual cycle**. It is controlled by the relative levels of estrogen and progesterone. The menstrual cycle may be divided into four phases: the **follicular phase**, **ovulation**, the **luteal phase**, and **menstruation**. As we describe each phase, we should look at Figure 12.7 to see how the hormone levels change.

Follicular Phase

The follicular phase begins when the **menstrual flow**, which sheds the uterine lining of the previous cycle, stops. GnRH secretion from the hypothalamus increases in response to the lower levels of estrogen and progesterone, whose concentrations fall off toward the end of each cycle. The higher concentrations of GnRH cause increased secretions of both FSH and LH. These two hormones work in concert to develop several ovarian follicles. The follicles begin to produce estrogen primarily, which at this point has a negative feedback effect and causes the GnRH, LH, and FSH concentrations to level off. Estrogen works to regrow the endometrial lining, stimulating vascularization and glandularization of the **decidua**.

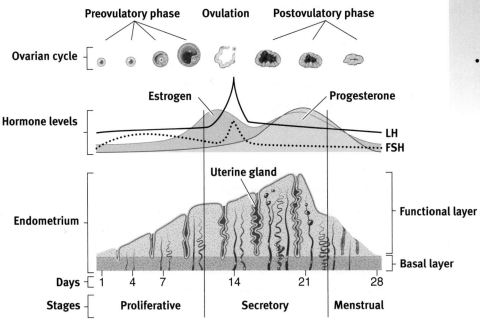

Figure 12.7

Ovulation

Estrogen is interesting in that it can have both negative and positive feedback effects. Late in the follicular phase, the developing follicles secrete more and more estrogen. Eventually, estrogen concentrations reach a level that paradoxically results in positive feedback, and GnRH, LH, and FSH levels spike. The **surge** in LH is important; it induces **ovulation**, the release of the ovum from the ovary into the abdominal cavity.

Luteal Phase

After ovulation, LH causes the ruptured follicle to form the corpus luteum. The corpus luteum secretes progesterone. From above, we know that although estrogen helps regenerate the uterine lining, it is progesterone that maintains it for implantation. Progesterone levels now begin to rise, while estrogen levels remain high. The very high levels of estrogen and progesterone cause negative feedback on GnRH, FSH, and LH. What is the purpose? To prevent the development of multiple ova in the same cycle; after all, we don't want to put all our eggs in one basket (*ba da bum!*).

Menstruation

If implantation does not occur, human chorionic gonadotropin (hCG, an LH analog; see Chapter 4) will not be made. Without hCG to stimulate the corpus luteum, progesterone levels decline and the uterine lining is sloughed off. The loss of high levels of estrogen and progesterone remove the block on GnRH so that the next cycle can begin.

Pregnancy

If fertilization has occurred, the corpus luteum will be maintained by the presence of hCG, which is secreted by the blastocyst, and the developing placenta. During the first trimester of development, it is the estrogen and progesterone secreted by the corpus luteum that keep the uterine lining in place. By the second trimester, hCG levels decline but progesterone and estrogen rise since they are now secreted by the placenta itself. The high levels of estrogen and progesterone serve as negative feedback mechanisms and prevent further GnRH secretion.

Menopause

Menopause, which usually occurs between the ages of 45 and 55, results from decreased responsiveness of the ovaries to FSH and LH. Fewer follicles will begin to develop each month, and some may fail to rupture. The decreased response to FSH and LH results in decreased levels of estrogen and progesterone. FSH and LH lose their feedback inhibition, so their plasma concentrations are usually increased in postmenopausal women. Many women report flushing, hot flashes, bloating, headaches, and irritability during menopause, as a result of these fluctuating hormone concentrations.

PINEAL GLAND

The pineal gland is located deep within the brain, where it secretes the hormone **melatonin**. The actual function of this hormone is unclear, although it is hypothesized that it may be involved in **circadian rhythms**. The evidence for this is projection of visual information from the eyes to this area of the brain, but the pineal gland is not directly involved in vision.

OTHER ENDOCRINE GLANDS

A brief mention of a few remaining organs with endocrine functionality will put us in good stead for Test Day. In the gastrointestinal tract, glandular tissue can be found in both the stomach and intestine. Many gastrointestinal peptides have been identified, and important ones include secretin, gastrin, and cholecystokinin (see Chapter 7). As we might expect for an organ system whose primary goal is to take food and break it down into its constituent components, the stimulation for release of most of these peptides is food intake.

In Chapter 11, we described the kidney's role in water balance. The renin–angiotensin–aldosterone system was mentioned as a way to increase salt and water reabsorption. The kidney also produces **erythropoietin**, which stimulates bone marrow to increase production of erythrocytes. It is secreted in response to low oxygen levels in the blood.

Two final organs that display endocrine function are the heart and the thymus. The heart releases **atrial natriuretic peptide (ANP)** to help regulate salt and water balance. The thymus, located directly behind the breastbone, releases **thymosin**, which is important for proper T-cell development and differentiation (Chapter 10). The thymus atrophies by adulthood. A full list of hormones and their actions can be found at the end of the chapter in Table 12.1

Mechanisms of Hormone Action ★★★★★★

Although we have described a number of hormones and their actions, we have not actually described the mechanism by which they effect those actions. Hormones are classified into three major groups: **peptide hormones**, **steroid hormones**, or **amino acid–derived hormones**. These distinctions are based on their chemical structure.

PEPTIDES

Peptide hormones are made up of amino acids. They range in size from quite small (ADH) to relatively large (insulin). They are all derived from larger precursor polypeptides that are cleaved by post-translational modifications (see Chapter 14). These smaller units will be transported to the Golgi, which, we know from Chapter 1, is the site of modification. These modifications activate the hormone and direct it to the correct location in the cell. Such hormones are released by exocytosis after having been packaged into vesicles.

Peptide hormones are charged, so they cannot cross the phospholipid cell membrane and instead bind to receptors on the exterior cell surface. They act as **first messengers**. Upon binding to their receptors, they stimulate the production of **second messengers**, such as cyclic AMP (cAMP). This conversion is catalyzed by the enzyme **adenylate cyclase**. cAMP can then bind to intracellular targets such as proteins or DNA to exert the hormone's ultimate effect. The connection between the hormone at the surface and the effect brought about by cAMP within the cell is known as a **signaling cascade**. At each step, there is the possibility of **amplification**. One hormone molecule may bind to multiple receptor molecules before it is degraded. Each receptor may activate several adenylate cyclases, each of which will make much cAMP. Thus, there is more signal after each step. The actions of cAMP are terminated by **phosphodiesterase**.

The effects of peptide hormones are usually shorter-lived, because they work through transient second messenger systems. It is quicker to turn them on and off, compared with steroid hormones, but their effects do not last without relatively constant stimulation.

STEROIDS

HOW ESTROGEN ACTS IN CELLS

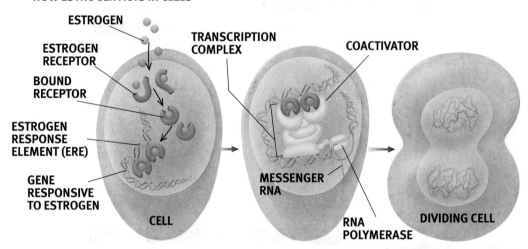

1. Estrogen binds to its receptor, which then binds to certain genes
2. A transcription complex forms and activates gene transcription
3. Cell behavior changes

Figure 12.8

As we have pointed out many times already, all steroid hormones (e.g., aldosterone, estrogen) are derived from cholesterol. Since they are derived from a nonpolar molecule, steroid hormones can easily cross the cell membrane. In fact, their receptors are usually intracellular or intranuclear. Upon binding to the receptor, they dimerize (pair up with another receptor–hormone complex). This dimer can then bind directly to DNA and alter its transcription (see Chapter 14), either increasing or decreasing transcription depending on the hormone and gene in question. The effects of steroid hormones are longer lived, as they alter the amount of mRNA and protein present in a cell; however, it takes longer to see the effect of steroid hormones, as the processes of transcription and translation are not immediate.

AMINO ACID DERIVATIVES

These hormones are less common than peptide and steroid hormones, but include some of the most important compounds that we mentioned in this chapter, including epinephrine, norepinephrine, and thyroxine. They are derived from one or two amino acids, usually with a few additional modifications. For example, thyroid hormone is made from tyrosine and includes the addition of several iodine atoms. Depending on the polarity of the molecule, they may either work through second messenger systems the way peptide hormones do (epinephrine falls in this category), or they may actually enter the cell and act like steroid hormones (thyroxine).

Table 12.1 Principal Hormones in Humans

Hormone	Source	Action
Growth hormone	Anterior pituitary	Stimulates bone and muscle growth
Prolactin	Anterior pituitary	Stimulates milk production and secretion
Adrenocorticotropic hormone (ACTH)	Anterior pituitary	Stimulates the adrenal cortex to synthesize and secrete glucocorticoids
Thyroid-stimulating hormone (TSH)	Anterior pituitary	Stimulates the thyroid to produce thyroid hormones
Luteinizing hormone (LH)	Anterior pituitary	Stimulates ovulation in females; testosterone synthesis in males
Follicle-stimulating hormone (FSH)	Anterior pituitary	Stimulates follicle maturation in females; spermatogenesis in males
Oxytocin	Hypothalamus; stored in posterior pituitary	Stimulates uterine contractions during labor, and milk secretion during lactation
Vasopressin (ADH)	Hypothalamus; stored in posterior pituitary	Stimulates water reabsorption in kidneys
Thyroid hormone	Thyroid	Stimulates metabolic activity
Calcitonin	Thyroid	Decreases the blood calcium level
Parathyroid hormone	Parathyroid	Increases the blood calcium level
Glucocorticoids	Adrenal cortex	Increase blood glucose level and decreases protein synthesis
Mineralocorticoids	Adrenal cortex	Increase water reabsorption in the kidneys
Epinephrine and Norepinephrine	Adrenal medulla	Increase blood glucose level and heart rate
Glucagon	Pancreas	Stimulates conversion of glycogen to glucose in the liver; increases blood glucose
Insulin	Pancreas	Lowers blood glucose and increases storage of glycogen
Somatostatin	Pancreas	Suppresses secretion of glucagon and insulin
Testosterone	Testis	Maintains male secondary sexual characteristics
Estrogen	Ovary/placenta	Maintains female secondary sexual characteristics
Progesterone	Ovary/placenta	Promotes growth/maintenance of endometrium
Melatonin	Pineal	Unclear in humans
Atrial natriuretic hormone	Heart	Involved in osmoregulation
Thymosin	Thymus	Stimulates T lymphocyte development

Conclusion

Our chapter contains a bevy of useful information. We have nearly completed our study of the organ systems; only the nervous system remains. The endocrine system is unique in that it is not a single organ or housed in a single location. Hormones that are made in a variety of localities can have wide-reaching effects throughout the entire organism. We need to be familiar with several points about each hormone for Test Day: name, effect, regulated by and regulator of, and chemical precursor. Table 12.1 should be our guide. The endocrine system allows for integration and execution of the homeostatic parameters that we saw in the previous chapter. For example, we learned that calcium is maintained within a narrow concentration range in the plasma by the antagonistic actions of calcitonin and parathyroid hormone. To do this, these hormones affected absorption, excretion, and bone remodeling. Vitamin D even became important when we discussed parathyroid hormone. The takeaway message for each of these hormones is that, although they have specific effects (e.g., decreasing blood glucose for insulin), they lead to manipulations that change the steady state of the whole organism. As we turn to the nervous system, we will also see how higher-level control can lead to system-wide coordination.

CONCEPTS TO REMEMBER

- ☐ The endocrine system is made up of organs throughout the body. They are defined by their ability to exert action at a distance.

- ☐ Hormones will be ineffective at sites where their receptors are absent.

- ☐ The hypothalamus is the master control gland. It directs the release of hormones from the anterior pituitary

- ☐ The anterior pituitary's hormones may be classified as direct (prolactin, endorphins, and growth hormone) or tropic (FSH, LH, ACTH, and TSH). Direct hormones exert their effects immediately, whereas the binding of tropic hormones to their receptors causes the release of another hormone (e.g., cortisol is released from the adrenal cortex by ACTH stimulation).

- ☐ The adrenal medulla makes epinephrine and norepinephrine, which are responsible for mediating the flight-or-fight sympathetic response (e.g., increased heart rate, greater blood flow to skeletal muscle).

- ☐ Parathyroid hormone and calcitonin are antagonistic hormones that control blood calcium levels. The former is secreted by the parathyroid glands, whereas the thyroid makes calcitonin. They alter absorption, excretion, and mobilization of calcium from bone.

- ☐ Insulin and glucagon are antagonistic hormones secreted by the islets of Langerhans that control blood glucose concentration.

- ☐ Estrogen exhibits both positive and negative feedback during the menstrual cycle.

- ☐ The presence of hCG maintains the corpus luteum, which is necessary for progesterone production during the first trimester.

- ☐ Hormones fall into one of three structural classes: steroid hormones (derived from cholesterol), peptide hormones (made up of amino acids), or amino acid derivatives (constituted of one or two amino acids with modifications).

Practice Questions

1. Which of the following associations between the hormone and its classification is FALSE?

   A. Cortisol—glucocorticoid
   B. Aldosterone—mineralcorticoid
   C. ADH—mineralcorticoid
   D. Androgens—cortical sex hormones

2. Which of the following hormones directly stimulates its target organ?

   A. ACTH
   B. TSH   *Thyroid stimulating hormone.*
   C. LH
   D. GH

3. Increased activity of the parathyroid gland leads to

   A. an increase in blood Ca^{2+} concentration.
   B. a decrease in the rate of bone resorption.
   C. a decrease in metabolic rate.
   D. a decrease in blood glucose levels.

4. Which of the following statements concerning growth hormone is NOT true?

   A. Overproduction of growth hormone in adults results in acromegaly.
   B. It promotes growth of bone and muscle.
   C. It is secreted by the hypothalamus. *(ant pituitary)*
   D. A deficiency in growth hormone results in dwarfism.

5. At which two points of the menstrual cycle are the levels of estrogen highest?

   A. Immediately before and after ovulation
   B. At ovulation and during the menstrual flow
   C. During the menstrual flow and pregnancy
   D. During pregnancy and after menopause

6. Iodine deficiency may result in

   A. acromegaly.
   B. cretinism.
   C. gigantism.
   D. hyperthyroidism.

7. Which of the following would NOT be seen during pregnancy?

   A. High levels of HCG in the first trimester
   B. High levels of estrogen and progesterone throughout the pregnancy
   C. Low levels of FSH in the first trimester
   D. High levels of GnRH throughout the pregnancy

8. Which of the following associations between the hormone and its role is FALSE?

   A. Estrogen—development of secondary sexual characteristics
   B. Progesterone—development and maintenance of endometrial walls
   C. LH—stimulate ovulation
   D. FSH—maturation of the ovarian follicles into the corpus luteum

9. Which of the following hormones is NOT derived from cholesterol?

   A. Aldosterone
   B. Testosterone
   C. Oxytocin
   D. Progesterone

10. Which of the following is TRUE regarding pancreatic somatostatin?

   A. Its secretion is increased by low blood glucose.
   B. It is always inhibitory.
   C. It is regulated by cortisol levels.
   D. It stimulates insulin and glucagon secretion.

11. Destruction of all beta cells in the pancreas would cause

   A. glucagon secretion to stop and a decrease in blood glucose.
   B. glucagon secretion to stop and an increase in blood glucose.
   C. insulin secretion to stop and an increase in blood glucose.
   D. insulin secretion to stop and a decrease in blood glucose.

12. Which of the following associations regarding aldosterone regulation is FALSE?

   A. Renin converts the plasma protein angiotensinogen to angiotensin I.
   B. Angiotensin I is converted to angiotensin II.
   C. Angiotensin II stimulates the adrenal cortex to secrete aldosterone.
   D. An increase in water reabsorption stimulates renin production.

13. A scientist discovers a new hormone that is relatively large in size and that triggers the conversion of ATP to cAMP. Which of the following best describes the type of hormone that was just discovered?

   A. Amino acid–derived hormone
   B. Peptide hormone
   C. Steroid hormone
   D. Tropic hormone

14. A patient presents to your office with muscle weakness, slowness in movement, and calcium deposits on his bones. A blood test reveals very low calcium levels in the blood. What is one treatment option for your patient?

   A. Increase calcitonin levels
   B. Increase PTH levels
   C. Increase mineralcorticoid levels
   D. Increase growth hormone levels

15. Oxytocin and vasopressin are

   A. produced and released by the hypothalamus.
   B. produced and released by the pituitary.
   C. produced by the hypothalamus and released by the pituitary.
   D. produced by the pituitary and released by the hypothalamus.

16. If the thymus gland is taken out in a three-year-old child, what problems will the child experience later in life?

   A. He will be prone to bacterial infections.
   B. He will be prone to viral and fungal infections.
   C. He will have dwarfism.
   D. He will have gigantism.

Small Group Questions

1. Many physiological parameters, such as blood Ca^{2+} concentration and glucose levels, are controlled by two hormones that have opposite effects. What is the advantage of achieving regulation in this manner instead of by using a single hormone that changes the parameters in one direction only?

2. At first glance, the signaling systems that involve cell surface receptors may appear rather complex and indirect, with their use of G proteins, second messengers, and often multiple stages of enzymes. What are the advantages of such seemingly complex response systems?

3. Discuss the sources and actions of parathyroid hormone and calcitonin in humans and describe the feedback mechanisms that control their release.

4. Suppose that two different organs, such as the liver and heart, are sensitive to a particular hormone. The cells in both organs have identical receptors for the hormone, and hormone-receptor binding produces the same intracellular second messenger in both organs. However, the hormone produces different effects in the two organs. Explain how this can occur.

5. The placenta secretes high levels of estradiol and progesterone during pregnancy. What would be the expected effect of these high hormone levels in the absence of pregnancy?

Explanations to Practice Questions

1. C

Let's take a look at each choice and eliminate the ones that correctly associate the hormone and its classification. Cortisol, along with cortisone, is a glucocorticoid secreted by the adrenal cortex. Aldosterone is a mineralcorticoid also secreted by the adrenal cortex. ADH, however, is not secreted by the adrenal cortex, but rather by the posterior pituitary, where it is stored after being synthesized by the hypothalamus. (C) is therefore the correct answer. Furthermore, ADH is a peptide hormone, not a steroid. For the sake of completion, we can confirm that androgens are cortical sex hormones also secreted by the adrenal cortex.

2. D

A hormone that directly stimulates its target organ is referred to as a direct hormone. Glancing at the answer choices, we notice that all of the hormones are secreted by the anterior pituitary gland. The direct hormones secreted by the anterior pituitary are growth hormone (GH), prolactin, and endorphins. From the given choices, only growth hormone is a direct hormone, which means that (D) is the correct answer. All of the other choices denote tropic hormones.

3. A

The parathyroid glands secrete parathyroid hormone (PTH), a hormone whose function is to increase blood calcium levels. An increase in activity of the parathyroid glands would lead to an increase in PTH levels, and therefore an increase in blood calcium levels (achieved mainly through an increase in the rate of bone resorption). (A) is thus the correct answer.

4. C

Growth hormone is a direct hormone secreted by the anterior pituitary. Among its many functions, the most important is the promotion of growth in bone and muscle.

An overproduction of growth hormone in children results in gigantism, whereas in adults it results in acromegaly (enlargement of the extremities of the face, such as the nose and ears). On the other hand, a deficiency of growth hormone results in dwarfism. From the answer choices, the only statement that is false is (C).

5. A

Estrogen levels increase right before ovulation, leading to a surge in LH, which stimulates the release of an egg (ovulation). Later, when the follicle develops into the corpus luteum, the levels of estrogen (and progesterone) increase to prepare for a possible pregnancy. The levels of estrogen are also high during pregnancy, when the placenta secretes high levels of estrogen and progesterone. (A) is therefore the correct answer.

6. B

Inflammation of the thyroid or iodine deficiency causes hypothyroidism in which the thyroid hormones are under-secreted or not secreted at all. Hypothyroidism in newborn infants is called cretinism, and is characterized by mental retardation, short stature, and coarse facial features. (B) is therefore the correct answer.

7. D

During the first trimester of pregnancy, the corpus luteum is preserved by human chorionic gonadotropin (HCG); hence, progesterone and estrogen secretion by the corpus luteum are maintained during the first trimester. During the second trimester, HCG levels decline but progesterone and estrogen levels rise, since they are now secreted by the placenta itself. High levels of progesterone and estrogen inhibit GnRH secretion, thus preventing FSH and LH secretion and the onset of a new menstrual cycle. From the given choices, the correct answer is (D).

8. D

Since we are looking for a false association, we have to analyze each choice and eliminate the ones containing correct definitions of their respective hormones. Estrogen contributes to the development of secondary sexual characteristics, so (A) can be eliminated. The same applies to (B), since it is true that progesterone contributes to the development and maintenance of endometrial walls. (C) is also true, because LH stimulates ovulation in females. (D), on the other hand, is a false statement. FSH does stimulate the maturation of ovarian follicles. However, it is LH, not FSH, which stimulates the development of the corpus luteum from an ovarian follicle. (D) is therefore the correct answer.

9. C

Steroid hormones are derived from cholesterol. This characteristic makes them lipophillic and allows them to diffuse freely across cell membranes. Among them, we can find glucocorticoids (cortisol and cortisone), mineralcorticoids (aldosterone), and cortical sex hormones (androgens). Androgens include estrogen, progesterone, and testosterone. Thus, the only hormone from the given choices that is not derived from cholesterol is oxytocin, which is a peptide hormone. (C) is therefore the correct answer.

10. B

Let's quickly refresh our knowledge of somatostatin. Pancreatic somatostatin secretion is increased by high blood glucose or amino acid levels, leading to both decreased insulin and glucagon secretion. Somatostatin is also regulated by the levels of cholecystokinin (CCK) and growth hormone (GH). Somatostatin is always inhibitory regardless of where it acts. Based on this, (B) is the correct answer.

11. C

Our task in answering this question is twofold: we have first to determine what beta cells in the pancreas produce, and second, what would be the effect of stopping this hormone from being secreted. Because of the nature of the answer choices, we can eliminate half of them immediately: a cessation in glucagon secretion would lead to a decrease in

blood glucose, whereas preventing insulin secretion would result in an increase in blood glucose. As such, we know for sure that (B) and (D) are incorrect. The beta cells in the pancreas produce and secrete insulin, as opposed to the alpha cells, which produce and secrete glucagon. Therefore, destruction of all beta cells in the pancreas would cause insulin secretion to stop, resulting in an increase in blood glucose levels. This is what occurs in type I diabetes. (C) is therefore the correct answer.

12. D

Let's begin with a quick review of aldosterone regulation, which is controlled by the renin-angiotensin system. When blood volume falls, the juxtaglomerular cells of the kidney produce rennin, an enzyme that converts the plasma protein angiotensinogen to angiotensin I. Angiotensin I is then converted to angiotensin II by an enzyme in the lungs; angiotensin II ultimately stimulates the adrenal cortex to secrete aldosterone. Aldosterone helps to restore blood volume by increasing sodium reabsorption at the kidney, leading to an increase in water reabsorption. This removes the initial stimulus for renin production. Thus, (A), (B), and (C) correctly describe the renin-angiotensin system. (D) is false because it implies that there is a positive feedback rather than a negative feedback mechanism between the increase in water reabsorption and renin production. As such, (D) is the correct answer.

13. B

We know from the question stem that the newly discovered hormone functions as a first messenger, converting ATP to cAMP, which functions as a second messenger, triggering a signaling cascade in the cell. Hormones that act via secondary messengers and are relatively large in size (short peptides or complex polypeptides) are peptide hormones, as (B) indicates.

14. B

The question stem is basically telling us that the patient has too much calcitonin in his blood, as indicated by the low levels of calcium, the muscle weakness and slowness in movement, and the calcium deposits on his bones. The best way to treat this problem is by increasing the PTH levels in his blood. PTH raises blood calcium levels by stimulating calcium release from bone and decreasing calcium excretion in the kidneys. (B) is therefore the correct answer.

15. C

Let's quickly review what we know about oxytocin and vasopressin. Oxytocin is produced by the hypothalamus and stored in the posterior pituitary; its primary function is to stimulate uterine contractions during labor and milk secretion during lactation. Vasopressin, also referred to as ADH, is made in the hypothalamus and stored in the posterior pituitary; its function is to increase water reabsorption in the kidneys. The only choice that correctly describes this is (C), the correct answer.

16. B

This question is asking us to determine the role of the thymus in a three-year-old child. The thymus gland secretes hormones such as thymosin during childhood. Thymosin stimulates T lymphocyte development and differentiation. The thymus atrophies by adulthood, after the immune system has fully developed. As such, removing the thymus gland in a child would leave him with undeveloped and undifferentiated T cells, which would make him prone to viral and fungal infections. This condition could be lethal. (B) is therefore the correct answer.

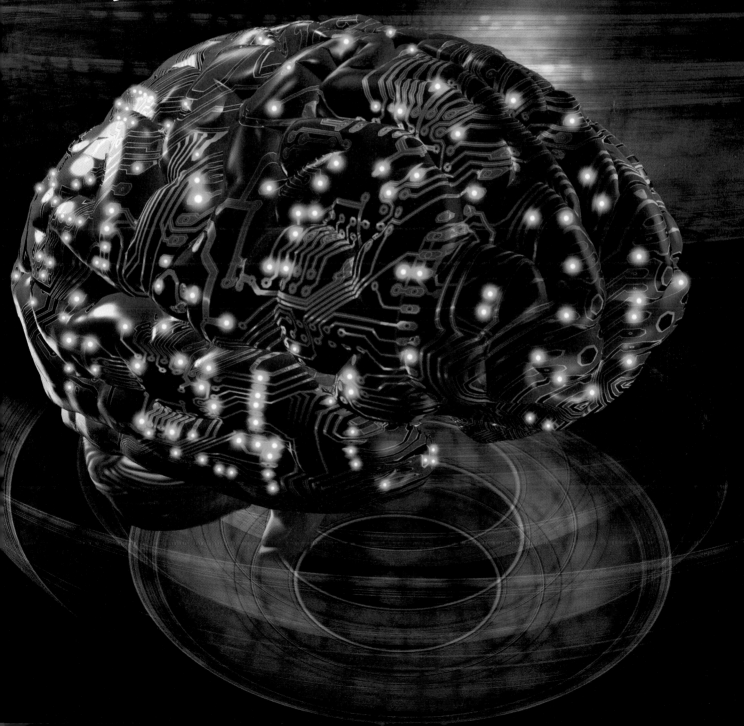

13

The Nervous System

You may have heard the one about the frog that allowed itself to be boiled to death. The story goes that a frog will immediately jump out of a pot of already boiling water, but will remain motionless if placed into cool water that is then heated to a boil very slowly. It's as if the frog's neurological system—its temperature and pain receptors—were unable to detect the increasing heat and the frog was completely unaware of the increasingly dangerous and ultimately deadly situation. Although the story has its origins in academic discussions of physiology published in the late 19th century (particularly one report of an experiment performed at Johns Hopkins University in 1882, in which a frog was boiled to death by raising the temperature by 0.12°C per minute) the supposed phenomenon has little scientific value today. We assure you that no National Institutes of Health–funded laboratories are slowly boiling frogs or other amphibians to their death (at least not for this particular objective). Rather, the story has taken on an almost allegorical significance, warning against everything from the slow encroachment of the police state or of communism, to moral relativism and the slow descent of all civilization toward its ultimate destruction.

Let's not worry, for the moment at least, whether we are being sufficiently vigilant to prevent ourselves from being slowly boiled to death in a pot of political or moral evil. Let's focus on what those 19th-century scientists were investigating: namely, the nervous system of the frog. Although we were not there in the lab working and observing alongside these scientists, we might imagine the questions they were asking and attempting to answer. *How does an organism sense its environment? What of its environment can an organism sense? How do organisms respond to the environment once they sense it? What are the thresholds for response?* And so on. These are fundamental questions about the nervous system, and, more than 100 years since these experiments, we are still asking them. We certainly have learned much about the nervous system, its anatomical and functional divisions, the nature of the action potential, and the system's central importance for the coordination of nearly every other organ system, but there is much, much more that we do not know. It has become something of a cliché to say that the brain is the final frontier of human exploration and discovery. And yet, in a real sense, this is true.

The nervous system regulates the overall response of an organism to its environment. The human brain alone contains 100 billion neurons and 10 trillion synaptic connections: all of this in a three-pound organ protected by the skull. The nervous system is responsible for the integration of all the sensory information we receive each day—from recognizing the sound of the honking taxi driver to knowing the taste of pistachio ice cream, to feeling the chill of the wind on our face. In addition, the nervous system is responsible for the control of all the muscular movement we described in Chapter 6 and glandular secretions, such as saliva (which is why your mouth becomes dry when you are nervous). In organisms such as humans, it is also capable of higher-level thinking and planning future goals. Its activities are coordinated through electrical and chemical messages. It truly is an amazing system. Let's get our synapses firing as we begin to probe carefully through the nervous system.

Neurons

STRUCTURE

Each neuron is specially designed to carry out its function. There are a variety of different types of neurons in the body, but they all share some features with which we should be familiar on Test Day. Let's take a look at Figure 13.1, which illustrates a prototypical neuron.

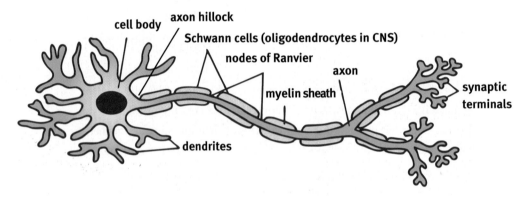

Figure 13.1

Starting on the left side of our diagram, we have the cell body. In the nervous system, we give this part of the cell a specialized name (**soma**). The nucleus, endoplasmic reticulum, and ribosomes that we discussed in Chapter 1 are all located within the soma. As we move away from the cell body, we see many processes. The majority of these are **dendrites**. Dendrites are structures made to receive information. They transmit this information to the cell body, where it is integrated at the **axon hillock**, the enlargement at the beginning of the axon. We will see the importance of the axon hillock in action potential generation in a few pages. The axon hillock provides a connection between the cell body and the **axon**, which is a nerve fiber that is specialized to carry an electrical message. Most mammalian neurons are insulated by myelin; this is to prevent signal loss. We see the same concept in the power cords on our appliances; in addition to preventing us from electrocuting ourselves, the cord wrapping prevents the electricity running in the wires from escaping. The myelin has the added benefit of increasing the speed of conduction in axons. Myelin is produced by **oligodendrocytes** in the central nervous system and **Schwann cells** in the periphery. If we look closely at our diagram, we notice small breaks in the myelin sheath at regular intervals along the axon membrane. These exposed areas of axon membrane are termed **nodes of Ranvier** and are critical to proper signal conduction, as we will soon see. Finally, as we reach the end of the axon, we come to the **nerve terminal** (**synaptic bouton**). This structure is enlarged and flattened to maximize neurotransmission to the next neuron and ensure proper production of neurotransmitter. Neurons are not physically connected to one another; rather, there is a slight space between two neurons. This space is known as the **synaptic cleft**, or simply, the **synapse**. Neurotransmitter released from the axon terminal traverses the synaptic cleft and binds to receptors on the second neuron. CEOs are much like neurons. They take in information from many sources (dendrites) and then integrate it together (axon hillock). Then, they carefully present a coordinated message (action potential traveling down the axon) that results in additional reports (neurotransmitters) distributed to division heads, directors, managers, and so on (muscles and glands), who are responsible for carrying out the company initiatives.

Real World

Sometimes the body mounts an immune response against its own myelin, leading to the destruction of this insulating substance (demyelination). Because myelin speeds the conduction of impulses along a neuron, the absence of myelin results in the slowing of information transfer. A common demyelinating disorder is multiple sclerosis (MS). In MS, the myelin of the brain and spinal cord is selectively targeted. Because so many different kinds of neurons are demyelinated, MS patients are riddled with a variety of symptoms such as weakness, lack of balance, vision problems, and incontinence.

[HOW IT WORKS]

MYELIN FORMATION

Long axons insulated with myelin carry signals between neurons faster than unmyelinated axons. Oligodendrocyte cells manufacture the fatty membrane and wrap the axon with 10 to 150 layers. Different factors can stimulate the myelination process; often astrocyte cells "listen in" on the signals traveling along axons and relay chemical messages to the oligodendrocytes. Below, a microscope shows axons in red being wrapped.

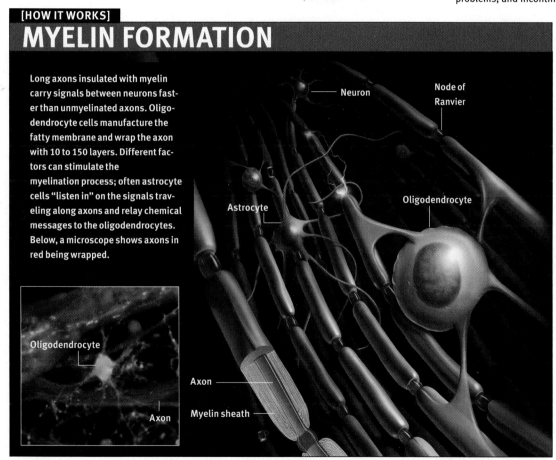

Figure 13.2

FUNCTION

Now that we have the basic anatomy of the neuron, we can discuss the physiology that underlies neuronal signaling. Neurons use all-or-nothing messages called

action potentials to relay information to and from the central and peripheral nervous systems. This might include transmitting to our brain the words we are reading in the sentence, as well as sending the information to the areas of our central nervous system that process language. Action potentials cause the release of neurotransmitter into the synaptic cleft. Let's see how they work.

Resting Potential

All neurons exhibit a **resting membrane potential**. If we recall our electricity definitions, this means that there is a potential (voltage) difference between the inside of the neuron and the extracellular space. Usually, this is about –70 mV (the inside of the neuron is negative relative to the outside). We should think about how this gradient is set up. Certainly, if the system were left to its own devices, it would want to equilibrate to 0 mV. Neurons use selective permeability to ions and the **Na^+/K^+ ATPase** to maintain a negative internal environment.

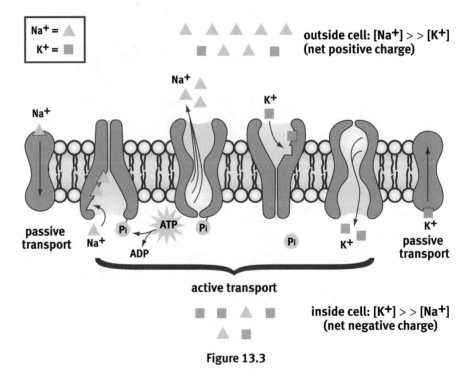

Figure 13.3

The neuron is like any other cell. It has a plasma membrane that is fairly impermeable to charged species. Remember that ions are unlikely to cross the non-polar barrier, because it is energetically unfavorable. Inside of the neuron, $[K^+]$ is high and $[Na^+]$ is low. Outside of the neuron, $[Na^+]$ is high whereas $[K^+]$ is low. The negative resting potential is generated by both negatively charged proteins within the cell and the relatively greater permeability of the membrane to K^+ compared with Na^+. If K^+ is more permeable and its concentration is higher inside, it will diffuse down its gradient out of the cell. What does this mean in terms of charge movement? K^+ is positively charged, so its movement out of the cell results in a cell interior that is negative. Put another way, if we assume that the membrane starts at zero, and we take away a positive one $(0 - +1)$, we end up with a negative one on the inside of the cell. Na^+ cannot readily enter at rest, so the negative potential is maintained. We can see that the gradients and selective permeability we learned about in Chapter 1 have proven their importance in yet another organ system.

The Na^+/K^+ ATPase is important for restoring this gradient after action potentials have been fired. They transport three Na^+ out of the cell for every two K^+ into the cell at the expense of one ATP. Why is ATP necessary? Both Na^+ and K^+ are moved against their gradients by this process; thus, they qualify as active transport. Each time the pump works, it results in the inside of the cell becoming relatively more negative, as two positive charges are moved in for every three that are moved out.

Action Potential Initiation

When we learned about muscular contraction in Chapter 6, we said that it occurred in an all-or-none fashion. Either the fiber completely responded or not at all. We alluded to the fact that this response was ultimately due to the function of the neuron, upon whose action muscle contraction depends. Because action potentials work in an all-or-none fashion, so, too, must muscles.

If we continue with the analogy of the CEO, we can understand that not all the information that she receives will be positive. Some may be negative, and she must determine, based on all the information, what the appropriate response for the company is. Similarly, neurons can receive excitatory and inhibitory input. The former type of input makes them more likely to fire an action potential, whereas the latter makes them less likely. As the information is integrated at the axon hillock, **depolarization** or **hyperpolarization** may occur. Inhibitory inputs cause hyperpolarization by making the cell more negative. Depolarization is caused by excitatory inputs and makes the cell less negative (relatively, more positive). If the axon hillock is depolarized to the **threshold value** (usually in the range of -55 to -40 mV), an action potential will be triggered.

The decision to initiate an action potential has been made, but how is it executed? Ion channels in the membrane open in response to the depolarization. Since they respond to voltage, they are known as **voltage-gated ion channels**. There are two types that are responsible for action potentials: Na^+ voltage-gated channels and K^+ voltage-gated channels. They are both present in each of the places we are about to discuss, but their activation is different.

Bridge

Remember that the Na^+/K^+ ATPase isn't present only in neurons. We saw it earlier in red blood cells as a way to control cell tonicity. The Na^+/K^+ ATPase is able to make both an osmotic and electrogenic contribution to the cell.

Key Concept

Na^+ wants to go into the cell because it is more negative inside (electrical gradient) and because there is less Na^+ inside (chemical gradient).

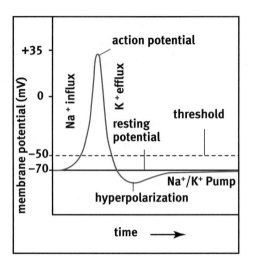

Figure 13.4

First, the Na⁺ channels respond to the depolarization. Where was the concentration of Na⁺ higher? Outside. In addition, the inside of the cell is negative. Thus, there is a strong **electric** and **chemical (electrochemical) gradient** for sodium to move into the cell. This makes the cell potential become positive as a result of the sodium ion influx. Sodium channels then rapidly close when the membrane potential reaches about +35 mV. We now have a cell that is positive in the region where the channels just opened and closed. Take a look at Part 1 of Figure 13.5 to see this. The bracketed area is where sodium channels have opened. We can see that the cell is now positive on the inside.

The positive potential inside the cell is the trigger for the voltage-gated potassium channels to open. If we examine the area of the cell in question now (same part of Figure 13.5 as before), we see that it is positive inside. We also know that potassium is high inside the cell. Just like there was for sodium, there is now an electrical and chemical drive to move potassium. The only difference is that potassium will be driven out of the cell. The movement of positive charges out of the cell will result in restoration of the negative membrane potential. This process is known as **repolarization**. Often, the efflux of K⁺ will cause an overshoot of the resting membrane potential and the membrane becomes more negative than that resting potential. We apply the term *hyperpolarization* to this situation.

Similar to what we observed in muscles, neurons exhibit **refractory periods**. During the **absolute** refractory period, no amount of stimulation will cause another action potential to occur. During the **relative** refractory period, there must be greater than normal stimulation to cause an action potential because the membrane is starting from a potential more negative than the resting value.

Impulse Propagation

All of the ion movements that we just discussed occurred only at the axon hillock. For a signal to be conveyed to another neuron, the action potential must travel down the axon and initiate neurotransmitter release. We term this movement **impulse propagation**. As the sodium from the axon hillock rushes in, it will cause depolarization in the regions surrounding it. This depolarization will result in the opening of sodium channels along the axon in a wavelike fashion. The depolarization of the membrane to +35 mV causes the sodium channels to slam shut just as the potassium channels begin to open. After the sodium depolarization wave, the potassium channels will cause a repolarization wave that resets the axon for the next action potential. Let's take a look at Figure 13.5 to see this drawn out.

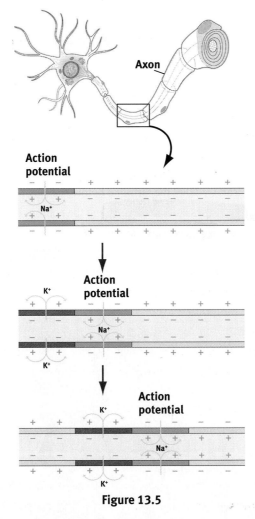

Figure 13.5

In Part 1, we can see that sodium influx has led to depolarization of the bracketed area. In Part 2, the sodium has caused the opening of neighboring voltage-gated sodium channels, causing depolarization there. Meanwhile, the first set of sodium channels has closed, and the potassium channels have opened, causing repolarization. The action potential is propagated by the ordered opening and closing of these channels.

Looking at Part 2 of Figure 13.5, we should consider why the action potential doesn't move backward (back up the axon). It is because that region of the axon is refractory immediately after it has fired an action potential. The functional consequence of this is the one-way flow of information in neuronal axons.

The speed at which action potentials move depends on the length and cross-sectional area of the axon: the longer the axon, the higher the resistance and the slower the conduction. The greater effect, though, is based on the diameter of the axon. Greater diameters allow for faster propagation as they decrease resistance. Certainly there is a tradeoff for this, and mammalian organisms have developed myelin to cope with it. Myelin is an extraordinarily good insulator, preventing the loss of the electric signal. The insulation is so good that the membrane is only permeable to ion movement at the nodes of Ranvier. Thus, the signal hops from node to node. Transmission that occurs in this manner is referred to as **saltatory conduction** (from the Latin for *to jump*).

Synapse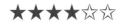

Our CEO is effective only if she has a company to run; our neuron is only useful if it has other cells to coordinate. The connection between two neurons is called a **synapse**. To make this clear, we label the terminal before the synapse (the neuron using its axon) the **presynaptic terminal** or **neuron**, and the neuron receiving information through its dendrites the **postsynaptic terminal**. If a neuron signals to a gland or muscle, as we saw in Chapter 6, that cell is termed an **effector cell**. Most synapses are **chemical** in nature; they use small molecules referred to as **neurotransmitters** to send messages from one cell to the next.

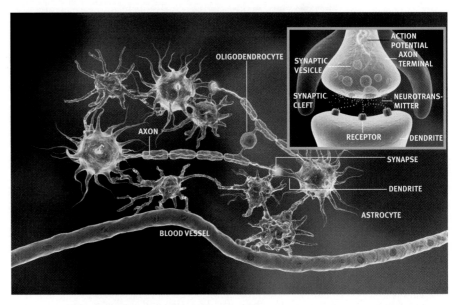

Figure 13.6

Neurons are like Boy Scouts: always prepared. At the nerve terminal, neurotransmitter is stored in membrane-bound vesicles. These vesicles wait for an action potential to come down the axon and depolarize the terminal membrane. They will then fuse with the presynaptic terminal and release the neurotransmitter into the synaptic cleft. This is an example of exocytosis, discussed in Chapter 1. Neurotransmitter release is calcium-dependent.

Once released into the synapse, the neurotransmitter molecules will diffuse across the cleft and bind to receptors on the postsynaptic membrane. This allows the message to be passed from one neuron to the next. As we stated earlier, neurons may be either inhibitory or excitatory; this distinction truly comes at the level of the neurotransmitter, when binding will result in either hyperpolarization or depolarization of the postsynaptic cell.

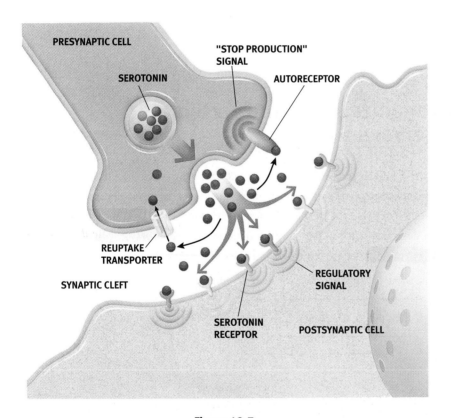

Figure 13.7

We don't want neurotransmission to continue indefinitely, so there must be a way to remove neurotransmitters from the synaptic cleft. In fact, there are several mechanisms, depending on the type of neurotransmitter involved. Some are broken down by enzymatic reactions (e.g., the action of acetylcholinesterase on acetylcholine, see Figure 13.8), some use **reuptake carriers** to be recycled into the presynaptic neuron (e.g., dopamine or serotonin as seen in Figure 13.7), and others may simply diffuse out of the area (e.g., nitric oxide).

Key Concept

It is critical to understand the difference between electrical and chemical transmission, and that neurons use both. Within a neuron, electricity is used to pass messages in an all-or-nothing fashion. Between neurons, chemical molecules are used to pass messages in a modulated manner that depends on how much neurotransmitter is released.

Real World

Many common drugs (either in clinical use or street drugs) modify processes that occur in the synapse. For instance, cocaine acts by blocking neuronal reuptake carriers, thus prolonging the action of neurotransmitters in the synapse by preventing neurotransmitter reentry into the nerve terminal. There are clinically useful drugs (e.g., used to treat glaucoma) that inhibit acetylcholinesterase, thereby elevating synaptic levels of acetylcholine. Nerve gases are extremely potent acetylcholinesterase inhibitors, which have been used in war and in recent terrorist activities. Nerve gas causes rapid death by preventing the action of skeletal muscle (most importantly, the diaphragm)—leading to respiratory arrest.

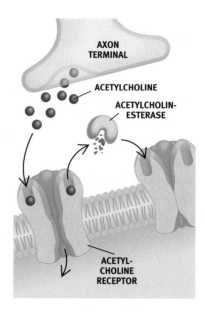

Figure 13.8

Organization of the Vertebrate Nervous System

★★★★☆

For the MCAT, we want to be able to describe the types of cells that make up the nervous system, as well as their interconnections. Neurons that carry information from the periphery to the brain or spinal cord are termed **afferent neurons**, whereas the cells that work in the opposite direction are **efferent neurons**. There are also **interneurons** that are only involved in local circuits. We will see examples of these in the next few pages, when we discuss reflex arcs.

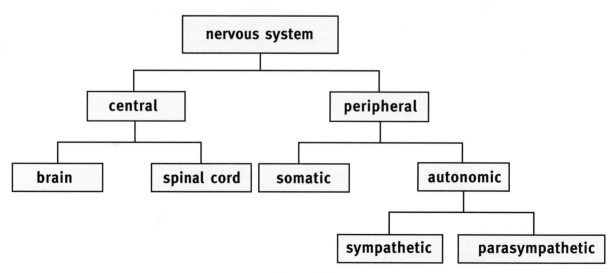

Figure 13.9

A single axon can carry only so much information, so the nervous system bundles many axons together into **nerves.** These nerves may be **sensory, motor,** or **mixed.** These terms refer to the type of information they carry. Mixed nerves carry both sensory and motor information. Much as the axons travel together, neuron cell bodies (somas) will also cluster. In the **peripheral nervous system**, these collections are known as **ganglia.** In the **central nervous system**, they are called **nuclei.** If we take a look at Figure 13.9, we can see the major divisions of the nervous system. The primary division is between the central (brain and spinal cord) and peripheral (all other structures) nervous systems. We will look at each system in turn.

CENTRAL NERVOUS SYSTEM

There are only two components to the central nervous system (CNS): the **brain** and the **spinal cord**.

Brain

The consistency of brain tissue is similar to that of gelatin. Since it is so delicate and vital for life, the brain is armored by the protective skull. It is responsible for integration of sensory information, coordination of motor movement, and cognition. The myelination that we saw around axons is also present in the brain. Its presence allows us to distinguish between **gray matter**, which is unmyelinated, and **white matter**, which is. We can divide the brain into the **forebrain**, the **midbrain**, and the **hindbrain**.

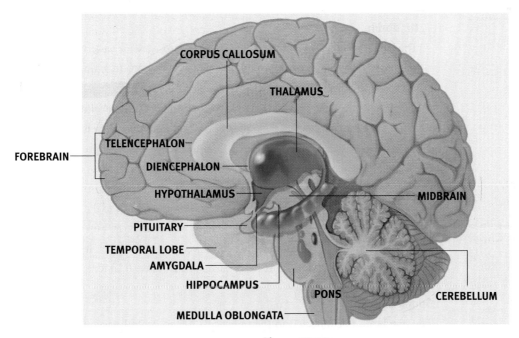

Figure 13.10

Forebrain

The forebrain is the most recently acquired part of the CNS in terms of evolutionary development. It is further broken down into the **telencephalon** and **diencephalon**. We can recognize the telencephalon from pictures of the brain. It consists of the left and right hemisphere. Each hemisphere can be further sectioned into the **frontal**, **parietal**, **occipital**, and **temporal** lobes. A large portion of the telencephalon is the **cerebral cortex**, a region of highly convoluted gray matter that can be seen on the surface of the brain. The cortex is responsible for the highest level functioning in the nervous system, including creative thought and future planning. It also integrates sensory information and controls movement. Each hemisphere is independent; however, they do communicate through a large connection called the **corpus collosum**.

Nestled below and inside the telencephalon is the diencephalon. It consists of the thalamus and hypothalamus. We thoroughly discussed the hypothalamus in the previous chapter in relation to the endocrine system. The thalamus is the St. Louis of the nervous system; it functions as the gateway to the brain. All ascending sensory information is passed through the thalamus before being relayed to the cortex.

Midbrain

The midbrain serves as a relay point between more peripheral structures and the forebrain. It passes sensory and visual information to the forebrain, while receiving motor instructions from the forebrain and passing them to the hindbrain.

Hindbrain

The hindbrain contains structures that are seen across a wide variety of organisms and are responsible for many of the involuntary functions (e.g., respiration) that we have previously discussed. It is made up of the **cerebellum**, **pons**, and **medulla**, which together are referred to as the brainstem. The cerebellum is a quality control agent. It checks that the motor signal sent from the cortex is in agreement with the sensory information coming from the body. It is what prevents us from falling over when we trip on a sidewalk curb. It rapidly realizes that the motor signal to take a step was not successfully carried out, as we tripped. Instead of letting us fall on our faces, the cerebellum helps the cortex to adjust to the new situation so that we catch ourselves, preventing scrapes and bruises, as well as embarrassment! The medulla is the most highly conserved part of the brain. It is responsible for modulating ventilation rate, heart rate, and gastrointestinal tone.

Spinal Cord

The hindbrain is connected to the other half of the central nervous system, the spinal cord. The spinal cord can be divided into four sections. From the base of the skull to the coccyx, the divisions are **cervical**, **thoracic**, **lumbar**, and **sacral**. Almost all of the structures below the neck receive sensory and motor innervation from the spinal cord. It is protected by the **vertebral column**, which, as it sounds, is a series of bones (vertebrae) that form a hollow column. The spinal cord runs through this column with nerves entering and exiting at each vertebra. In addition to integrating and distributing nerve signals for the brain, the spinal cord can participate in simple reflex arcs of its own. Like the brain, we can see both gray and white matter in the spinal cord cross-section. The gray matter is deep to the white matter. As before, the white matter contains axons. In the spinal cord, these are the axons of motor and sensory neurons. The sensory neurons bring information in from the periphery and enter on the dorsal (back) side of the spinal cord. The cell bodies of these sensory neurons are found in the **dorsal root ganglia**. Motor neurons exit the spinal cord ventrally.

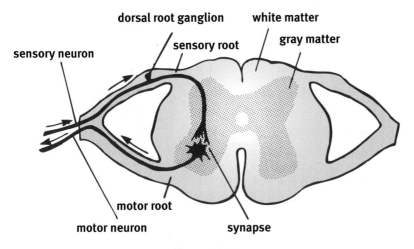

Figure 13.11

PERIPHERAL NERVOUS SYSTEM

Glancing back at Figure 13.9, we can see that the peripheral nervous system has a few more components, including 12 pairs of cranial nerves and 31 pairs of spinal nerves. We can divide peripheral innervation between the **somatic** (SNS) and **autonomic** nervous system (ANS). We have previously mentioned both of these divisions in relation to the musculoskeletal system.

Somatic Nervous System

The SNS is responsible for voluntary movement. We described the interface between the neuron and muscle as the neuromuscular junction. Release of acetylcholine from the nerve terminal onto the muscle leads to contraction (Chapter 6). The acetylcholine binding to its receptor on the muscle ultimately leads to muscle depolarization. The SNS is also responsible for providing us with reflexes, which are automatic. They do not require input or integration from the brain to function. There are two types of reflex arcs: **monosynaptic** and **polysynaptic**. Reflexes usually serve a protective purpose. For example, we'd pull our hand away from a hot stove before our brain processes that it is hot.

Monosynaptic

In a monosynaptic reflex arc, there is a single synapse between the sensory neuron that received the information and the motor neuron that responds. A classic example is the **knee-jerk** reflex (see Figure 13.12). When the patellar tendon is stretched, information travels up the sensory neuron to the spinal cord, where it interfaces with the motor neuron to contract the quadriceps muscle. The net result is a straightening of the leg, which lessens the tension on the patellar tendon. We should notice that the reflex is responding to a potentially dangerous situation. If the patellar tendon is stretched too far, it may tear, damaging the knee joint. This reflex helps to protect us.

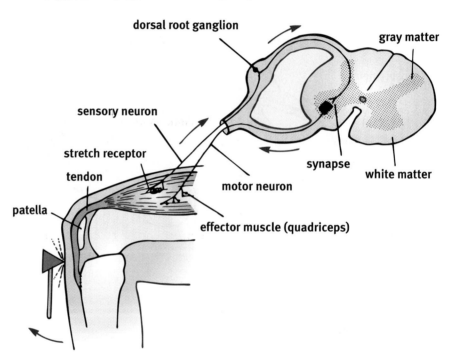

Figure 13.12

Polysynaptic

In a polysynaptic reflex arc, there is at least one interneuron between the sensory and motor neuron. A real-life example is your reaction to stepping on a tack, which involves the **withdrawal reflex.** The foot that steps on the tack will be stimulated to jerk up; this is a monosynaptic reflex. However, if we are to maintain our balance, we need our other foot to go down and plant itself on the ground. For this to occur, the motor neuron that controls the opposite (downward-moving) leg must be stimulated. Interneurons in the spinal cord provide the connection from the incoming sensory information on the leg being jerked up to the motor neuron for the supporting leg.

Autonomic Nervous System

We briefly mentioned the autonomic nervous system in several chapters, most recently in the endocrine chapter when we described the "fight-or-flight" and "rest-and-digest" responses. Let's now take a look at the physical underpinnings of this system. The ANS is sometimes referred to as the involuntary nervous system, as it requires no conscious control. From Chapter 6, we know that cardiac and smooth muscle are both innervated by the autonomic nervous system. Smooth muscle is found throughout the body, including the blood vessels, the bronchi, the bladder, and the gastrointestinal tract. It is no surprise to us, then, that the autonomic nervous system exerts great control over blood pressure, ventilation dynamics, urination, and digestion.

The primary difference between the SNS and ANS is that the ANS is a two-neuron system. A motor neuron in the SNS goes directly to the muscle without synapsing. In the ANS, the neurons play a game of telephone; two neurons work in series to transmit messages. The first neuron is known as the **preganglionic neuron**, whereas the second is the **postganglionic neuron**. The preganglionic neuron's soma is in the CNS, whereas its axon travels to a ganglion in the PNS. Here, it synapses on the cell body of the postganglionic neuron, which then affects the target tissue (because it can be glandular, too).

Although the ANS can regulate each organ individually, it can also have coordinated effects. These can be divided into **sympathetic** and **parasympathetic**.

Sympathetic Nervous System

This is the part of the ANS that is responsible for "fight-or-flight". If our bothersome bear from the previous chapters makes another surprise appearance, we would want to increase blood flow to the heart and skeletal muscle, while decreasing it to the GI tract and kidneys. In addition, increasing breathing rate and heart rate would ensure an adequate supply of oxygen to meet the demands of the rapidly contracting skeletal muscles. Finally, our pupils would dilate, so we could keep our eyes on that bear as we escaped. Preganglionic neurons use acetylcholine, whereas postganglionic neurons in the sympathetic nervous system use norepinephrine. Preganglionic sympathetic neurons can also cause the release of epinephrine from the adrenal medulla.

Parasympathetic Nervous System

The parasympathetic nervous system is the calm brother of the sympathetic nervous system. Once we get away from that bear, we can eat a nice pizza. We then would want increased blood flow to the organs of digestion and excretion with a concomitant decrease in flow to the skeletal muscle and heart. Moreover, since pizza eating is not a highly aerobic activity, heart rate and ventilation

Key Concept

The first neuron in the autonomic nervous system is called the preganglionic neuron and the second is the postganglionic neuron.

Mnemonic

The ANS controls many functions within the body, but think in big picture terms. Autonomic means *automatic*. If it is a body function we don't have to think about, it probably has at least some autonomic input. From there, we can decide whether it is sympathetic (flight-or-fight) or parasympathetic (rest-and-digest).

rate would decrease. The **vagus nerve**, which is one of the 12 cranial nerves, is responsible for many of the parasympathetic effects in the thoracic and abdominal cavities. The parasympathetic nervous system uses acetylcholine as a neurotransmitter at both preganglionic and postganglionic neurons.

Special Senses

We have divided our discussion of neurons into sensory and motor. Sensory neurons come in three varieties: **interoceptors**, **proprioceptors**, and **exteroceptors**. The word root in each of them clues you in to what they monitor. Interoceptors monitor internal environment parameters such as blood volume, blood pH, and partial pressure of CO_2 in the blood. Proprioceptors are important for our position sense. When we get up in the middle of the night to grab a cookie and glass of milk, proprioceptors help our brains grasp the relative position of our bodies in the dark. Exteroceptors are responsible for monitoring the external environment such as light, sound, touch, taste, pain, and temperature. Furthermore, **nociceptors** sense pain and relay that information to the brain.

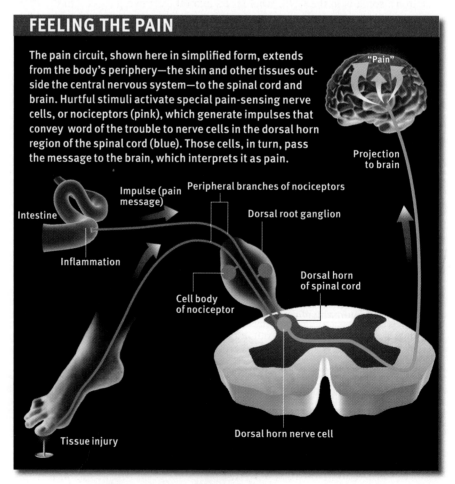

FEELING THE PAIN

The pain circuit, shown here in simplified form, extends from the body's periphery—the skin and other tissues outside the central nervous system—to the spinal cord and brain. Hurtful stimuli activate special pain-sensing nerve cells, or nociceptors (pink), which generate impulses that convey word of the trouble to nerve cells in the dorsal horn region of the spinal cord (blue). Those cells, in turn, pass the message to the brain, which interprets it as pain.

"Pain"

Projection to brain

Impulse (pain message)

Peripheral branches of nociceptors

Intestine

Dorsal root ganglion

Inflammation

Cell body of nociceptor

Dorsal horn of spinal cord

Tissue injury

Dorsal horn nerve cell

Figure 13.13

THE EYE

The eye is a specialized organ used to detect light (in the form of photons). Most of the exposed portion of the eye is covered by a thick layer known as the **sclera**. This is commonly known as the white of the eye and does not cover the cornea. The eye is supplied with nutrients and oxygen by the **choroid**, which is directly beneath the sclera. The innermost layer of the eye is the **retina**, which contains the actual cells (**photoreceptors**) that transduce the light into electrical information the brain can process.

Looking at our own eyes, we know that the sclera is not continuous around the eye. In the front, there are several structures that allow light to pass into the eye and onto the retina. Light first passes through the **cornea**, a transparent structure that bends and focuses it. Light rays then move through the **pupil**. The muscular, pigmented **iris** can adjust the amount of light entering the eye by altering the diameter of the pupil; the more light available, the greater the degree of constriction. After the pupil, the light is passed through the **lens**, which does the final focusing. **Ciliary muscles** can adjust the thickness of the lens, which focuses the image on the retina. Once light has been focused by these three structures, it will impinge on the photoreceptors of the retina and be turned into an electrical signal.

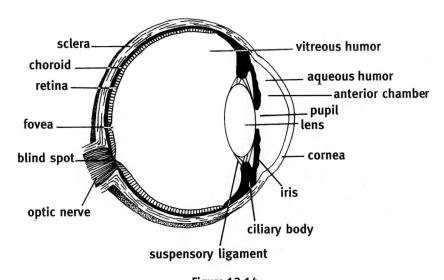

Figure 13.14

There are two main types of photoreceptors: **rods** and **cones**. Rods are responsible for transmission of black-and-white images, and respond to low-intensity illumination. This makes them useful for night vision. Cones come in three varieties and manage color images. Each type of cone contains a pigment that absorbs a different wavelength of light; these wavelengths correspond to the colors red, green, and blue. Rods have only one pigment, **rhodopsin**, which explains their ability to respond only to black and white.

Real World

Color-blindness is a result of lacking one, two, or three of these sets of cones. Total color blindness is most commonly due to a complete lack of cones.

Real World

Some people develop a plumbing problem in the eye and cannot adequately drain aqueous humor. This disease is called glaucoma. Because of the draining problem, pressure builds in the anterior chamber and is transmitted to the vitreous humor, leading to increased pressure on the optic nerve. If the pressure is not relieved, this condition can permanently damage the optic nerve and lead to blindness.

After excitation by light, the photoreceptors send a signal to the **bipolar cells**, which relay the information to the **retinal ganglion cells**. The axons of the ganglion cells bundle to form the **optic nerve**, which then exits the back of the eye. Because the optic nerve takes up space on the back of the eye, displacing photoreceptors, there is a **blind spot** at the site of exodus. Since we have two eyes, this is rarely a problem, as each eye compensates for the blind spot of the other.

The eye is filled with fluid to simplify the transmission of light to the retina. Aqueous humor is secreted near the iris at the base of the eye. It then travels to the anterior chamber, where it will exit and eventually enter the venous blood.

THE EAR

The ear transduces sound waves (mechanical disturbances of pressure) into electrical signals that can be interpreted by the brain. In addition, it houses certain nerves that help coordinate balance.

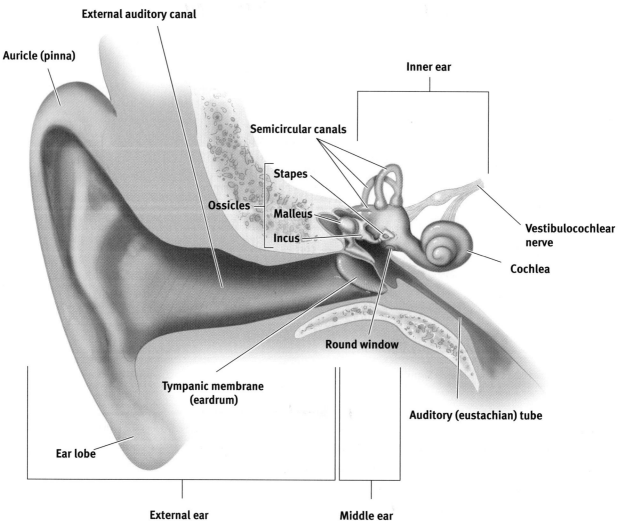

Figure 13.15

When listening to our favorite song on our MP3 players, quite a bit happens so that we hear the lyrics and the melody. The speaker generates longitudinal waves. The **outer ear**, which consists of the auricle and auditory canal, collects the waves and channels them to the **tympanic membrane**. The tympanic membrane is the beginning of the **middle ear**, which also includes the ossicles (**malleus, incus**, and **stapes**). The tympanic membrane vibrates due to sound waves pushing on it, and the ossicles move back and forth. These three bones then transmit the information through the **oval window** to the fluid-filled inner ear, which is made up of the **cochlea** and **semicircular canals**. The movement of the ossicles on the oval window creates fluid waves in the inner ear that depolarize the **hair cells** of the cochlea. This is the transduction mechanism that generates an electrical signal the nervous system can interpret. The action potentials from the hair cells travel along the **auditory nerve to the brain**.

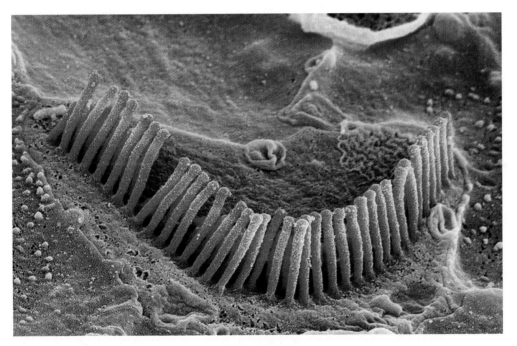

Figure 13.16

The semicircular canals are important for balance. There are three per ear, one oriented in each plane (think X-, Y-, and Z-axes). The canals are filled with a fluid called **endolymph**, whose movement through the canals puts pressure on the hair cells inside (see the hair cells in Figure 13.16). There is a canal in each dimension, so the brain can integrate the signal from each canal and maintain balance, as well as interpret sudden acceleration and deceleration.

THE CHEMICAL SENSES

Taste and smell are the two chemical senses, so named because they take chemical molecules from the environment and turn them into electrical signals. This is termed **olfaction** and **gustatation** for smell and taste, respectively.

Taste

Taste receptors, or taste buds, are located on the tongue, soft palate, and epiglottis. Taste buds are composed of approximately 40 epithelial cells. The outer surface of a taste bud contains a taste pore, from which microvilli, or taste hairs, protrude. The receptor surfaces for taste are on the taste hairs. Interwoven around the taste buds is a network of nerve fibers that they stimulate. These neurons transmit gustatory information to the brainstem via three cranial nerves. There are four kinds of taste sensations: sour, salty, sweet, and bitter. Although most taste buds will respond to all four stimuli, they respond preferentially, i.e., at a lower threshold, to one or two of them.

Smell

Olfactory receptors are found in the olfactory membrane, which lies in the upper part of the nostrils over a total area of about 5cm^2. The receptors are specialized neurons from which olfactory hairs, or cilia, project. These cilia form a dense mat in the upper nasal mucosa. When odorous substances enter the nasal cavity, they bind to receptors in the cilia, depolarizing the olfactory receptors. Axons from the olfactory receptors join to form the olfactory nerves. The olfactory nerves project directly to the olfactory bulbs in the base of the brain.

Conclusion

You should pat yourself on the back. All of the organ systems have been covered! Now let's examine that pat on the back. It required your sight to read the sentence instructing you to pat your back. The signal was then sent to the area of the brain that processes vision, which passed it off to the language centers. Once the meaning was understood, an impulse was sent along a motor neuron to cause your muscle to contract in such a way that you could actually pat yourself on the back. Then, sensory neurons told your brain that you had accomplished the action. Maybe you should get another pat on the back just for successfully going through all those connections! The nervous system is a highly integrated one; millions upon millions of cells allow for our appropriate interactions in the everyday world. If we dig even deeper to examine what else was going on during your back patting, we can understand that your

Real World

Have you ever gone into a room with a very strong smell that was hardly noticeable after a while? Olfactory receptors can be overpowered, and after constant stimulation will desensitize to a given stimulus. This desensitization is a hallmark of much of the nervous system.

heart was beating and your lungs were drawing air. Even as your nervous system directed some of its attention and energy to accomplishing a specific task (patting your back), it never lost sight of the big picture: whole-body coordination of every organ system to maintain life. Congratulate your autonomic nervous system for doing such an excellent job. Hopefully you haven't tired your brain out by learning how it works! Let's move on to a more microscopic topic: genetics.

CONCEPTS TO REMEMBER

☐ The basic unit of the nervous system is the neuron, a polarized, electrically excitable cell.

☐ The resting potential of a neuron is established as a result of the chemical gradients of sodium and potassium ions, as well as their relative permeabilities to the membrane.

☐ An action potential requires rapid sodium efflux followed by slower potassium influx. Voltage-gated ion channels are responsible for allowing the ions to cross the plasma membrane.

☐ Depolarization of the nerve terminal will cause an influx of calcium ions that leads to vesicle fusion and exocytosis of neurotransmitters.

☐ Neurotransmitter activity in the synaptic cleft may be terminated by degradation, reuptake, or diffusion out of the synapse.

☐ The central nervous system consists of the brain and spinal cord. The peripheral nervous system includes the 12 pairs of cranial nerves and 31 pairs of spinal nerves.

☐ Sensory information enters the spinal cord on the dorsal side, whereas motor signals leave from the ventral surface.

☐ The autonomic nervous system is responsible for involuntary actions, and the somatic nervous system is capable of carrying out voluntary movements.

☐ The autonomic nervous system may be further subdivided into two antagonists: the sympathetic and parasympathetic nervous system.

☐ The special senses (sight, hearing, smell, and taste) use special receptors to transmit the sensory information to the central nervous system.

Practice Questions

1. Resting membrane potential depends on

   A. the differential distribution of ions across the axon membrane.
   B. active transport.
   C. selective permeability.
   D. all of the above.

2. All of the following are associated with the myelin sheath EXCEPT

   A. faster conduction of nervous impulses.
   B. nodes of Ranvier forming gaps along the axon.
   C. increased energy output for nervous impulse conduction.
   D. saltatory conduction of action potentials.

3. The all-or-none law states that

   A. all hyperpolarizing stimuli will be carried to the axon terminal without a decrease in size.
   B. the size of the action potential is proportional to the size of the stimulus that produced it.
   C. increasing the intensity of the depolarization increases the size of the impulse.
   D. once an action potential is triggered, an impulse of a given magnitude and speed is produced.

4. Which of the following would NOT be observed in a patient with a cerebellar lesion?

   A. Memory impairment
   B. Inability to balance
   C. Inability to coordinate hand and eye movements
   D. Inability to time rapid movements

5. By increasing the intensity of the stimulus, the action potential will

   A. increase in amplitude.
   B. increase in frequency.
   C. increase in speed.
   D. both B and D.

6. Which of the following pairings is correct?

   A. Sensory nerves—afferent
   B. Motor nerves—afferent
   C. Sensory nerves—ventral
   D. Motor nerves—dorsal

7. When a sensory receptor receives a threshold stimulus, it will do all of the following EXCEPT

   A. become depolarized.
   B. transduce the stimulus to an action potential.
   C. inhibit the spread of the action potential to sensory neurons.
   D. cause the sensory neurons to send action potentials to the central nervous system.

8. Which of the following structures focuses light on the retina?

   A. Cornea
   B. Vitreous humor
   C. Lens
   D. Both A and C

9. A specific disease affects only the rods present in a patient's retina. Which of the following will you most likely observe about the patient?

A. He can no longer see colors.

B. He can see very well in the dark.

C. His levels of rhodopsin are almost nonexistent.

D. He cannot detect more than one wavelength of light.

10. When the potential across the axon membrane is more negative than the normal resting potential, the neuron is said to be in a state of

A. depolarization.

B. hyperpolarization.

C. repolarization.

D. hypopolarization.

11. Which of the following statements concerning the somatic division of the peripheral nervous system is INCORRECT?

A. Its pathways innervate skeletal muscles.

B. Its pathways are usually voluntary.

C. Some of its pathways are referred to as reflex arcs.

D. Its pathways always involve three neurons.

12. In the ear, what structure transduces pressure waves to action potentials?

A. Tympanic membrane

B. Organ of Corti

C. Oval window

D. Semicircular canals

Small Group Questions

1. Tetraethylammonium (TEA) is a drug that blocks voltage-gated K^+ channels. What effect would TEA have on the action potentials produced by a neuron? If TEA could be applied selectively to a presynaptic neuron that releases an excitatory neurotransmitter, how would it alter the synaptic effect of that neurotransmitter on the postsynaptic cell?

2. The nerve gas sarin inhibits the enzyme acetylcholinesterase, which is normally present in the neuromuscular junction and is required to break down acetylcholine. Based on this information, what are the likely effects of this nerve gas on muscle function?

Explanations to Practice Questions

1. D

The polarization of the neuron at rest is the result of an uneven distribution of ions between the inside and outside of the cell. This difference is achieved through the active pumping of ions in and out of the neuron (e.g., Na^+/K^+ pump) and the selective permeability of the membrane, which allows only certain ions to cross. As such, (D) is the correct answer.

2. C

Let's quickly review the role of myelin in the nervous system. Myelin is a white, lipid-containing material surrounding the axons of many neurons in the central and peripheral nervous systems. Myelin is produced by glial cells (oligodendrocytes in the central nervous system and Schwann cells in the peripheral nervous system) and is arranged on the axon discontinuously. The gaps between the segments of myelin are called nodes of Ranvier. Myelin increases the conduction velocity by insulating segments of the axon so that the membrane is permeable to ions only at the nodes of Ranvier. Because of these nodes, the action potential jumps from node to node, a process known as saltatory conduction. Going back to the question, we can now safely select (C) as the correct answer. Myelin sheaths do not increase the energy output of nervous impulse conduction; rather, they speed conduction.

3. D

The action potential is often described as an all-or-none response. This means that whenever the threshold membrane potential is reached, an action potential with a consistent size and duration is produced. Neuronal information is coded by the frequency and number of action potentials, not the size of the action potential. From the given answers, only (D) correctly describes the all-or-none response of a neuron.

4. A

A lesion in the cerebellum would affect some or all of its functions. A healthy cerebellum helps to modulate motor impulses initiated by the motor cortex, and is important in the maintenance of balance, hand–eye coordination, and the timing of rapid movements. Generally, alcohol affects the cerebellum, so an intoxicated person transiently exhibits signs typical of a cerebellar lesion. From the given choices, only (A) does not describe an effect that would be produced from an impaired cerebellum. The hippocampus is the brain structure involved in memory. (A) is therefore the correct answer.

5. B

Neuronal information is coded by the frequency and number of action potentials, not the size of the action potential. Thus, increasing the intensity of the stimulus will increase the frequency of the action potential. The nervous system distinguishes a gentle touch versus a needle poke, not by the magnitude of the action potential, but rather by its frequency. (B) is therefore the correct answer.

6. A

Glancing at the answer choices, we notice that all of them are dealing with sensory or motor neurons, so let's quickly review these two categories. Sensory neurons bring information from the outside (skin, eyes, ears, etc.) to the nervous system, and they are therefore called afferent neurons. Additionally, sensory neurons synapse in the dorsal spinal cord. Motor neurons, on the other hand, take information from the nervous system to effector organs (e.g., muscles), and are therefore efferent. Also, they synapse in the ventral spinal cord. Based on this, we can safely select (A) as the correct answer.

7. C

Let's quickly review what happens when a sensory receptor receives a threshold stimulus. Since the stimulus is strong enough, we can assume that the receptor becomes depolarized, allowing it to transduce the stimulus to an action potential. The action potential will then be carried by sensory neurons to the central nervous system. Therefore, from the given choices, the only incorrect statement is found in (C). If a receptor is stimulated, it will promote the spread of the action potential to sensory neurons.

8. D

Light is focused on the retina by the cornea and the lens. The lens in the eye is a converging (convex) lens. The cornea also acts as a converging lens. As such, both the cornea and the lens help to focus light on the retina. (D) is thus the correct answer.

9. C

The rods detect low-intensity illumination and are important in night vision. The rod pigment, rhodopsin, absorbs one wavelength. If a patient's rods were affected, we would expect him to have a really difficult time seeing anything in the dark and his levels of rhodopsin would drop sharply. The only choice that matches this prediction is (C), the correct answer.

10. B

When the potential across the axon membrane is more negative than the normal resting potential, the neuron is referred to as hyperpolarized. Hyperpolarization occurs right after an action potential and is caused by too much potassium exiting the neuron. (B) is therefore the correct answer.

11. D

The somatic division of the peripheral nervous system innervates skeletal muscles and is responsible for voluntary movement. Some of the pathways in this part of the nervous system are reflex arcs, which are reflexive responses to certain stimuli that involve only a sensory and a motor neuron. These neurons synapse in the spinal cord (they do not involve the brain). The pathways of the somatic division of the peripheral nervous system can involve two, three, or more neurons, depending on the type of signal. The correct answer therefore is (D).

12. B

The cochlea includes the organ of Corti, which contains specialized sensory cells called hair cells. Vibration of the ossicles exerts pressure on the fluid in the cochlea, stimulating the hair cells to transduce the pressure into action potentials, which travel via the auditory nerve to the brain for processing. (B) is therefore the correct answer.

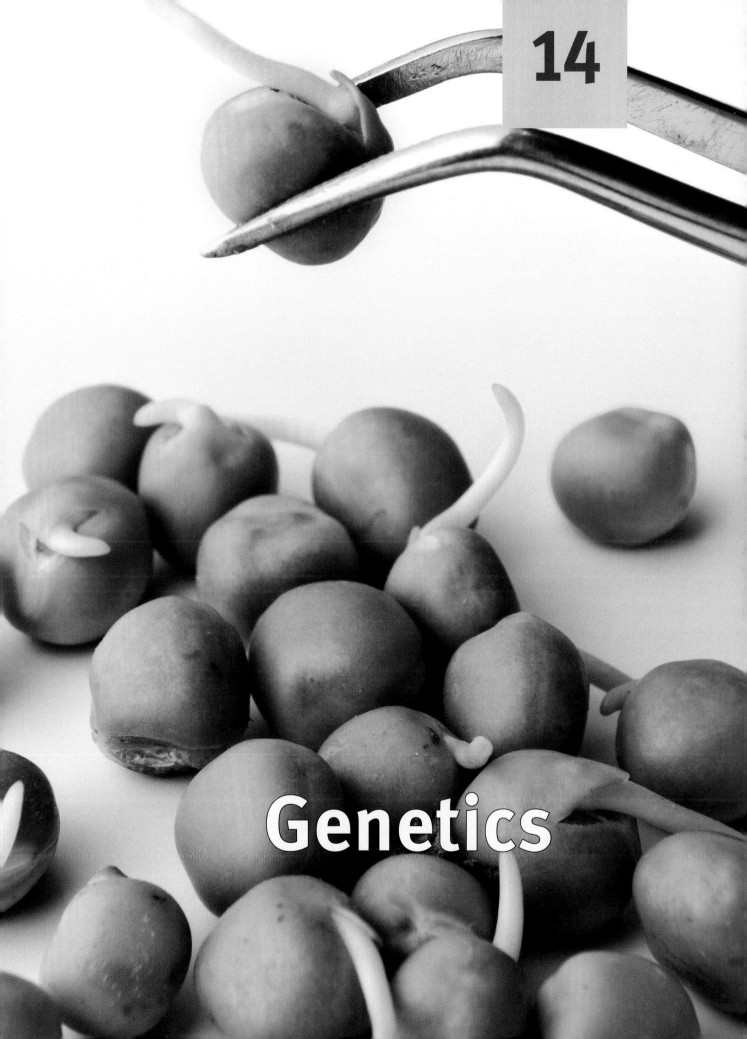

Genetics

There is a saying: *The family that prays together, stays together*, implying that families united through religious or spiritual activity will experience less familial conflict and strife. For hundreds of years, European royalty practiced a notion at once quite similar and radically different, which we might characterize as, *The family that breeds together, leads together*. European royal families, for generations, have practiced what is known as royal intermarriage. For purposes of establishing or continuing political alliances, maintaining bloodline purity, or smoothing out diplomatic relations, marriages between and within royal families were arranged, resulting in such an interweaving of bloodlines that eventually most European royalty was (is) genetically related.

Such marriage unions led to rather severe restrictions on the gene pool—all the alleles represented in the royal family line(s). Offspring of parents who were also related to each other through blood lineage came to have greater similarities in their genotypes, and certain alleles became so frequent that their phenotypic expression became almost a hallmark of royal descent. For example, the House of Habsburg was perhaps the most infamous for its inbreeding practices and members of this royal family bore the unmistakable mark of their restricted genes through a jaw malformation that even came to be known as the Habsburg lip. Medically termed *prognathism* (Greek for *forward jaw*), the condition is a misalignment of the upper and lower jaws (the maxilla and mandible, respectively). The Habsburg family portraits present individuals with prominent, forward-thrusting lower jaws and chins, characteristic of mandibular prognathism. The genetic condition has more than just aesthetic implications; it can lead to serious disfigurement and disability. Charles II of Spain suffered from the worst case of the Hapsburg lip on record; his lower jaw protruded so much further out than his upper jaw that he was not able to chew his food.

Every physical characteristic of every living organism (and virus) is determined by a set of codes called genes. **Genes** are the heritable traits that can be passed on from one generation to the next. Coded for by DNA (the focus of our next chapter), they are organized onto **chromosomes**. We know from the ABO and Rh blood antigen system (Chapter 9) that there may be alternative forms of a gene. These different forms are known as **alleles**. Two final terms we should be familiar with are **genotype** and **phenotype**. Genotype is the actual allelic distribution of genes in an organism; phenotype is the outward appearance of an organism and depends on the genotype. How this control occurs will be a central theme of this chapter.

Mendelian Genetics ★★★★☆

A monk named Gregor Mendel developed several of the tenets of genetics in the 1860s based on his work with pea plants. By crossing only **true-breeding** plants

MCAT Expertise

The MCAT commonly tests the difference between genotype and phenotype. If we are given the genotype of an organism, we should be able to predict the phenotype. However, if we are given the phenotype, we cannot always predict the genotype because of the presence of dominant and recessive alleles.

(those whose offspring only ever have the same traits as the parents) with different traits, he was able to determine the laws of inheritance.

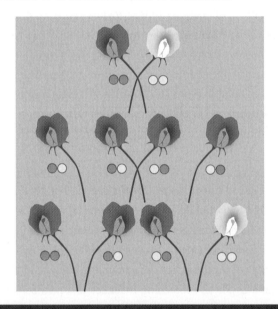

Seeking Variation

MENDEL'S FACTORS: Early 20th-century scientists rediscovered the ideas of Gregor Mendel, who experimented with pea plants during the 1850s and 1860s to derive detailed laws of inheritance. Mendel posited the existence of discrete factors carrying trait information and observed that each individual would carry two copies—one from each parent—of a given factor. Although both were present, only one of the copies would dominate and produce the visible trait.

Figure 14.1

MENDEL'S FIRST LAW: LAW OF SEGREGATION

There are four basic tenets to Mendel's first law.

- Genes exist in alternative forms (alleles).
- An organism has two alleles for each gene, one inherited from each parent.
- The two alleles segregate during meiosis, resulting in gametes that carry only one allele for any inherited trait.
- If two alleles in an individual organism are different, only one will be fully expressed, and the other will be silent. The expressed allele is said to be **dominant**, and the silent allele, **recessive**.

In genetics problems, including those on the MCAT, dominant traits are assigned capital letters and recessive alleles are denoted by lowercase letters. If both copies of the allele are the same, that individual is said to be **homozygous.** If they are different, the individual is **heterozygous** for that trait.

Monohybrid Cross

A cross in which only one trait is being studied is said to be **monohybrid** (*mono–* means *one*). Gregor Mendel used pea plants with either purple or white flowers. The **Parent** or **P generation** refers to the individuals being crossed; the offspring are the **Filial** or **F generation**. The F distinction can be applied to multiple generations by using numeric subscripts. If we think of our grandparents as the P generation, then our parents are F_1, and we are F_2.

In Mendel's experiments, the purple flowers were determined to be homozygous dominant. This genotype can be designated as PP. The white flowers were homozygous recessive; their genotype would be written pp. When crossed, the genotype of the F_1 generation will be 100% Pp; we will show this graphically in a moment. What does this mean in terms of the color (phenotype) of our F_1 flowers? They will all be purple, because purple is dominant to white.

Punnett Square

For the MCAT, we will want to be able to draw and analyze a Punnett square, which is a diagram that predicts the relative genotypic and phenotypic frequencies that will result from a crossing of two individuals. The alleles of the two parents are arranged on the top and side of the square, with the genotypes of the progeny being represented at the intersection of these alleles (see Figure 14.2). The genotypes of the progeny will be the sum of the parental alleles.

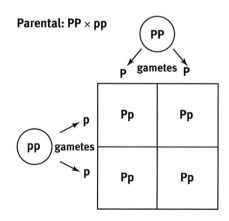

Parental: PP × pp

F$_1$ genotypes: 100% Pp (heterozygous)

F$_1$ phenotypes: 100% purple flowers

Figure 14.2

If the F_1 generation crosses with itself (**self-cross**); the resulting offspring (F_2 generation) will be more phenotypically and genotypically diverse than their parents. First, note that the F_1 generation in Figure 14.2 is 100% Pp; all the flowers are purple heterozygotes. Now, if we take two of these individuals and cross them, we will get the Punnett square shown in Figure 14.3. The genotypic percentages will be 25% PP, 50% Pp, and 25% pp. Phenotypically, we get a 3:1 distribution, because both the homozygous dominant and heterozygous dominant will result in a purple flowering plant. We should clearly notice that, unlike the F_1 generation, in which the phenotype and genotype had the same percentages (100% percent), in the F_2 generation, there is a 1:2:1 distribution (homozygous dominant: heterozygous dominant: homozygous recessive) genotypically and a 3:1 distribution (purple: white) phenotypically. These ratios are, of course, theoretical and will not always hold true. They represent the probabilities of certain outcomes but not with complete certainty. Usually, the more offspring a couple has, the closer their phenotypes will be to the expected ratios.

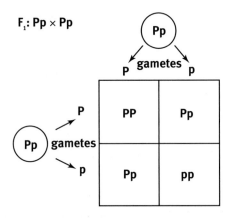

F$_2$ genotypes: 1:2:1; 1PP: 2Pp:1pp

F$_2$ phenotypes: 3:1; 3 purple:1 white

Figure 14.3

These ratios are standard Mendelian inheritance patterns that we should be familiar with for Test Day. Knowing them will save us time, translating into more questions and more points.

Test Cross

Monohybrid crosses are useful but they aren't quite as interesting if we already know what the outcome should be, as we did above. After all, it's more exciting to be the detective on a case than to be a simple fact checker. **Test crosses** allow us to be intrepid explorers. They are used to determine unknown genotypes. Let's take a look at Figure 14.4, and then discuss how it works.

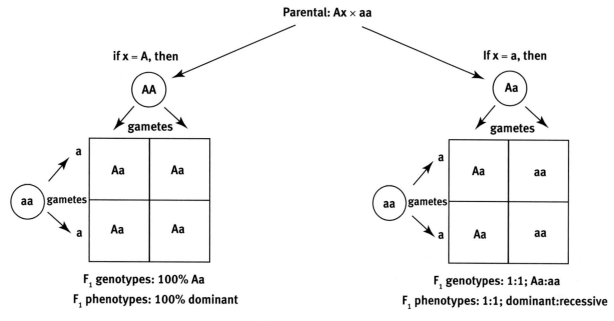

Parental: Ax × aa

if x = A, then

AA

gametes

aa gametes

	a	a
a	Aa	Aa
a	Aa	Aa

F₁ genotypes: 100% Aa
F₁ phenotypes: 100% dominant

If x = a, then

Aa

gametes

aa gametes

	a	a
a	Aa	aa
a	Aa	aa

F_1 genotypes: 1:1; Aa:aa
F_1 phenotypes: 1:1; dominant:recessive

Figure 14.4

A fact that helps us with test crosses (and will help us on Test Day) is that only with a recessive phenotype (e.g., white flower) can we be sure of the genotype (pp). We cannot be sure if a dominant phenotype is heterozygous or homozygous, since both result in the same outcome. We can determine the phenotype (and be good detectives) by crossing the unknown plant with a plant that has the recessive phenotype. If all the offspring (100%) are of the dominant phenotype, we would predict that the unknown parent is homozygous dominant for the trait (PP). If, instead, we get roughly a 1:1 distribution (50% purple and 50% white), we would expect that the unknown parent is heterozygous dominant (Pp). Since we are determining the genotype of the parent based on its offspring, test crosses are sometimes called **back crosses**. This makes sense, as we are working *back*ward.

MENDEL'S SECOND LAW: LAW OF INDEPENDENT ASSORTMENT

Dihybrid Cross

We can extend what we just learned to a situation in which we examine the inheritance of two genes using a **dihybrid cross** (*di–* means *two*). Mendel's **law of independent assortment** is named; simply, it means that each gene's inheritance (assortment) is independent of (unrelated to) the inheritance of other genes.

Suppose you buy detergent so that you can do your laundry during your MCAT study session (multitasking is important!). While standing at the checkout line, you also decide to buy gum. The two purchases are entirely independent of each other. Buying detergent does not make you more or less likely to buy gum.

Key Concept

Can we think of why we wouldn't use a homozygous dominant organism for the test cross? It is because we wouldn't be able to tell the genotype of the test animal. Phenotypically, all of the offspring would be the same, because they would have at least one dominant allele from the homozygous dominant parent. Using a recessive individual allows us to work backward and determine genotype from phenotype (which isn't always possible).

We might say that these two purchasing decisions are unlinked. For genes that are **unlinked**, we can stick with Mendel and independent assortment. On the other hand, we will soon see cases in which genes are **linked** and the inheritance of one *does* affect the other.

Take a quick glance at Figure 14.5 before we walk through the details. The next few paragraphs will explain how the statistics for the genotypes and phenotypes are derived. We want to have these sorts of numbers memorized on Test Day to save us time.

Parental: **TTPP × ttpp**

F_1 genotypes: **100% TtPp**

(self-cross) $F_1 × F_1$: **TtPp × TtPp**

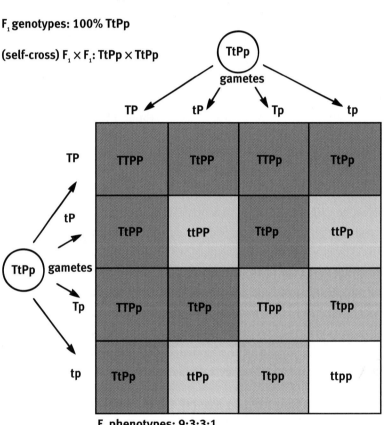

F_2 phenotypes: **9:3:3:1**

9 tall purple:3 tall white:3 dwarf purple:1 dwarf white

Figure 14.5

From Mendel's example, we will add another trait besides flower color: height. Recall from the monohybrid cross that purple was dominant to white. Similarly, the tall phenotype (T) is dominant to the dwarf one (t). As a quick check of our skills, what would the genotype of a short, white flowering plant be? ttpp. Remember that to generate the F_1 progeny, we crossed two true breeding plants. Here, this would be one tall, purple plant (TTPP) and one dwarf, white plant (ttpp). Similar to what we saw with the monohybrid cross, all of the offspring will be the same: heterozygous tall, heterozygous purple plants (TtPp). The genotypes and phenotypes are both 100% for a certain plant type. Now we can have some fun. We can take the heterozygous progeny and cross them again. This is what we see in Figure 14.5. The result will be plants that distribute in a 9:3:3:1 phenotypic ratio (nine tall, purple/three tall, white/three dwarf, purple/one dwarf, white), which is typical for a Mendelian dihybrid cross.

Statistical Analyses

Recall gametes from Chapter 5. Each pea plant in the F_1 generation is capable of producing four possible gametes, because the genes are independent of one another. The four gametes are **TP**, **Tp**, **tP**, and **tp**. We can calculate the given likelihood of a genotype in the progeny by multiplying the likelihood that one parent donated a specific gamete by the likelihood that the other parent donated a specific gamete. We multiply them because we are looking for the probability that *both* alleles will be incorporated.

If we wanted to generate a homozygous tall, homozygous purple plant (TTPP), we would need a TP from each parent. The likelihood of this is $\frac{1}{4}$ in each case. Multiplying these together, we get $\frac{1}{16}\left(\frac{1}{4}\times\frac{1}{4}\right)$. What does this mean to us? That 1 pea plant out of 16 will have this genotype (and the corresponding phenotype).

Let's look at a more interesting case. Say that we wanted to get a heterozygous purple, heterozygous tall plant. We could cross TP × tp, Tp × tP, tP × Tp, or tp × TP. Each of these would result in our desired genotype. We need to do the multiplication for each case. Every time, the likelihood of each gamete being selected is still $\frac{1}{4}$. We then multiply this by $\frac{1}{4}$, which is the chance of the desired allele from the other parent. As before, we get $\frac{1}{16}$; however, now we have 4 situations that could lead to this result. Since any of these combinations would work equally well, we sum these values $\frac{1}{16}+\frac{1}{16}+\frac{1}{16}+\frac{1}{16}=\frac{4}{16}=\frac{1}{4}$. Thus, $\frac{1}{4}$ of our plants will be heterozygous tall and heterozygous purple. We get $\frac{1}{4}$ as a result of the laws of statistics; we must sum the independent chances that we achieve the desired result. Like all statistical analyses, these rules work best with a large sample size.

Problem Solving

We may be asked on the MCAT to solve problems that involve crosses between organisms of known phenotype but unknown genotype. Let's walk through a hypothetical example now. Suppose that we have a tall, purple plant of unknown genotype crossed with a tall, white plant of unknown genotype. The offspring are 62 tall, purple plants, 59 tall, white plants, 20 dwarf, purple plants, and 21 dwarf, white plants. We would like to know the genotypes of the parents. On the MCAT, it is best to examine each trait separately, and then assign the overall genotype.

Key Concept

Each trait assorts individually in a 3:1 ratio, as in a monohybrid cross. There are nine purple, tall plants and three purple, dwarf plants, for a total of 12 purples; and there are three white, tall plants and one white, dwarf plant, for a total of four whites. Hence, the purple/white ratio is 12:4 = 3:1. Likewise, the tall/dwarf ratio is 3:1.

Let's start with color. We know the white plant will be pp, because white is recessive to purple. We also know that the other parent must be heterozygous for color, because there are white offspring in the F_1 generation. Thus, the other parent is Pp.

Now we can examine the height. Because there are dwarf offspring in the F_1 generation, and both parents are phenotypically tall, they *must* both be heterozygous tall (Tt). If either (or both) were homozygous, all the progeny would be tall.

Thus, one parent is heterozygous purple and heterozygous tall, whereas the other is homozygous white and heterozygous tall.

We might consider that we could have analyzed this problem mathematically. An approximately 1:1 purple to white ratio exists (62 + 20 to 59 + 21), which is what we expect from crossing a heterozygous dominant trait (purple flower) with a homozygous recessive one (white flower). For height, we have a 3:1 tall to dwarf ratio (62 + 59 to 20 + 21); this is the standard distribution for a heterozygous organism crossed to another heterozygous individual. However, on the MCAT we should be efficient and perform only the math that is required. It wasn't necessary here, and on Test Day we could address a problem like this without actually crunching the numbers.

The Chromosomal Theory of Inheritance

As we previously mentioned, genes are organized in a linear fashion onto chromosomes. From Chapter 4, we should remember that **diploid** species have homologous pairs of chromosomes. One allele is located on one chromosome, whereas the other allele is located on the paired (homologous) chromosome.

SEGREGATION AND INDEPENDENT ASSORTMENT

Now that we have a firm grip of Mendel's laws (perhaps by the kinetochores), we should briefly review meiosis, as Mendel's laws are the functional consequence of it. Before meiosis I, cells undergo genome replication. The daughter DNA strand is held to the parent strand at the centromere. Together, they are known as sister chromatids. Homologous pairs of chromosomes line up during metaphase I and then separate during anaphase I. Recall that the name given to meiosis I is the **reductional division**, as cells are haploid afterward. Homologous pairs separate, although the sister chromatids remain attached until meiosis II. Since this is the step during which homologous chromosomes separate, independent assortment occurs during meiosis I.

Bridge

What is the value of segregation and independent assortment? It allows for greater genetic diversity in the offspring.

NONINDEPENDENT ASSORTMENT AND GENETIC LINKAGE

Let's recall that our laundry detergent and sum example demonstrated independent purchases; buying one didn't cause you to buy the other. We will now take a look at nonindependent assortment of genes. Buying detergent may not make you purchase gum, but it does make it more likely that you will buy fabric softener because the two are typically located in the same aisle. Similarly, two genes that are closely related (in terms of distance from one another on a chromosome) may be inherited together.

Genetic linkage is a direct result of the organization of genes along chromosomes; linked genes are located on the same chromosome. During meiosis I, homologous chromosomes segregate into different cells. If two genes are located on the same chromosome, they tend to segregate together. The degree of genetic linkage can be tight and complete, with no recombinant phenotypes. Linkage can also be weak, for instance when the number of recombinants in the F_1 progeny approaches the number expected from independent assortment. Tightly linked genes recombine at a frequency close to zero percent; weakly linked genes recombine at frequencies approaching 50 percent (i.e., the percentage expected from independent assortment).

RECOMBINATION FREQUENCIES: GENETIC MAPPING

Let's detail how we can determine the degree of linkage between two genes. We already stated that the frequency of recombination can range from 0% (completely linked) to 50% (completely unlinked). The process that leads to recombination is the physical exchange of DNA between homologous chromosomes that are paired during meiosis. This process is termed **crossing over** (Figure 14.6). Genes that were initially linked may be unlinked by crossing over. Of course, if recombination occurred between sister chromatids, no change in linkage frequency would be observed because sister chromatids are genetically identical.

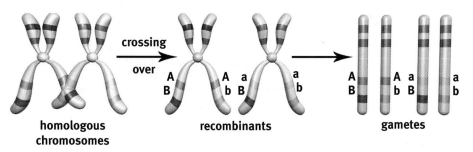

homologous chromosomes — crossing over — recombinants — gametes

Figure 14.6

The distance between gene loci on a chromosome determines the degree of genetic linkage. The chance that a crossover and exchange event will occur between two points is generally directly proportional to the distance between the genes. In other words, the further apart two genes are, the more likely it is that there will be a recombination event between them.

By analyzing **recombination frequencies,** we can construct a **genetic map**. A genetic map is a diagrammatic representation that shows the relative distance between the genes on a chromosome. By convention, one **map unit** corresponds to a 1% chance of recombination occurring. Thus, if we had two genes that were 25 map units apart, we would expect for 25% of the total gametes we examined to show recombination somewhere between these two genes. Recombination frequencies can be added in a crude approximation. For example, let's say we have genes *XYZ* that sit linearly on the chromosome. If we know the distance between *X* and *Y*, as well as the distance between *Y* and *Z*, the sum of these two numbers should provide us with the approximate recombination frequency for *X* and *Z*.

We can see a specific example illustrating this in Figure 14.7. We are shown that the recombination frequency of *X* and *Y* is 8%. We draw this in Step 1 of the diagram. Now, we are told that the recombination frequency of X and Z is 12%. As we see in Step 2 of Figure 14.7, Z could be in either of two spots, since we haven't yet determined if the gene order is *ZXY* or *XYZ*. We'll need to use the distance between *Y* and *X* as an arbiter. From the first two data points (*X* to *Y* and *X* to *Z*), they are either 20 map units (*ZXY* orientation) or four map units apart change to (*XYZ* orientation). Checking against what we have been given (*YZ* is four map units), we conclude that *XYZ* (or *ZYX*) is the correct orientation in Step 3. These sorts of questions require a little bit of mental math, but if we know how to approach them, they will result in quick points on Test Day.

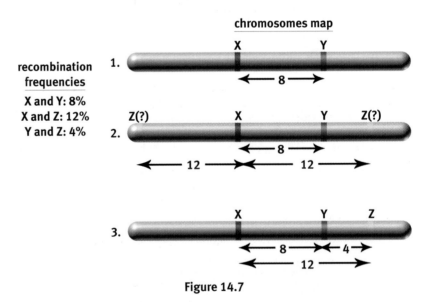

Figure 14.7

Variations on Mendelian Genetics

Although it would certainly be nice if all systems followed Mendelian genetics, that isn't the case. We have actually already seen an exception with the ABO blood group system in Chapter 9. Mendelian genetics is based on the premise that there is a clear relationship between phenotype and genotype. We expect 100% of recessive phenotypes to have homozygous recessive genotypes; we also expect 100% of dominant phenotypes to be either heterozygous or homozygous dominant. In reality, we must be wory of four specific situations: **incomplete dominance**, **codominance**, **penetrance and expressivity**, and **inherited disorders**.

INCOMPLETE DOMINANCE

Our pea plant flowers, were either white or purple, depending on the genotype. There was a clear 3:1 phenotypic ratio that we could predict in the F_2 generation; this proportion was based on the purple coding allele being dominant to the white coding allele. In some cases, however, neither allele is dominant (**incomplete dominance**); the resulting phenotype is a mixture of the two parental phenotypes. This occurs in another flower, the snapdragon, which has two alleles for color, red and white. We would expect the plants to be either red or white, depending on which allele is dominant. When we cross a homozygous red plant with a homozygous white plant, however, we get 100% pink plants in the F_1 generation. If we further self-cross these progeny, we find a 1:2:1 distribution (red to pink to white). If red were fully dominant, we would expect the Mendelian phenotype ratio of 3:1 (red to white). The pink color results from the combined effects of both alleles. See this data illustrated in Figure 14.8.

CODOMINANCE

Two conditions must be met for codominance to occur: first, there must be multiple coding alleles for a gene; second, more than one of these alleles must be dominant when expressed with a recessive allele. In situations of codominance, when two dominant alleles are both present, they will be expressed simultaneously. An important point to note is that the resulting phenotype is not an intermediate of the two alleles (incomplete dominance); it is, in fact, complete expression of both phenotypes.

When we studied the ABO blood system in Chapter 9, we were actually looking at a codominant system. Blood types A (I^A) and B (I^B) are both dominant to O (i). We can see that there are three coding alleles in the human population, but we know from Mendel's laws and our understanding of the chromosomal theory of inheritance that we will only have two alleles in any particular individual. People with type A blood have either $I^A I^A$ or $I^A i$ alleles; type B blood is the result of $I^B I^B$ or $I^B i$ alleles; type

> ### Key Concept
> Note that this 1:2:1 distribution for incomplete dominance is distinct from the 3:1 that we saw with classic monohybrid crosses.

> ### Bridge
> Type A individuals carry the A antigen on their RBCs and have circulating anti-B antibodies. Type B folks carry the B antigen and have circulating anti-A antibodies. Type O individuals have neither antigen and both antibodies. Type ABs have both antigens but neither antibody. That makes type O individuals universal donors and type AB individuals universal recipients.

snapdragons
R = allele for red flowers
r = allele for white flowers
Parental: RR × rr (red × white)

	R	R
r	Rr	Rr
r	Rr	Rr

F_1 genotypic ratio: 100% Rr
F_1 phenotypic ratio: 100% pink

F_1: Rr × Rr (pink × pink)

	R	r
R	RR	Rr
r	Rr	rr

F_1 genotypic ratio: 1RR:2Rr:1rr
F_2 phenotypic ratio: 1 red:2 pink:1 white

Figure 14.8

O blood only occurs with two recessive alleles ii. What happens when we combine the two codominant alleles? The genotype will be $I^A I^B$, and our individual will have type AB blood. We should emphasize that type AB blood is not an intermediate phenotype (what we would expect if A and B were incompletely dominant); instead, type AB blood is a fourth phenotype generated from the full expression of both the A and B alleles.

PENETRANCE AND EXPRESSIVITY

Penetrance and expressivity both reveal the complex interplay between genes and the environment. Penetrance of a genotype is defined as the number of individuals in the population carrying the allele who actually express the phenotype. Huntington's disease is an example of a disease that is not **fully penetrant**; it is an autosomal dominant disorder, yet 5% of people who have the dominant allele will not express symptoms of the disease. Diseases that exhibit this phenomenon may be further be described by the degree of penetrance. We would say that Huntington's disease is **highly penetrant**, because 95% of individuals with the affected allele will exhibit disease symptoms.

A related, but distinct, concept is expressivity, which is defined as the varying expression of disease symptoms despite identical genotypes. Whereas penetrance is all or nothing in each individual (i.e., disease present or absent), expressivity is more of a gray area. The disease neurofibromatosis type 2 (NF2) is an autosomal dominant disease, as a result of the mutation of the gene *merlin*. Interestingly, there is a range of phenotypes associated with carrying the affected allele. Some patients are not affected at all, whereas others have debilitating tumors of the auditory nerve, which is needed for hearing and balance (Chapter 13). The disease shows variable expressivity because there is a range of presentations between none and severe. Although we don't need to remember these specific diseases for the MCAT, we should be able to recognize *penetrance* and *expressivity* when we see them in a question.

INHERITED DISORDERS

Recessive

If a condition is recessive, two copies of the recessive allele must be present for the disease phenotype to be present. Heterozygotes are **carriers** of the disease. The normal allele protects them from the affected one. Homozygous recessive individuals are usually the result of mating between two carriers. Offspring of these carriers will exhibit the expected 3:1 phenotypic ratio that we saw in our initial monohybrid cross earlier in the chapter. That is, one out of four children will be expected to have the disease. Some recessive disorders, such as albinism, may be mild or have little functional consequence, whereas others may be **lethal**. An example of a more detrimental disease would be **cystic fibrosis** (CF). CF is caused by the deletion of a specific amino acid residue in a chloride channel. Individuals who are homozygous affected have problems with secretions like mucus and sweat. Their thick respiratory mucus predisposes them to infection with certain bacteria. Recessive diseases are capable of remaining in the gene pool, because carriers are not subject to the disease phenotype. CF heterozygotes have no problem in terms of secretions and will not be subject to natural selection on this basis. The majority of recessive lethal gene mutations are **early-acting**; that is, they cause death before the individual reproduces, usually during embryonic development or early childhood. We might expect these genes eventually to be selected against (Chapter 15); however, in several cases it has been shown that carrying a mutation (but not being homozygous for it) may confer a survival advantage. For example, individuals who are heterozygous for sickle cell anemia exhibit natural resistance to malaria. The incidence of the sickle cell gene is significantly higher in individuals of African descent; it is hypothesized that this is due to malaria being pandemic in Africa, which places selective pressure on the sickle cell allele.

Dominant

Lethal alleles may also be dominant. In a dominant disease, only one copy of the allele is required for the phenotype to be expressed. An example of a dominant lethal disease is the Huntington's disease, which was discussed above. Because the effects of Huntington's disease gene aren't expressed until middle age, most of its victims have already had children by the time of diagnosis; assuming the other parent is normal, 50 percent of the children are predicted to inherit the Huntington's disease gene. This is an example of a **late-acting** mutation, because the lethality does not occur until the individual has passed on his or her genes.

SEX DETERMINATION

All of our previous discussion has concerned the **autosomes**. We will now turn our attention to the **sex chromosomes**. In sexually divergent species, a variety of mechanisms are responsible for determining sex. For the MCAT, we want to be experts on how this process occurs in mammals, and, more specifically, humans. Humans have 22 pairs of autosomes and 1 pair of sex chromosomes. Females have two homologous X chromosomes, whereas males have an X and a Y chromosome (heterologous).

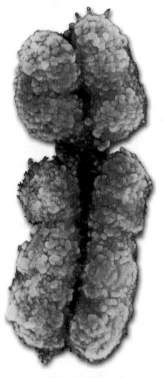

Figure 14.9a

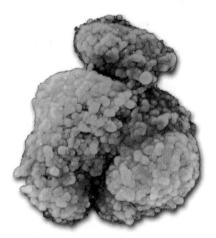

Figure 14.9b

During meiosis, these two chromosomes pair up for segregation purposes. We should know from Chapter 4 that these chromosomes will separate during meiosis I, which is when homologous pairs of autosomes part ways. The sex of a zygote is determined by the father, because the mother will always contribute an X chromosome. Approximately 50% of sperm contain the X chromosome and 50% contain the Y chromosome. The changes of being genotypically male (XY) or genotypically female (XX).

Key Concept

The odds of a child being a boy or a girl are 50:50. That means that regardless of how many sons or daughters a couple might have, the odds of having a boy or girl the next time around remains 50%. Each fertilization is an independent event!

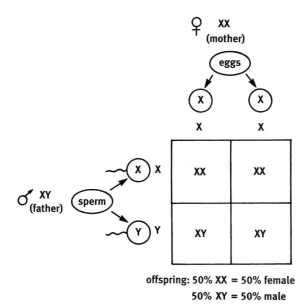

offspring: 50% XX = 50% female
50% XY = 50% male

Figure 14.10

SEX LINKAGE

Females have two X chromosomes, and so may be heterozygous or homozygous for a genetic condition that is carried on the X chromosome. Males have only one X chromosome. If that chromosome has a mutation, the male will be affected. Such males are said to be **hemizygous**. Because there is never an extra X allele in males to compensate for a genetic mutation, **X-linked recessive** diseases appear much more commonly in males. We will use hemophilia as a model disease to look at sex-linked inheritance. There are few X-linked dominant diseases and the Y chromosome is very small, so diseases of this sort aren't likely to be tested. However, if we were given a hypothetical situation on the MCAT involving a mutation on the Y chromosome, who would we predict to be affected? Males only. Moreover, if a man were affected, every one of his sons would have the disease, because he contributes his Y to each of them.

The ratios for sex-linked diseases depend on both parents. First, if the female is homozygous normal, none of the children will be affected. Why? All the sons will receive a normal X from the mother. Each daughter will receive a normal X as well.

Mnemonic

Remember SEX-linked is X-linked (unless told otherwise)..

Because the diseases are recessive, it is irrelevant what the daughter receives from the father.

Let's now say that we have a carrier female and a normal male. This is shown in Figure 14.11a. First, we note that all of the daughters will be phenotypically normal (nonhemophiliac). They each receive a normal X from their father, and so are protected from the disease. Genotypically, there is a 50:50 chance that they receive the affected allele from the mother. Thus, 50% of the daughters will be carriers and the other 50% will be homozygous normal. Now, for the sons. Each son gets a Y from the father, so the mother determines the presence of the disease. Like the daughters, there is a 50:50 chance of receiving each chromosome from the mother. Because the sons have only one X chromosome, they are either affected or normal; none of the sons can be carriers. We see that 50% will be hemophiliacs and 50% will be normal. Because there is an equal likelihood of having a male or female child, the overall distribution is 25% female homozygous normal (XX), 25% female heterozygous carrier (XX_h), 25% male normal (XY), and 25% male hemophiliac (X_hY).

a. Cross between a carrier female (X^hX) and a normal male (XY)

	X^h	X
X	X^hX	XX
Y	X^hY	XY

offspring
25% X^hX = 25% carrier female
25% XX = 25% normal female
25% X^hY = 25% hemophiliac male
25% XY = 25% normal male

b. Cross between a carrier female (X^hX) and a hemophiliac male (X^hY)

	X^h	X
X^h	X^hX^h	X^hX
Y	X^hY	XY

offspring
25% X^hX^h = 25% hemophiliac female
25% X^hX = 25% carrier female
25% X^hY = 25% hemophiliac male
25% XY = 25% normal male

Figure 14.11

Key Concept

The male completely determines the sex of the child. This has certain implications for sex-linked diseases. Because they are usually on the X chromosome, a male cannot pass a sex-linked disease to his sons.

Now let's examine what happens if we have a carrier mother and an affected father. This is diagrammed in Figure 14.11b. Starting with the daughters, we see that they will receive an affected allele from their father. The distribution of alleles from the mother has not changed from above; however, as a result of the affected allele from the father, 50% of the daughters will be hemophiliacs and 50% will be carriers. For the males, the analysis is the same as above because the father still only contributes the Y chromosome to his sons. Again, there is an equal likelihood of having a male or female child, so the overall distribution is 25% female homozygous affected (X_hX_h), 25% female heterozygous carrier (XX_h), 25% male normal (XY), and 25% male hemophiliac (X_hY).

Pedigree Analysis ★★★★★★

The ratios that we have determined throughout the chapter have depended on our ability to perform test crosses. Certainly, it would be unethical for scientists to perform these crosses on humans; instead, we use crosses that have already naturally occurred, and analyze the outcomes. We diagram these crosses in **pedigrees**. When we see a pedigree on Test Day, we will need to remember it's conventions. Males are represented by squares, and females are depicted with circles. If the shape is shaded, the individual is affected with the disease. Unshaded individuals are unaffected. If the disease in question is recessive, a carrier may (but will not always) be shown by half-shaded shape. For sex-linked traits, female carriers are always half-shaded if they have been identified as such.

Figure 14.12a shows the pedigree for an autosomal recessive trait, and 14.12b for a sex-linked recessive trait. For practice, try to determine the genotypes of all the individuals shown below

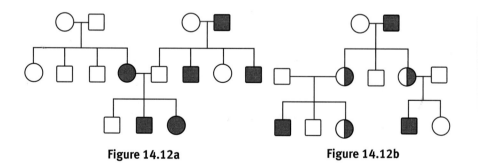

Figure 14.12a   **Figure 14.12b**

> **MCAT Expertise**
>
> When analyzing a pedigree, look for the recessive phenotype (because you will know the genotype) and work from there. If only males are affected, suspect sex linkage.

Chromosomal Aberrations ★★★☆☆☆

The proper segregation and assortment of genes depend on having both the correct number of chromosomes and chromosomes that are structurally normal. Failure to meet either of these criteria may result in genetic abnormalities in the offspring.

NUMERICAL ABNORMALITES

In humans, the diploid number is 46. Individuals with variations from this number are referred to as **aneuploid**. The most common cause for aneuploidy is **nondis-junction**. If during meiosis I homologous chromosomes, or during meiosis II sister chromatids, fail to separate, extra genetic material will be present in the gamete. If we consider a secondary spermatocyte that fails to disjoin correctly for chromosome 21, we will get one gamete with two copies of chromosome 21 and one gamete with zero copies of chromosome 21. There will also be two normal gametes, each with one copy. Remember that the primary spermatocyte will have generated two secondary spermatocytes. If the other secondary spermatocyte does disjoin correctly, it will generate two gametes with normal genetic complements.

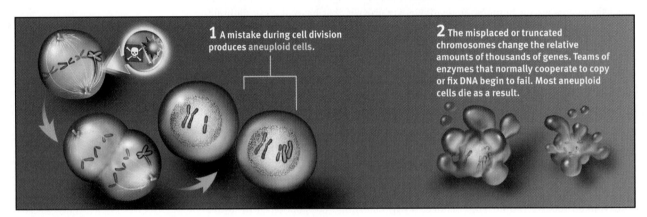

1 A mistake during cell division produces aneuploid cells.

2 The misplaced or truncated chromosomes change the relative amounts of thousands of genes. Teams of enzymes that normally cooperate to copy or fix DNA begin to fail. Most aneuploid cells die as a result.

Figure 14.11

If these sperm were to fuse with a genetically normal egg, there would be four possible results. Two out of four times, there would be no effect due to fusion with the normal haploid gametes. The diploid number would be restored. In one out of four cases, there would be an extra 21st chromosome (2N+1). This is referred to as **trisomy**, more specifically trisomy 21, because that is the chromosome that is affected. The last gamete would result in **monosomy** (2N-1), more accurately monosomy 21. Trisomy 21 results in Down syndrome.

Other than trisomy 21, aberrations in the number of autosomes usually result in spontaneous abortion before birth; the sex chromosomes are much more resilient. Females may be born with a single X chromosome (**XO**); they are known as Turner syndrome females and are characterized by short stature, sterility, and few to no secondary female sexual characteristics. Females may also be born with an extra X chromosome (**XXX**) and are referred to as **metafemales** or **superfemales**. They may be mentally retarded and sterile. Males are also subject to extra sex chromosomes.

An XXY genotype (**Klinefelter male**) results in a tall male who develops breasts and undescended testes, and is also usually sterile. Finally, some males may have an **XYY** genotype and may be taller than the average male. Generally, the presence of extra sex chromosomes is not incompatible with life.

CHROMOSOMAL BREAKAGE

Chromosomes may be damaged spontaneously or by environmental factors (e.g., x-rays, chemotherapeutic drugs). If a chromosome loses material, it has a **deletion**. The fragment that was lost may join to the homologous chromosome, resulting in a **duplication**, or it may join another chromosome, which leads to a **translocation**. If the genetic material finds its original home, but reinserts itself in the opposite orientation, it has undergone an **inversion**. If these changes occur in the germ line cells, they may be passed on to the offspring. In fact, approximately 5% of Down syndrome cases result from a specific type of translocation (Robertsonian) rather than meiotic nondisjunction.

Conclusion

Genetics is a commonly tested topic with which we will want to be familiar for the MCAT. Mendel began the work of genetics by studying pea plants and showing the independent assortment of genes. We must understand the stereotypical ratios of monohybrid and dihybrid crosses. Ultimately, Mendel described the basics of genetics but was later corrected on several counts. Genes can be inherited together if they are linked which depends on physical distance between the genes. In addition, allelic systems that show codominance, incomplete dominance, penetrance, or variable expressivity do not usually show a complete agreement between genotype and phenotype. In these cases, we must carefully analyze the genotypes to determine the deviations that are present. Furthermore, we described diseases as either dominant or recessive, depending on how many alleles were necessary to cause the phenotype. Sex-linked diseases are primarily due to mutations on the X-chromosome. They are usually inherited from the mother. Our final pages took us through alterations that could occur in chromosome structure or number. As we mentioned at the outset, genes (and therefore, chromosomes) are made of DNA. Our next chapter will examine nucleic acids and molecular genetics in great detail.

Real World

Chronic myeloid leukemia (CML) is associated with a specific chromosomal abnormality called the Philadelphia chromosome. The Philadelphia chromosome represents a reciprocal translocation from chromosome 22 to chromosome 9. The presence of the Philadelphia chromosome is a reliable marker for CML.

CONCEPTS TO REMEMBER

- [ ] Genes are the heritable units of organisms. They are composed of DNA and organized into chromosomes.

- [ ] Mendel's first law describes gene variants (alleles) and that an individual carries two alleles for each gene. One of these alleles is inherited from each parent.

- [ ] Mendel expanded on his work by showing that genes are inherited independently of one another. That is to say, the segregation of one gene does not affect the segregation of another during gametogenesis.

- [ ] Genes may segregate together because of the degree of linkage between them; the physical distance between genes is directly related to the chance of recombination.

- [ ] Recombination can unlink genes by exchanging material between homologous chromosomes.

- [ ] Codominant systems, such as the ABO blood antigens, result from the existence of multiple alleles with at least two alleles being dominant to a third. The resulting phenotype is unique.

- [ ] In incomplete dominance, the resulting phenotype is an intermediate of the parents' phenotypes.

- [ ] Traits may be either recessive or dominant. A recessive trait requires two affected alleles for the phenotype to be expressed. A dominant trait requires only one.

- [ ] Sex-linked traits are primarily associated with the X-chromosome and usually are recessive. Males are disproportionately affected.

- [ ] Variations in chromosomal number can result in disease. Aneuploidy of the sex chromosomes exhibits a milder disease course relative to aneuploidy of the autosomes.

Practice Questions

(handwritten margin notes)

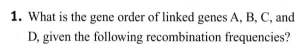

1. What is the gene order of linked genes A, B, C, and D, given the following recombination frequencies?

   freq AB: 6%   freq CD: 17%

   freq BC: 18%   freq AC: 12%

   freq AD: 5%   freq BD: 1%

   A. ACDB
   B. BDAC
   C. CBDA
   D. DBAC

2. In humans, the allele for black hair (B) is dominant to the allele to brown hair (b), and the allele for curly hair (C) is dominant to the allele for straight hair (c). When a person of unknown genotype is crossed against a straight-brown-haired individual, the phenotypic ratio is:

   25% curly black hair
   25% straight black hair
   25% curly brown hair
   25% straight brown hair

   What is the genotype of the unknown parent?

   A. BbCC
   B. bbCc
   C. Bbcc
   D. BbCc

3. Which of the following is TRUE concerning a sex-linked recessive disorder that is lethal in infancy?

   A. Females are unable to carry the gene.
   B. It will cause death in both males and females.
   C. It will cause death only in males.
   D. Male children of male carriers will be carriers.

4. Assuming classical Mendelian inheritance, how can one differentiate between a homozygous dominant individual and one who is heterozygous for the dominant trait?

   A. By crossing each individual with a known homozygous dominant and examining the offspring
   B. By crossing each individual with a known homozygous recessive and examining the offspring
   C. By crossing each individual with a known heterozygote and examining the offspring
   D. Both B and C

5. The distance between linked genes is directly proportional to

   A. the frequency of crossing over.
   B. the frequency of nonsense codons.
   C. the length of polypeptide chains.
   D. the ratio of AT:GC.

6. If a male hemophiliac (X^hY) is crossed with a female carrier of both color blindness and hemophilia (X^cX^h), what is the probability that a female child will be phenotypically normal?

   A. 0%
   B. 25%
   C. 50%
   D. Same as for a male child

7. If a test cross on a species of plants reveals the appearance of a recessive phenotype in the offspring, what must be true of the phenotypically dominant parent?

A. It must be genotypically heterozygous.
B. It must be genotypically homozygous.
C. It could be either genotypically heterozygous or homozygous.
D. It must have the same genotype as the testcross control parent.

8. Which of the following definitions is FALSE?

A. Penetrance—the percentage of individuals in the population carrying the allele who actually express the phenotype associated with it.
B. Expressivity—the degree to which the phenotype associated with the genotype is expressed in the entire population.
C. Incomplete dominance—occurs when the phenotype of the heterozygote is an intermediate of the phenotypes of the homozygotes.
D. Codominance—occurs when multiple alleles exist for a given gene and more than one of them is dominant.

9. In pea plants, the allele for round seeds (R) is dominant to the allele for wrinkled seeds (r), and the allele for yellow seeds (Y) is dominant to the allele for green seeds (y). A doubly heterozygous, round, yellow-seeded plant is crossed with a green, wrinkled-seeded plant. What percentage of the F_1 generation are recombinants?

A. 0%
B. 25%
C. 50%
D. 100%

Questions 10 to 12 are based on the pedigree below. The genotypes of individuals a, b, c, d, and e are unknown. (Shading is not indicated in these individuals.)

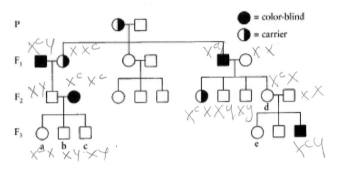

10. What are the genotypes of a, b, and c in the F_3 generation?

A. X^cY, X^cX, and X^cX, respectively
B. X^cX, X^cY, and X^cY, respectively
C. X^cY, X^cX^c, and X^cX^c, respectively
D. X^cX^c, X^cY, and X^cY, respectively

11. What is the genotype of d in the F_3 generation?

A. X^cX^c
B. X^cX
C. XX
D. X^cY

12. What is the genotype of e in the F_3 generation?

A. X^cX
B. X^cX^c
C. XX
D. Either X^cX or XX

13. Which of the following definitions is INCORRECT?

A. Trisomy—the zygote has three copies of a chromosome
B. Nondisjunction—failure of homologous chromosomes or of sister chromatids to separate
C. Translocation—the event by which a chromosomal fragment joins with its homologous chromosome
D. Inversion—the event by which a chromosomal fragment joins with its original chromosome, but in reverse position

14. In a species of plants, a homozygous dominant red flower (RR) is crossed with a homozygous recessive yellow flower (rr). If the F_1 generation is self-crossed and the F_2 generation has a phenotype ratio of red:orange:yellow of 1:2:1, which event accounts for these results?

A. Codominance
B. Incomplete dominance
C. Penetrance
D. Expressivity

Small Group Questions

1. Why are lethal dominant alleles much less common than lethal recessive alleles?

2. Regarding hair color in rabbits, the B and b alleles are both dominant to w, but B is incompletely dominant to b. BB individuals have black hair, bb individuals have tan hair, and ww individuals have white. What would be the observed phenotypic ratios in the offspring of a Bb mother and a bw father?

Explanations to Practice Questions

1. B

This is a simple gene-mapping problem. Because there is a one-to-one correspondence between the frequency of recombination and the distance between genes on a chromosome, if we are given the frequencies, we can determine gene order. Remember that one map unit equals 1 percent recombination frequency. The easiest way to begin is to determine the two genes that are farthest apart, i.e., the genes that have the highest recombination frequency. In this case, genes B and C recombine with a frequency of 18%; this means that B and C are 18 map units apart on the chromosome:

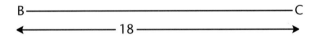

The recombination frequency for C and D is 17%; C and D are 17 map units apart. D can either be 17 units to the right of C or 17 units to the left. To determine where D is, we need to look at the recombination frequency for B and D; if D were to the right of C, the BD frequency would be 18 + 17 = 35%. However, we are told that D is, in fact, 1%, indicating that D is to the left of C:

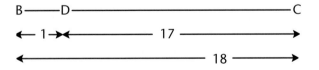

Now, we need to find out where A fits into the picture. The AC frequency is 12%; if A were 12 map units to the right of C, the AD frequency would be 17 + 12 = 29%. In fact, the AD frequency is 5%, indicating that A is 5 units to the right of D and 12 units to the left of C. The BD frequency + the AD frequency should equal the AB frequency, which is in fact the case: 1% + 5% = 6%.

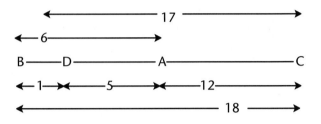

So, the gene order is BDAC, choice (B). If we had drawn out the chromosome in the reverse order, CADB, that would have also been correct. However, since this is not one of the answer choices, we deduce that we should reverse CADB to BDAC.

2. D

In this dihybrid problem, a doubly recessive individual is crossed with an individual of unknown genotype; this is known as a test cross. The straight- and brown-haired individual has the genotype bbcc, and can thus produce gametes of only one class, bc. Looking at the F_1 offspring, there is a 1:1:1:1 phenotypic ratio. The fact that both the recessive and dominant traits are present in the offspring means that the unknown parental genotype must contain both recessive alleles (b and c). The unknown parental genotype must therefore be BbCc. If you want to double check the answer, you can work out the Punnett square for the cross BbCc x bbcc: BbCc can produce four different types of gametes, BC, Bc, bC, and bc, whereas bbcc can produce only bc gametes as previously mentioned. So, the unknown parental genotype is BbCc, choice (D).

	BC	Bc	bC	bc
bc	BbCc	Bbcc	bbCc	bbcc
bc	BbCc	Bbcc	bbCc	bbcc
bc	BbCc	Bbcc	bbCc	bbcc
bc	BbCc	Bbcc	bbCc	bbcc
	↓	↓	↓	↓
	25% black curly	25% black straight	25% brown curly	25% brown straight

3. C

A sex-linked recessive gene is one that is carried on the X chromosome and can be passed only from fathers to daughters and from mothers to both sons and daughters. An early-acting lethal sex-linked recessive will kill all males in infancy, because males are XY and lack a dominant allele to mask the effects of the recessive lethal code. Males cannot be carriers of the lethal gene, as there will be no males of reproductive age with this gene to pass it on to offspring. Therefore, the gene will be inherited only from female carriers, who will pass the lethal gene to 50% of their offspring (all of their sons will die in infancy). A female can never be homozygous, because that would mean that she inherited one of the lethal alleles from her father—but that is impossible because all afflicted males die in infancy. Hence, there will be no female deaths as a result of the lethal allele. Thus choices (A), (B), and (D) can be ruled out. A cross between a female carrier and a normal male will produce 25% carrier daughters, 25% normal daughters, 25% homozygous sons (who will die in infancy), and 25% normal sons. So the correct answer is choice (C): all males with the early-acting sex-linked lethal recessive allele will die.

4. D

To differentiate between a homozygous dominant and a heterozygous dominant for a trait that exhibits classic dominant/recessive Mendelian inheritance, one must perform a cross that results in offspring that reveal the unknown parental genotype; this is known as a test cross. If we cross the homozygous dominant with a homozygous recessive, we will get 100% phenotypically dominant offspring; if we cross the heterozygous dominant with the homozygous recessive, we will get 50% phenotypically dominant and 50% phenotypically recessive offspring. Thus, using a homozygous recessive as a test crosser will allow us to distinguish between the two. We can also use a known heterozygote as the test crosser because when this is crossed with the homozygous dominant, 100% phenotypically dominant offspring are produced, and when it is crossed with the heterozygote, the phenotypic ratio of the offspring is 3:1 dominant: recessive. Hence, the correct answer is choice (D), because both choices (B) and (C) are viable options. Crossing both dominants with a known homozygous dominant, as in choice (A) will produce 100% phenotypically dominant offspring for both crosses, not allowing us to distinguish between the homozygote and the heterozygote.

5. A

Linked genes can recombine at frequencies between 0 and 50% to produce recombinants. The recombinant chromosomes arise through the physical exchange of DNA between homologous chromosomes paired during meiosis (during crossing over). The degree of genetic linkage is a measure of how far apart two genes are on the same chromosome. The probability of a crossover and exchange occurring between two points is generally directly proportional to the distance between the points. For example, pairs of genes that are far apart from each other on a chromosome have a higher probability of being separated during crossing over than pairs of genes that are located close to each other. Thus, the frequency of genetic recombination between two genes is related to the distance between them. Choice (A) is therefore the correct answer.

6. C

We are told that the female in this cross is a carrier of two sex-linked traits: color blindness and hemophilia. We are also told that the genes for these traits are not found on the same X chromosome, as indicated by her genotype, X^cX^h. Doing the cross, we obtain the following results:

	X^c	X^h
X^h	X^cX^h	X^hX^h
Y	X^cY	X^hY

Offspring

25% female hemophiliac
25% female carrier of both traits
　　　(phenotypically normal)
25% male hemophiliac
25% male color-blind

So, of the female offspring, half, or 50%, will be phenotypically normal. Choice (C) is thus the correct answer.

7.　A

Since homozygous recessive organisms always breed true (i.e., the genotype of the offspring can be predicted with 100% accuracy), they can be used to determine the genotype of another parent. In a process known as test cross or back cross, an organism with a dominant phenotype of unknown genotype (Ax) is crossed with a phenotypically recessive organism (genotype aa). In a test cross, the appearance of the recessive phenotype in the progeny indicates that the phenotypically dominant parent is genotypically heterozygous. Choice (A) is therefore the correct answer.

8.　B

Glancing at the answer choices, we notice that we are tested on four basic definitions, so our task is to read each one of them and cross out the ones that are correct. Penetrance is indeed the percentage of individuals in the population carrying the allele who actually express the phenotype associated with it, so choice (A) can be eliminated. Expressivity, however, is the degree to which the phenotype associated with the genotype is expressed in individuals who carry the gene. Since choice (B) talks about the entire population, rather than the individuals who are actual carriers, it is a false statement, and therefore the correct answer. Just to confirm, choices (C) and (D) contain correct definitions about incomplete dominance and codominance, so they can be safely eliminated.

9.　C

This is a basic dihybrid cross between a heterozygous, round, yellow-seeded plant (RrYy) and a green, wrinkled-seeded plant (rryy). RrYy produces four classes of gametes: RY, Ry, rY, and ry; rryy can produce only ry gametes. Here is the Punnett square:

	RY	Ry	rY	ry
ry	RrYy	Rryy	rrYy	rryy
ry	RrYy	Rryy	rrYy	rryy
ry	RrYy	Rryy	rrYy	rryy
ry	RrYy	Rryy	rrYy	rryy

The F_1 genotypic ratio is 1 RrYy:1 Rryy:1 rrYy:1 rryy. Phenotypically, the F_1 generation is one round yellow to one round green to one wrinkled yellow to one wrinkled green. Thus, 25% of the offspring are RrYy, which is one of the parental genotypes, and 25% of the offspring are rryy, which is the other parental genotype. Hence, 50% of the offspring have nonparental, or recombinant, genotypes.

10.　B

Color blindness is a sex-linked recessive trait; females carrying the allele can pass it on to both sons and daughters, whereas males can pass it on only to their daughters. We are told that the genotypes of individuals a, b, c, d, and e on the pedigree are unknown. The parents of a, b, and c are a normal male (XY) and a color-blind female (X^cX^c). Using a Punnett square,

	X^c	X^c
X	X^cX	X^cX
Y	X^cY	X^cY

we see that all female offspring are carriers and all male offspring are color-blind. Therefore, *a*'s genotype is X^cX, and *b* and *c* share the genotype X^cY.

11. B

The parents of *d* are a color-blind male (X^cY) and a normal female (XX). In the F$_3$ generation, *d* is a female. In such a mating, all daughters will be carriers because they inherit one of their Xs from their father, whose X chromosomes all have the trait for color blindness. Therefore, the genotype of *d* is X^cX, making choice (B) the correct answer.

12. D

In order to determine the genotype of *e*, we must first know the genotype of *d*. The parents of *d* are a color-blind male (X^cY) and a normal female (XX). In such a mating, all daughters will be carriers because they inherit one of their Xs from their father. Thus, *e*'s parents are a carrier female (X^cX) and a normal male (XY). Using a Punnett square,

	X^c	X
X	X^cX	XX
Y	X^cY	XY

we see that 50% of daughters are carriers and 50% are normal. Hence, the genotype of *e* is unknown; it could be either X^cX or XX, making choice (D) the correct answer.

13. C

Glancing at the answer choices, we notice that they all test us on our knowledge of chromosomal aberrations. Let's quickly go through each choice, eliminating the ones containing correct definitions.

Trisomy can be thought of as a type of nondisjunction, which results in the zygote having three copies of a chromosome; a typical example is Down syndrome, which often has a trisomy of chromosome 21. Choice (A) can be

therefore crossed out. Nondisjunction is indeed the failure of homologous chromosomes to separate during meiosis I or of sister chromatids to separate during meiosis II; we can eliminate choice (B) as well. Choice (C) is incorrect; in translocation, the chromosomal fragment joins with a nonhomologous chromosome; if the fragment joins with its homologous chromosome, the event is referred to as duplication. Choice (C) must be the answer we want. We can quickly verify that choice (D) contains the correct definition of inversion, and indeed, it does.

14. B

Some progeny in the second generation are apparently blends of the parental phenotypes. The orange color is the result of the combined effects of the red and yellow heterozygotes. An allele is incompletely dominant if the phenotype of the heterozygote is an intermediate of the phenotypes of the homozygotes. Choice (B) is therefore the correct answer.

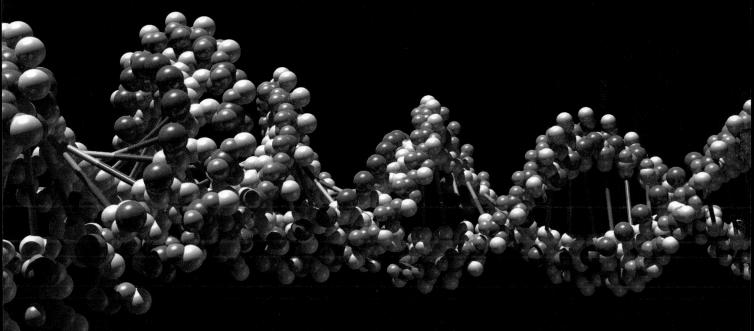

15

Molecular Genetics

In the world of molecular genetics, the devil truly is in the details. Seemingly small changes to the genetic code can result in disastrous, life-altering, life-threatening, even life-incompatible alterations to protein structure and function. As protein function necessarily depends on protein structure, protein structure necessarily depends upon the genetic code. One of the clearest examples of this—and a clear example of the dire results of even the smallest errors in the genetic system—is the molecular basis for the pathophysiology of sickle cell disease, also called sickle cell anemia. A disease most prevalent in people of tropical or subtropical origin, sickle cell anemia is a genetic disorder that results in abnormally shaped red blood cells. Rather than having the normal, flexible, biconcavity, these red blood cells assume a shape that is rigid and sickle-shaped (like the curved blade used to cut tall grasses).

Sickle cell disease is caused by a point mutation in the gene for the β-globin chain of hemoglobin. In this particular mutation, a thymine nucleotide is substituted for an adenine nucleotide, resulting in the substitution of valine for glutamic acid at the sixth position from the amino terminus of the β-globin chain. Individuals with sickle cell disease are homozygous for the mutated allele, which is autosomal recessive. The substitution of a nonpolar amino acid for an acidic (charged) amino acid has no effect on the secondary, tertiary, and even quaternary structure of hemoglobin: under normal physiological conditions, this is a totally benign mutation! However, under low-oxygen conditions, the deoxy form of hemoglobin exposes a hydrophobic patch on the protein, with which the nonpolar valine residue can interact by way of hydrophobic interactions. These interactions cause the hemoglobin molecules (called hemoglobin S, for the sickle cell mutation) to aggregate and form precipitates that distort the shape of the red blood cell and decrease its elasticity.

Under conditions of low oxygen tension, the aggregation of hemoglobin and the resulting shape change lead to damage of the erythrocyte membrane. Repeated sickling causes accumulated membrane damage and significantly decreased elasticity. These damaged cells do not return to their normal shape even after oxygen levels have been restored. When these abnormally shaped cells pass into the microvasculature (i.e., the capillaries), they can get stuck, blocking off blood supply to the tissue and causing ischemic tissue damage and high levels of pain.

The last chapter introduced us to genes as the fundamental units of heredity. We briefly noted that they are composed of **deoxyribonucleic acid (DNA)**. We saw that in order for traits to be inherited, the genes that code for the traits must be passed from one generation of individuals to the next. This ultimately means that the genetic code itself (DNA) must be transmitted. Each cell in the human body contains the complete blueprint for all the proteins necessary for life and which make each person unique. In Chapter 4, we noted that DNA replication is critical for cell division and reproduction. The self-replicating nature of DNA, and its ability to direct protein production, form the central dogma of molecular genetics (see Figure 15.1). This chapter will take us through the complete process from DNA to RNA to protein, and in some cases (e.g., retroviruses) backward from RNA to DNA and ultimately to protein. We will primarily examine the eukaryotic mechanisms of gene replication, although a review of some bacterial and viral genetics is included for Test Day completeness.

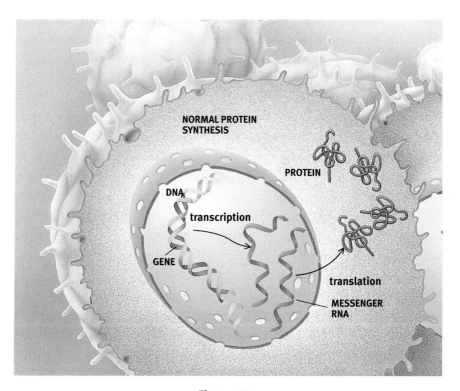

Figure 15.1

DNA

Like many other biological molecules that we have examined, DNA is a polymer. Its basic unit is a **nucleotide**, which has three basic parts: a **deoxyribose sugar**, a **nitrogenous base**, and a **phosphate group** (see Figure 15.2). The sugar forms the core to which the other two components are bound. There are four nitrogenous bases in two categories: **cytosine** and **thymine** are single-ringed **pyrimidines**, whereas **adenine** and **guanine** are double-ringed **purines**. Take a glance at the sidebar for a quick way to remember this distinction on Test Day.

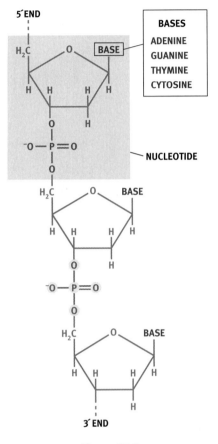

Figure 15.2

DNA nucleotides may be combined to form **polynucleotides**. The ordering and bonding between them is regular. The deoxyribose sugar has both a 3′-OH and a 5′-OH group. It gets the name *deoxy–* because the 2′ position has an –H rather than an –OH. The 3′ group is bound to the 5′ group of the next sugar. The three-dimensional structure of DNA has the chain formed by the sugars and phosphates, with the nitrogenous bases being put off to the side. This has important functional consequences that we will see momentarily.

Looking at Figure 15.3, we can see several features of DNA. First, two linear molecules are wound together in a spiral orientation, making it a **double-stranded helix**. The sugar phosphate chain that we mentioned in the last paragraph is oriented to the outside of the helix, whereas the nitrogenous bases are forced into the middle of the DNA molecule. This allows for base pairing through hydrogen bonding of the side chains, giving greater stability to the overall molecule. A pairs with T, forming two hydrogen bonds; and C with G, making three hydrogen bonds. Note that a pyrimidine pairs with a purine in each case.

Key Concept

Because of complementary base pairing in DNA, the amount of A will equal the amount of T, and G will equal C in double-stranded organisms. Also, because G is triple bonded to C, the higher the G/C content of DNA, the more tightly bound the two strands will be.

Key Concept

If A–T forms two hydrogen bonds and C–G forms three hydrogen bonds, what does this mean about the relative stability of DNA strands that are A/T-rich versus those that are C/G-rich? Because H-bonds are *inter*molecular interactions, you can use heat to melt the two strands of DNA apart. This is the basis of the polymerase chain reaction. This A/T versus C/G ratio tells us how high this temperature needs to be, with more C/G requiring a higher temperature.

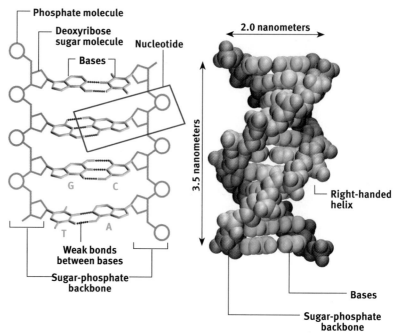

Figure 15.3

Key Concept

One of the most common MCAT topics to be tested is the 5′→3′ nature of DNA. This may be in the form of a discrete or passage-based question. It may be on transcription, translation, or general base pairing. The bottom line is that DNA and RNA work in a 5′→3′ direction. This fact is likely to earn you a quick point on Test Day.

We can see in Figure 15.3 that the two strands are **antiparallel**; that is, one strand has a **5′→3′ polarity**, whereas its complementary strand has a **3′→5′ polarity**. The directionality of DNA is one of its most important features; the enzymes that replicate and transcribe DNA can only move 5′→3′. We will discuss the functional consequences of this shortly. The 5′ end of DNA has an –OH or phosphate group bound to the number 5 carbon of the terminal sugar, while the 3′ end has a –OH on the number 3 sugar. The combination of all these properties gives us the **Watson-Crick model** of DNA.

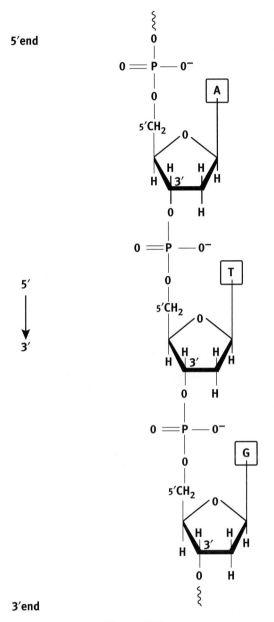

5′end

5′

3′

3′end

Figure 15.4

Watson, Crick, and Wilkins (another one of their colleagues) were awarded the 1962 Nobel Prize in Physiology or Medicine for their discovery of DNA, along with the elucidation of its structure and significance. It was revealed later that Rosalind Franklin was actually the scientist who had created the X-ray images of DNA used by Watson and Crick. Unfortunately, she died by the time this information became public.

DNA REPLICATION (EUKARYOTIC)

For both reproduction and replacement purposes, cells must be able to replicate the genome. We will focus on eukaryotes for the MCAT, although prokaryotes use a similar process.

Semiconservative Replication

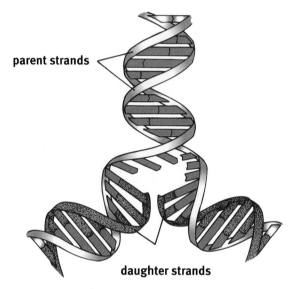

parent strands

daughter strands

Figure 15.5

Chapter 4 introduced us to the idea that DNA undergoes **semiconservative replication**. Each new helix contains a strand from the parent DNA molecule and a newly synthesized strand (see Figure 15.5). Because the DNA helix is tightly bound together, the helix must first unwind to allow replication to occur. This allows each of the parent strands to act as a template for generation of a daughter strand. In the days before printing presses, monks used to carry out the same process with ancient tomes. They would copy a book from an existing manuscript (parent strand), generating a new one (daughter strand). Like DNA, this would allow for further dissemination of the material contained in the books. This process also ensures that each of the new helices is identical.

Origin of Replication

The human genome has about 3 billion base pairs; it is truly amazing to think that all of those base pairs are in every single one of our cells (with the exception of gametes, which have half the genetic complement). Because there are so many bases, DNA unwinds in multiple places to allow for efficient replication to occur. Each of these points is named an **origin of replication** (see Figure 15.6). The generation of new DNA proceeds in both directions, creating **replication forks**, so named because each looks like a fork in the road.

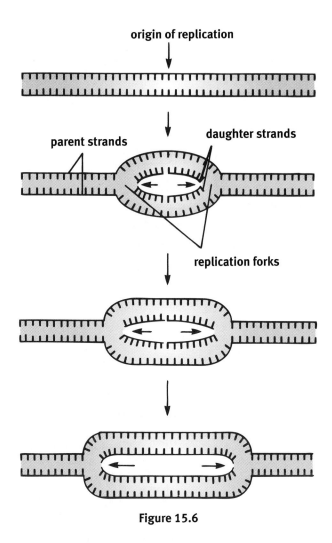

origin of replication

parent strands

daughter strands

replication forks

Figure 15.6

Unwinding and Initiation

Now that we know where the helix dissociates, we can describe the enzymes that carry this process out. **Helicase** unwinds the helix, generating single-stranded regions of DNA. DNA isn't particularly fond of being unwound; recall that we described the hydrogen bonding that occurs between the two strands. To keep the two strands from reassociating, **single-strand binding proteins** (SSB) enter and stabilize the single strands. Think of two large magnets; we have to work to pull them apart, just as helicase has to pull apart the two strands of the DNA helix. And if we don't keep them apart, they will reassociate. As helicase unwinds DNA, it causes positive supercoiling that strains the DNA helix. So, **DNA gyrase** (a topoisomerase), relieves overwound DNA by introducing negative supercoils. We can illustrate supercoiling by thinking of the old-fashioned cord between the phone and the handset. It has coils in it already; however, as we know from experience, the cord may wrap around itself further. These coils are known as **supercoils**.

Bridge

Remember that bacteria have topoisomerases as well. Some of our antibiotics poison these as their mechanism of actions. Because the topoisomerases of bacteria are somewhat different from ours, we aren't hurt. We also use topoisomerase poisons in cancer treatment. In this case, we want to stop cell division, so we prevent DNA replication (which is required for cell division) by keeping it from unwinding.

DNA polymerase is the enzyme responsible for adding the individual nucleotides to the growing strand. However, it won't work unless it recognizes where to begin. It requires an RNA **primer** that is several nucleotides long. **Primase** (an RNA polymerase) is the enzyme that generates the RNA primer. When children learn to read, they must first understand the alphabet, and may use a reading primer to help them. DNA polymerase needs the RNA primer to understand how to generate the new strand. The first nucleotide incorporated binds to the 3′ end of the primer chain.

Synthesis

As we alluded to already, synthesis occurs in the 5′→3′ direction. A number of different enzymes collectively referred to as **DNA polymerases** catalyze this process. Helicase moves forward, unwinding the DNA helix. SSBs bind to prevent reassociation, and DNA gyrase introduces negative supercoils to prevent torsional strain on the helix. Free nucleotide triphosphates (in the 5′ position) will pair with the parent strand, and DNA polymerase will cut the phosphodiester linkage to incorporate the new base. Free pyrophosphate (PP_i) will also be generated.

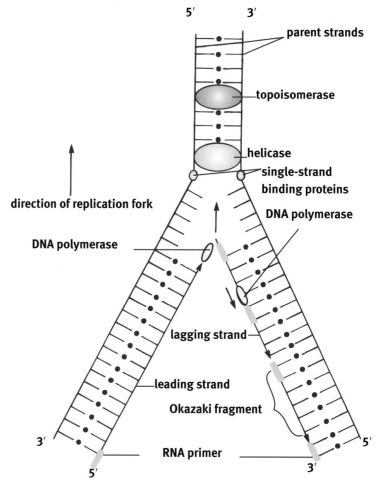

Figure 15.7

Due to the directionality of DNA polymerase, certain constraints arise. Remember that the two strands of the helix are antiparallel to each other. In each replication, there will be a 3′→5′ strand whose complement will be coded 5′→3′. This presents no problem to the DNA polymerase, which can form the complement strand, known as the **leading strand**, in a continuous fashion. The complementary parent strand at the replication fork will have a 5′→3′ polarity. If DNA polymerase were to sit down directly and work, it would necessarily have to produce the daughter strand in the 3′→5′ direction, because it would have to read the parent strand 5′→3′. We already know that DNA polymerase cannot do this. How do we solve this problem? DNA polymerase can only produce daughter strand DNA in the 5′→3′ direction, so small sections known as **Okazaki fragments** (around 1000 base pairs) are produced at a time. The primer is introduced as far forward as possible, and then instead of working forward toward the point of the replication fork (which occurs in the leading strand), DNA polymerase works back toward the origin of replication. This strand is known as the **lagging strand**. Since the replication fork is moving in the other direction, synthesis occurs piecemeal so that the ultimate direction of replication is the same and both new strands can be generated at the same time. To be clear, the leading strand is produced continuously 5′→3′. The lagging strand is produced discontinuously through the formation of Okazaki fragments, which are produced 5′→3′. The summation of Okazaki fragments is in the 3′→5′ direction. The small gaps between the Okazaki fragments are also filled with nucleotides and the sugar phosphate backbone is added by **DNA ligase** (see Figure 15.6).

Key Concept

As we said before, replication is subject to the 5′→3′ rule. This means that one strand, the lagging, is synthesized discontinuously. In the past, the MCAT has used this fact to ask which strand is more likely to be subject to errors. Not surprisingly, it is the lagging strand, as the replication machinery has to hop on and off more often.

RNA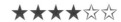

Ribonucleic acid (RNA) is similar to DNA in many ways, with three major exceptions. It uses ribose instead of deoxyribose as a sugar; it is usually **single stranded**; and the base uracil replaces thymine. There are multiple types of RNA, each of which have different functions. RNA is found in both the nucleus and the cytoplasm, where it participates in **transcription** and **translation**, respectively. We will discuss four types of RNA: **mRNA**, **tRNA**, **rRNA**, and **hnRNA**. The name of each type clues us in to its function.

Key Concept

DNA:
- Double stranded
- Sugar = deoxyribose
- Base pairing: A/T, G/C
- Found in nucleus only

RNA:
- Single stranded
- Sugar = ribose
- Base pairing: A/U, G/C
- Found in nucleus and cytoplasm

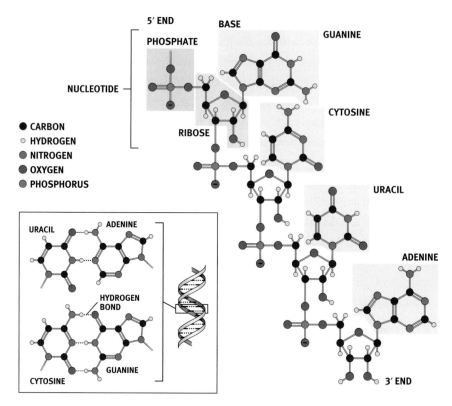

Figure 15.8

MESSENGER RNA (mRNA)

Messenger RNA is created during transcription. It carries the genetic message from the nucleus to the cytoplasm so that it can be translated into a protein. In eukaryotes, mRNA is **monocistronic**, meaning that each mRNA molecule translates into only one product. In prokaryotes, particularly bacteria, messages may be **polycistronic** and different proteins can be formed by starting translation at different positions on the mRNA.

TRANSFER RNA (tRNA)

Once the message arrives at the ribosome, amino acids must be linked into the nascent polypeptide chain. tRNA, found in the cytoplasm, carries out this function. There are 20 amino acids, each of which is selected by a different **codon**, so there is a different tRNA for each amino acid.

RIBOSOMAL RNA (rRNA)

Ribosomal RNA is synthesized in the nucleolus. It forms an integral part of the ribosomes that are used for protein assembly in the cytoplasm.

HETEROGENEOUS NUCLEAR RNA (hnRNA)

We will soon describe how mRNA is generated. Its immediate precursor is heterogeneous nuclear RNA, which is larger and includes riboproteins in its structure.

> ### Key Concept
>
> mRNA is the messenger. The DNA codes for proteins but can't carry out any of the enzymatic reactions itself. Proteins can carry out the ultimate reactions necessary for life but need to know how to build themselves in order to perform the right chemistry. mRNA takes the work orders from the DNA to the ribosomes to create the proteins.

Protein Synthesis (Eukaryotic)   ★★★★★☆

TRANSCRIPTION

Although the DNA contains the actual coding sequence for a protein, the machinery to generate that protein is in the cytoplasm. DNA cannot leave the nucleus, as it will be quickly degraded. So, it must use RNA to transmit its message. The encoding of mRNA is known as **transcription**.

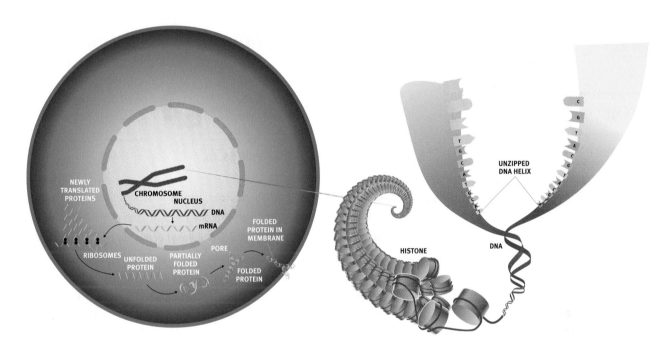

Figure 15.9

Transcription begins in a manner analogous to DNA replication. We must unwind the DNA helix so that we can access the gene of interest. However, we use only one strand to generate the growing RNA molecule. This template strand is also called the **antisense strand** because its nucleotide sequence is antiparallel and complementary to the RNA strand produced from it. Like DNA replication, this process can only occur in the 5′→3′ direction; it is catalyzed by **RNA polymerase**. Base pairing is the same as that in DNA with the exception that uracil substitutes for thymine in the RNA chain. We might wonder how the transcription machinery knows where to begin work, as there are 3 billion base pairs in the genome and over 30,000 genes. Specialized DNA regions known as **promoters** signal where to begin transcription. There are also **termination sequences**, which signal RNA polymerase to dissociate from DNA, thereby stopping transcription. The DNA double helix re-forms, and the newly formed RNA is hnRNA (pre-mRNA).

POST-TRANSCRIPTIONAL PROCESSING

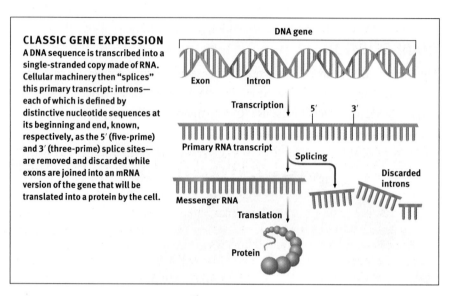

CLASSIC GENE EXPRESSION
A DNA sequence is transcribed into a single-stranded copy made of RNA. Cellular machinery then "splices" this primary transcript: introns—each of which is defined by distinctive nucleotide sequences at its beginning and end, known, respectively, as the 5′ (five-prime) and 3′ (three-prime) splice sites—are removed and discarded while exons are joined into an mRNA version of the gene that will be translated into a protein by the cell.

Figure 15.10

Before an hnRNA strand can leave the nucleus, it must undergo three processes to become a messenger RNA that is capable of interacting with the ribosomal subunits in the cytoplasm (see Figure 15.10). First, a 5′-guanosyl cap must be added to stabilize the starting end of the transcript. Second, we need to put a poly-adenine (poly-A) tail on to protect the 3′ end of our message. The last piece of the puzzle is to remove the **introns**. Eukaryotic genes contain coding (**exons**) and noncoding (**introns**) regions. We want our message to include only the coding regions so that the proper protein will be made. The processing of hnRNA to mRNA occurs in the nucleus. You can think of introns as the commercials in a television show. If you were to tape the show in that antiquated VCR your friends make fun of, you might choose to pause recording during the commercials, so that only the show itself (exons) gets taped.

THE GENETIC CODE

We know that DNA and RNA share the same language; they both code using nitrogenous bases. Proteins are made of amino acids, which are not nitrogenous bases. We use the genetic code as a Rosetta Stone to advance from an RNA-coded message to a protein during translation.

There are four letters in the genetic alphabet (A, C, T/U, and G) and 20 words (amino acids) in the protein language. The different nucleotide letters can be put together to form words (e.g., ACC). These mRNA words are then translated into the words of amino acids, the language of proteins (e.g., ACC corresponds to threonine). If each nucleotide word consisted of only two nucleotides, the maximum number of words that could be formed would be 16 (4^2). However, since there are 20 naturally occurring amino acids (i.e., 20 words in the protein language), 16 nucleotide words would be insufficient. Using three genetic letters to form each word, however, would be sufficient. With three nucleotides, we can make 64 words (4^3). As you will immediately recognize, there is actually an excess of genetic words. This is the **degeneracy** or **redundancy** of the genetic code. There are multiple three-letter nucleotide words that can code for the same amino acid. This **triplet** word is known as a **codon** (see Table 15.11). With few exceptions, the genetic code is universal.

NATURE'S CODE

IF A GENE SEQUENCE is a "sentence" describing a protein, then its basic units are three-letter "words," or "codons," each of which translates into one of 20 amino acids or a "stop translating" signal. Cellular machinery transcribes DNA genes into RNA versions—whose nucleotide building blocks are represented by the letters A, C, G and U—and then translates the RNA genes, codon by codon, into a corresponding amino acid sequence. Nature's exact amino acid definitions (*below*) were worked out during the early 1960s. But the significance of patterns in the code would not be fully appreciated for several decades.

SYNONYMS AND SIMILARITIES

Many of the 64 possible three-letter codons specify the same amino acid, providing alternative ways for genes to spell out most proteins. These synonymous codons tend to differ by just a single letter, usually the last, forming a pattern of blocks. Codons for amino acids with similar affinities for water also tend to differ by their last letter, and codons sharing the same first letter often code for amino acids that are products or precursors of one another. These features, as it turns out, are crucial to the survival of all organisms and may even help speed their evolution.

First Nucleotide Position	Second Nucleotide Position			
	U	**C**	**A**	**G**
U	UUU Phenylalanine UUC Phenylalanine UUA Leucine UUG Leucine	UCU Serine UCC Serine UCA Serine UCG Serine	UAU Tyrosine UAC Tyrosine UAA STOP UAG STOP	UGU Cysteine UGC Cysteine UGA STOP UGG Tryptophan
C	CUU Leucine CUC Leucine CUA Leucine CUG Leucine	CCU Proline CCC Proline CCA Proline CCG Proline	CAU Histidine CAC Histidine CAA Glutamine CAG Glutamine	CAU Arginine CAC Arginine CAA Arginine CAG Arginine
A	AUU Isoleucine AUC Isoleucine AUA Isoleucine AUG Methionine	ACU Threonine ACC Threonine ACA Threonine ACG Threonine	AAU Asparagine AAC Asparagine AAA Lysine AAG Lysine	AAU Serine AAC Serine AAA Arginine AAG Arginine
G	GUU Valine GUC Valine GUA Valine GUG Valine	GCU Alanine GCC Alanine GCA Alanine GCG Alanine	GAU Aspartate GAC Aspartate GAA Glutamate GAG Glutamate	GAU Glycine GAC Glycine GAA Glycine GAG Glycine

Figure 15.11

TRANSLATION

Now that we have a proper RNA message in the cytoplasm, and we understand the system of conversion from genetic words (codons) to protein words (amino acids), we can put together a protein sentence. This process is known as **translation**. Translation requires the mRNA, tRNA, ribosomes, amino acids, and energy.

tRNA

The genetic code tells us which amino acid and codon go together, but it doesn't actually do the heavy lifting. It is up to tRNA to shuttle the correct amino acid

Bridge

We can think of DNA as being responsible for genotype, and proteins as being responsible for phenotype.

Key Concept

The base pairing between the codon and anticodon is both complementary and antiparallel: the 5′ end of the codon lines up with the 3′ end of the anticodon. Be advised that the convention is that both codons and anticodons are *always* written in 5′→3′ order. That means that the codon AUG would bind to the anticodon CAU. (If it helps you to visualize this: 5′-AUG-3′ binds to 5′-CAU-3′ in an antiparallel fashion.) We must feel comfortable with this convention or we'll end up missing easy points on the MCAT.

Key Concept

Although the most common energy currency of the cell is ATP, the formation of the aminoacyl-tRNA complex actually uses energy generated from GTP (a similar molecule). This seems like a minor point, but it is one of those exceptions that the MCAT likes to test, and can lead to a higher score on Test Day.

Key Concept

Note that AUG is both the start codon and the only codon for methionine. The first AUG that the ribosome encounters will not only start polypeptide synthesis but also put a methionine in that position. Thus, all polypeptide chains start with methionine, although it is commonly removed during post-translation modifications. Further AUG sequences in the mRNA simply add another methionine to the chain.

to the ribosome when it is needed. In order to do this, tRNA needs to be able to recognize both the codon and the amino acid that it is carrying. This is reflected in tRNA's three-dimensional structure. On one end, there are nucleotides that are complementary to the codon; they are known as the **anticodon**. On the opposite pole of the molecule, tRNA is bound to the amino acid that corresponds to the codon in question. Each tRNA has a CCA nucleotide sequence where the amino acid binds. We might wonder how the tRNA knows which amino acid to select if the CCA sequence is conserved between all tRNAs. Each tRNA has a helper **tRNA synthetase**, an enzyme that binds the amino acid to the tRNA using GTP. The result is an **aminoacyl-tRNA complex**.

Ribosomes

Way back in Chapter 1, we referred to ribosomes as the factories of the cell. Now we are going to see them in action. Ribosomes are composed of two subunits, each of which is made up of ribosomal proteins and rRNA. There is a large and small subunit, and they only bind together during protein synthesis. The purpose of the ribosome is to take the actual message and the charged aminoacyl–tRNA complex to generate the protein. To do so, they have three binding sites. One is for the mRNA; the other two are for the tRNA. The binding sites for tRNA are the **A site**, which holds the aminoacyl-tRNA complex, and the **P** site, which binds to the tRNA attached to the growing polypeptide chain.

Polypeptide Synthesis

Once we have all the requisite components, we can actually make a protein. This process can be divided into three stages: **initiation**, **elongation**, and **termination**. As we describe each step, let's look at Figure 15.12 to help us follow the intricacies.

Initiation

Synthesis begins with mRNA seeking out a small ribosome. They bind in the presence of **initiation factors** and the small ribosome slides along the mRNA until it reaches a start codon (AUG). The initiation aminoacyl–tRNA complex, **methionine tRNA** (with the anticodon 5′-CAU-3′), base pairs with the start codon. At this point, the large ribosomal subunit joins the complex, completing the ribosome. The tRNA is in the **P site** at this point, because it is a part (and the only part) of the growing polypeptide chain.

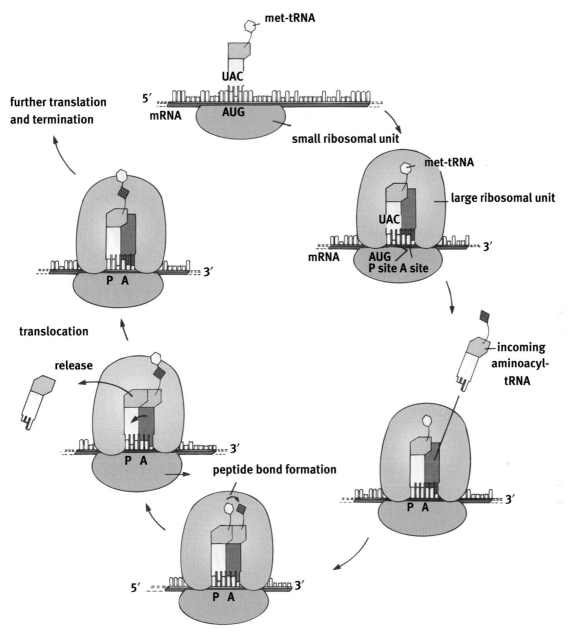

Figure 15.12

Elongation

Once the complex has been formed, the ribosome can slide along the mRNA, adding new amino acids as it goes. Hydrogen bonds form between the mRNA codon in the A site and the complementary tRNA anticodon. This fills the A site. We now have a charged aminoacyl–tRNA in both the A site and the P site. The enzyme, **peptidyl transferase**, uses the energy that was stored in the amino-acyl–tRNA complex when the amino acid was loaded (remember, this was from GTP) to catalyze the formation of a peptide bond. The aminoacyl–tRNA used for this is the one in the P site. The bond is made between the single amino acid in the A site and the methionine in the P site. Now the tRNA in the P site is free and there is still an aminoacyl–tRNA in the A site. This aminoacyl–tRNA has its own amino acid that is now bound to a methionine. **Translocation** is necessary to add the next amino acid residue. The ribosomal assembly slides in a $5' \rightarrow 3'$ direction along the mRNA. This moves the next codon into place in the A site. At the same time, the uncharged tRNA in the P site is expelled, and the aminoacyl–tRNA that is carrying our nascent chain moved from the A site to P site. The process is ready to begin again with an empty A site (see Figure 15.12).

Termination

Translation has its own set of stop signs. If the codon in the A site is UGA, UAA, or UAG, it is known as a **termination codon**. Instead of a new aminoacyl–tRNA binding to the A site, a protein called **release factor** binds to the termination codon, causing a water molecule to be added to the polypeptide chain. The polypeptide chain will then be released from the tRNA in the P site, and the two ribosomal subunits will dissociate. To save time, as well as increase the amount of protein that may be made from a single transcript, several ribosomes may translate a message at the same time. This is known as a **polyribosome**.

POST-TRANSLATIONAL MODIFICATIONS (PTM)

The new polypeptide is subject to modification just as hnRNA was after transcription. It will fold into a secondary structure based on the lowest energy conformation. Often during this process, the polypeptide will be cleaved or have sugars added to it. We saw an example of this in Chapter 12 with insulin, which is cleaved from a larger peptide to its active form. Other modifications include phosphorylation, carboxylation, and methylation.

MUTATIONS

We mentioned mutations briefly in the previous chapter as a way to increase genetic diversity (at the always present risk of killing the organism). Let's take a glance at the types of mutations and how they occur. They may be classified as **base pair mutations**, **base pair insertions**, or **base pair deletions**. Base pair mutations are also called **point mutations**, whereas insertions and deletions are both also known as **frameshift mutations**.

Types of Mutations

Point Mutations

A point mutation occurs at a single nucleotide residue. Depending on where it is in the genome, it may have no effect at all (perhaps if it is in a noncoding region), to a highly detrimental effect (sickle cell anemia). Even if the mutation occurs in a coding region, it may still have no effect. Such mutations are termed **silent mutations**. Looking back at the genetic code chart, can we think of why such mutations exist? It is because the genetic code is degenerate. For example, the amino acid glycine requires only the first two nucleotides of the codon to ensure that it be inserted into the polypeptide chain. The final nucleotide could be A, C, U, or G, and therefore, a "mutation" in this position would be irrelevant. Thus, a mutation at this nucleotide position will have no effect. Changes in either the second or first nucleotide can be more detrimental. A point mutation at the first or second position in the codon may result in a **missense mutation**, in which one amino acid is substituted for another.

Figure 15.13

Sickle cell anemia results from the mutation of the second nucleotide in the codon resulting in a GUG instead of a GAG (see Figure 15.12). The resultant hemoglobin S (mutant hemoglobin) is generated with a valine instead of a glutamic acid. Figure 15.14 shows red blood cells affected with sickle cell anemia. Notice that the classic biconcave shape is no longer present, all due to a single amino acid swap.

Key Concept

Silent mutations are a result of the degeneracy of the genetic code. It makes sense that those amino acids that are used most commonly are redundant. That way, if the third position gets changed, no effect will be seen in the organism.

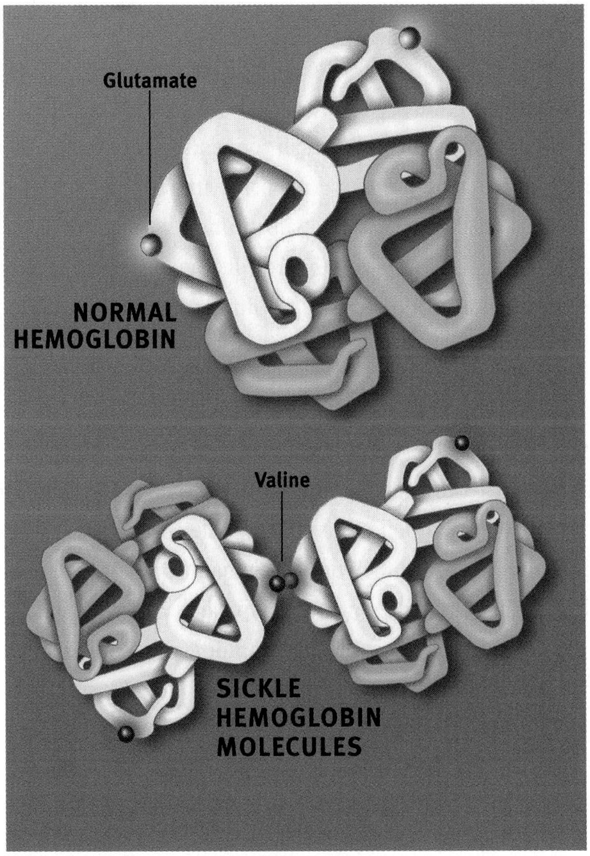

Real World

A **nonsense mutation** is a mutation that produces a premature termination of the polypeptide chain by changing one of the codons to a stop codon. Nonsense mutations can have disastrous effects. Thalassemia is a genetic disease in which erythrocytes are produced with little or no functional hemoglobin, leading to severe anemia. Thalassemia can be caused by a variety of different mutations: Point mutations can change a codon into a stop codon, and frame-shift mutations (insertions and deletions) can introduce a stop codon in the altered reading frame.

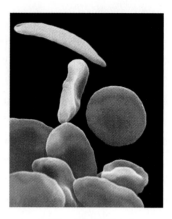

Figure 15.14

Frame Shift Mutations

Codons consist of three nucleotides; this is referred to as the **reading frame**. Insertion or deletion of nucleotides will shift the reading frame, usually resulting in either changes in the amino acid sequence or premature truncation of the protein (due to the generation of a nonsense mutation). The effects are usually much more serious than a base pair substitution. For example, cystic fibrosis is caused by a frame shift mutation that results the loss of a phenyl-alanine at position 508 in the polypeptide chain, resulting in a defective chloride ion channel. The disease is characterized by infertility, increased incidence of bacterial infections, and decreased life span.

Mutagenesis

New mutations may be introduced in a variety of ways. DNA polymerase is subject to making mistakes, albeit at a very low rate. In addition, ionizing radiation such as ultraviolet rays from the sun can damage DNA. DNA is also capable of damaging itself. Elements known as **transposons** can remove and insert themselves into the genome. If they insert in the middle of a coding sequence, the gene will be disrupted.

How Sunlight Can Cause a Permanent Mutation

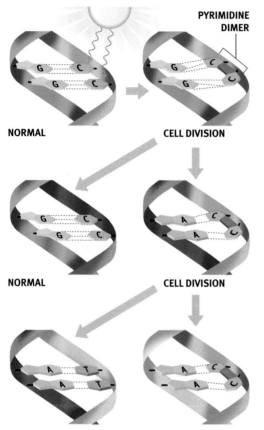

PYRIMIDINE DIMER

NORMAL   CELL DIVISION

NORMAL   CELL DIVISION

ULTRAVIOLET LIGHT can break chemical bonds in adjacent pyrimidine bases, often at a point on the DNA strand where two cytosines (C) occur. New bonds then form (red), linking the disrupted bases together in a so-called pyrimidine dimer.

REPLICATION requires that a cell separate the paired DNA strands (green and blue), each of which is used as a template to construct a new strand (purple)—by mating guanine (G) with cytosine and adenine (A) with thymine (T). The strand unaffected by sunlight produces normal DNA (left), but the strand containing the pyrimidine dimer pairs disturbed Cs with As instead of matching them properly with G s.

CONTINUED REPLICATION repeats the error, mating the dimer once more with a pair of As (right). On the opposite strand (left), these As are matched with Ts, creating a genetic mutation. The dimer may eventually be eliminated by "excision repair," but the C-to-T mutation is permanent. When such a mutation falls within a cancer-related gene, the cell becomes prone to malignancy.

Figure 15.15

Key Concept

Remember, a mutation will be inherited only if it occurs in the germ (sex) cell line. Mutations limited to somatic cells will not be passed on to the next generation. They may, however, have an important role in the development of tumors.

Viral Genetics

★★★★☆☆

Viral genomes come in a variety of shapes and sizes. Some are made of only a few genes, whereas others have several hundred. In addition, they may be made of either DNA or RNA, and they may be single- or double-stranded. Viruses are specific in terms of host selection and may even be cell specific within that host. For example, herpes simplex type 1 infects only neurons.

SINGLE-STRAND
RNA VIRUS

DOUBLE-STRAND
RNA VIRUS

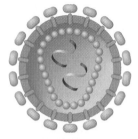

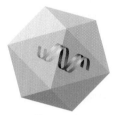

HUMAN IMMUNODEFICIENCY VIRUS
(CAUSES AIDS)

REOVIRUS
(PATHOGEN OF PLANTS
AND ANIMALS)

DOUBLE-STRAND
DNA VIRUSES

SINGLE-STRAND
DNA VIRUS

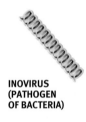

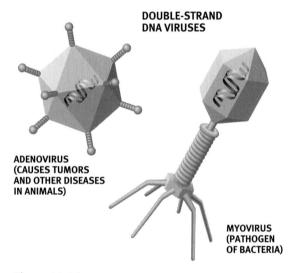

INOVIRUS
(PATHOGEN
OF BACTERIA)

ADENOVIRUS
(CAUSES TUMORS
AND OTHER DISEASES
IN ANIMALS)

MYOVIRUS
(PATHOGEN
OF BACTERIA)

Figure 15.16

INFECTION OF HOST CELL

We know from Chapter 1 that viruses cannot reproduce on their own, violating a key tenet of the Cell Theory. Instead, they must invade a host cell and hijack its machinery. Viruses may only infect cells that have receptors that recognize the viruses' protein coat (**capsid**). Otherwise, the cell is essentially invisible to the virus. Depending on the virus, different amounts of material will be inserted into the cells. Viruses such as HIV fuse and completely insert, whereas bacteriophages only insert the genetic material, leaving their capsids outside.

GENOME REPLICATION AND TRANSCRIPTION

DNA-Containing Viruses

The DNA-containing viruses have it a bit simpler than the RNA-containing ones. Because their genome is DNA, just like the cells, they can enter the nucleus and make use of the DNA and RNA polymerases found there without extra work. A few DNA viruses carry out replication in the cytoplasm. These viruses must bring with them their own DNA and RNA polymerases because the host's are restricted to the nucleus, which these particular viruses never enter.

RNA-Containing Viruses

When the viral genome is RNA, the process is slightly different and occurs in the cytoplasm. Our cells do not have enzymes to replicate RNA. Some viruses will bring **RNA replicase** with them. Others will wait for the enzyme to be translated from their own genome, which acts as mRNA for this purpose.

There is a special subclass of RNA viruses known as **retroviruses**. These viruses create a DNA copy from RNA using an enzyme called **reverse transcriptase**. It is called reverse transcriptase because it creates DNA from RNA rather than the other way around (normal transcription). These viruses then integrate the newly synthesized DNA into the host genome. This is clever, because the host will then transcribe and translate the DNA as if it were its own. Moreover, the only way to remove the offending virus genome from the cell now is to kill the cell. This is one reason why diseases such as HIV are particularly difficult to treat. The following figure shows the integration of HIV into the genome.

A SELF-COPYING COMMANDO

Efforts to devise vaccines and new treatments for HIV depend on knowledge of the virus's life cycle. HIV invades host cells and commandeers their machinery to make more copies of itself. First, a protein called Envelope on the virus must bind to CD4 and CCR5 proteins on the cell surface (*1*). As the virus fuses with the cell, it empties its contents into the cytoplasm (*2*). A viral enzyme, reverse transcriptase, then copies the virus's RNA genome into double-stranded DNA (*3*), often making errors that generate diversity in the virus copies. Another viral enzyme,

integrase, inserts the copy into the host DNA (*4*). Cell machinery transcribes the viral genes back into RNA (including RNA that can serve as templates for proteins) that travels to the cytoplasm, where ribosomes produce the encoded proteins (*5*). Viral RNA and proteins then move toward the cell membrane, where they gather into a budding virus particle (*6*). In the immature new virus copy, the HIV protease enzyme modifies viral protein chains, enabling the particles, or "virions," to mature into a form that is ready to infect a new cell (*7*).

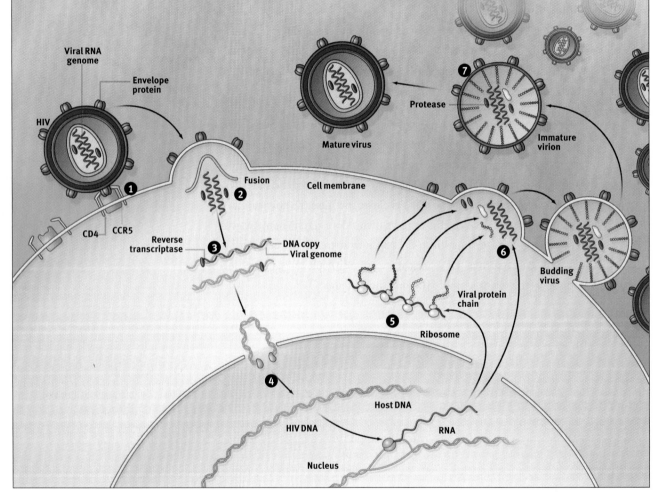

Figure 15.17

TRANSLATION AND PROGENY ASSEMBLY

Using the ribosomes, tRNA, amino acids, and enzymes of the host, the transcribed genes are now translated into protein. These proteins are usually structural and allow for creation of new viral particles (**virions**). A single virus may create hundred or thousands of new virions.

PROGENY RELEASE

Viral progeny may be released in two ways. The host cell may lyse as a result of being filled with viral particles. The viral invasion may also initiate apoptosis (cell suicide), and in the process release viral progeny. Cell lysis commonly happens when a large number of virions are formed in the cell. The disadvantage of this for the virus is that it cannot continue to use the cell for its life cycle. When a virus instead leaves the cell by fusing with its plasma membrane, the process is known as **extrusion**. It is similar to budding, and allows the virus to keep the host cell alive. A virus in this state is said to be in a **productive cycle** (see Figure 15.18).

host cell membrane

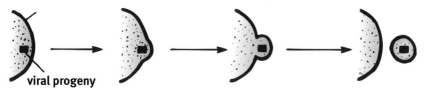

viral progeny

Figure 15.18

BACTERIOPHAGE

Bacteriophages are viruses that specifically target bacteria. As mentioned earlier, they simply insert their DNA while keeping their viral envelopes and other structures outside the cell, by boring a hole in the bacterial surface. Depending on growth conditions and the specific phage, the virus may enter a **lytic** or **lysogenic** cycle. These two phases are similar to the lysis and productive cycle that we saw previously.

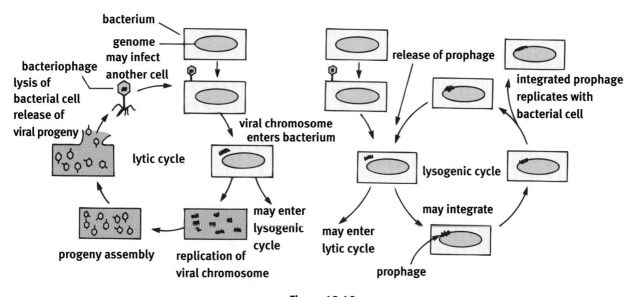

Figure 15.19

Lytic Cycle

During a lytic cycle, the virus makes maximal use of the cell's machinery with little regard to damaging the cell. Once the host is swollen like a balloon with new virions, the cell lyses and other bacteria can be infected. Bacteria in the lytic phase are termed *virulent*.

Lysogenic Cycle

In the event that the virus does not lyse the bacteria, it may integrate into the host genome as a provirus. One of the clever aspects to this system is that as the bacteria reproduces, so will the virus, because it is a part of the host's genome. Although the virus may remain indefinitely integrated into the host genome, at some point, environmental factors (radiation, light, or chemicals) will cause the provirus to leave the genome and revert to a lytic cycle (see Figure 15.19). Although phages seem quite deadly to bacteria (and make no mistake, they can be), there may be some benefit to having them integrated in the lysogenic cycle. Infection with one strain of phage generally makes the bacteria less susceptible to other phages (superinfection). Since the provirus is relatively innocuous, there may be some evolutionary advantage to this association.

Bacterial Genetics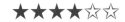

BACTERIAL GENOME

Our last set of organisms to consider are bacteria. Remember from Chapter 1 that bacteria are prokaryotes. They are single-celled organisms containing a circular DNA genome and no membrane-bound organelles. The genome localizes to the nucleoid region of the cell.

Many bacteria contain extrachromosomal material known as **plasmids**. We mentioned these in Chapter 1 as a way for bacteria to gain antibiotic resistance. A specialized subset of plasmids known as **episomes** is capable of integrating into the genome. When we discussed transcription and translation in eukaryotes, we noted that they were separate events. This distinction is in both time and space. Transcription occurs in the nucleus, whereas translation occurs in the cytoplasm. Transcription occurs well before translation, because the hnRNA must be processed and translocated to the cytoplasm before translation occurs. This is not the case in bacteria. Because there are no membrane-bound organelles, the two processes are not physically separate. In fact, they occur almost simultaneously. Recall that we saw that eukaryotic mRNA is monocistronic, meaning each mRNA can code only for one protein. Bacteria may produce polycistronic messages in which multiple proteins are coded in the same mRNA molecule.

REPLICATION

Because the bacterial chromosome is a single circular molecule, containing far fewer genes than eukaryotic chromosomes, bacteria do not need as many origins of replication. In fact, they have only one. Replication occurs in both directions at the rate of approximately 500 bases per second. A commonly used laboratory strain of *E. coli* only has about 4.5 million base pairs (compared with 3 billion in humans), so it doesn't take long for the entire genome to be duplicated.

GENETIC VARIANCE

In Chapter 4, we described the details of sexual and asexual reproduction. Under favorable growth conditions, bacteria utilize binary fission, a method of asexual reproduction, to increase their numbers rapidly. What was the important consequence of this? Each daughter cell would be genetically identical. We showed that sexual reproduction would allow for greater genetic diversity, which helps species survive less-than-ideal situations by introducing new, potentially advantageous phenotypes. Bacteria have three mechanisms to increase genetic diversity: **transformation**, **conjugation**, and **transduction**.

Transformation

Transformation results from the integration of a foreign chromosome fragment (plasmid) into the host genome. The result is a bacterium that is genetically unique from the cell that it just was and any daughter cells that it produced before adding the plasmid to its genome.

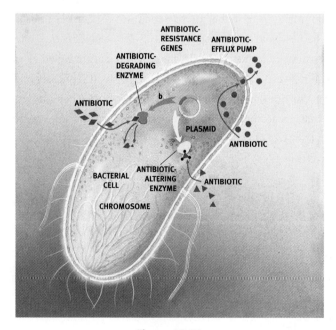

Figure 15.20

Conjugation

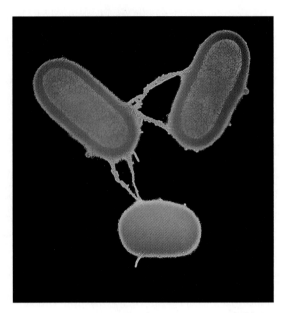

Figure 15.21

Conjugation is the bacterial form of mating (sexual reproduction). It involves two cells forming a **cytoplasmic bridge** between them that allows for the transfer of genetic material. The transfer is one way, from the **donor male (+)** to the **recipient female (−)**. The bridge is made from appendages called **sex pili** that are found on the donor male. To form the pili, bacteria must contain plasmids known as **sex factors**. The best-studied sex factor is the F factor in *E. coli*. Bacteria possessing this plasmid are termed F+ cells; those without it are called F− cells. During conjugation between an F+ and an F− cell, the F+ cell replicates its F factor and donates the copy to the recipient, converting it to an F+ cell (see Figure 15.22). Plasmids that do not induce pili formation may transfer into the recipient cell along with the sex factor.

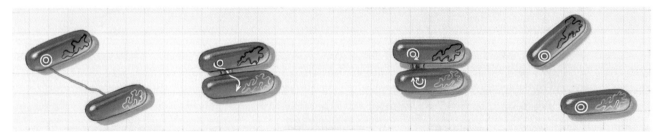

Figure 15.22

The sex factor is a plasmid, but through processes such as transformation it can become integrated into the host genome. In this case, when conjugation occurs, the entire genome replicates since it now contains the sex factor. The donor cell will then attempt to transfer its entire genome into the recipient. Usually the bridge collapses before the full DNA sequence can be moved. Cells that have undergone this change are referred to by the abbreviation **Hfr** for high frequency of recombination.

Transduction

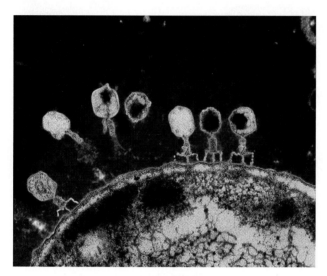

Figure 15.23

Transduction is an accidental method of genetic recombination, but this doesn't mean that it isn't useful. When bacteriophages integrate into the host genome, they do not always perfectly excise. In fact, they may be removed from the circular chromosome and take whole bacterial genes with them. These bacterial genes will then be packaged along with the viral genome, since the cellular machinery doesn't distinguish between them. The phage can then go infect a new bacterium, and when it integrates into the genome, the new host bacterium will receive the new gene (see Figure 15.24).

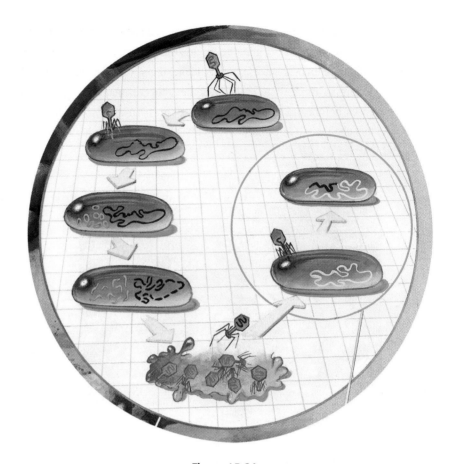

Figure 15.24

GENE REGULATION

Unlike eukaryotes, which separate their biochemical functions into distinct compartments (and thereby add a level of control), prokaryotes use regulation primarily at the transcriptional level to regulate metabolism.

In prokaryotes (and eukaryotes, as well), the ability to transcribe a gene is based on RNA polymerase's access to the genome. **Operons** direct this process. They are made up of **structural genes**, an **operator gene**, and a **promoter gene** (Figure 15.25).

Starting from the right side of Figure 15.25, we can identify each of these. The structural gene codes for the protein of interest—for example, lactase, an enzyme that digests the disaccharide lactose. Next is the operator site. It consists of a nontranscribable region of DNA that is capable of binding a repressor protein. The promoter site is similar in function to that seen in eukaryotes: It provides a place for RNA polymerase to bind. The sequence farthest to the left codes for a protein known as the **repressor**. This protein can bind to the operator sequence and acts as a roadblock. RNA polymerase cannot get from the promoter to the structural gene because the operator region has a giant repressor in the way.

These systems come in two flavors: **inducible** and **repressible**. Inducible systems require the presence of a compound known as an **inducer** to cause transcription of the structural gene. Repressible systems are the opposite. They are constantly transcribing unless a **corepresssor** is present. Let's take a look at each system in more detail.

Inducible Systems

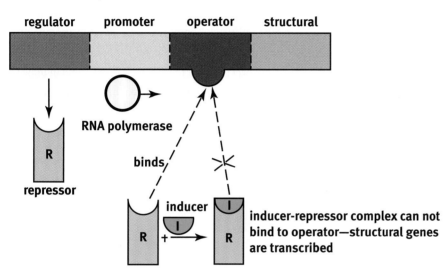

Figure 15.25

In these systems, the repressor is always made. It binds tightly to the operator sequence, and thereby prevents transcription of the structural genes. To remove the block, an inducer must bind the repressor protein so that RNA polymerase can move down the gene. Inducible systems operate on a principle analogous to competitive feedback for enzyme activity. As we raise the level of inducer high, most of the repressor will be bound to it, rather than the operator sequence. This system is useful because it allows gene products to be produced only when they are needed. An example is the *lac* operon, which codes for enzymes that allow a bacterium to digest lactose in place of glucose (see Figure 15.26). Because this is more energetically expensive, bacteria use this option only when lactose is high and glucose is low. Thus, the correct genes are induced by the situation.

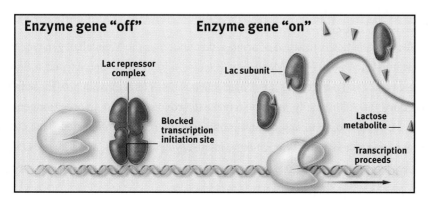

Figure 15.26

Key Concept

What sort of systems would you want to be inducible? Why make a system inducible at all? Recall that gene expression (from transcription to the final protein product) is energetically expensive. Any cell looks to do it at a minimum level of energy expenditure while maintaining maximal output. Inducible systems in bacteria are one way to do this, by preventing gene expression when it is unnecessary.

Repressible Systems

Serving as the antithesis to inducible systems, repressible systems allow constant production of a protein product. In contrast to the inducible system, the repressor made by the regulator region is inactive until it binds to a co-repressor. The complex can then bind to the operator region and prevent further transcription. Repressible systems behave on the principle of negative feedback. Often the final structural product can serve as a co-repressor. Thus, as its levels get higher, it can bind the repressor and the complex will attach to the operator region to prevent further transcription of the same gene. An example is the *trp* operon (see Figure 15.27). Bacteria produce the amino acid tryptophan under a repressible system. When tryptophan is high in the local environment, there is no need to make it internally. Tryptophan serves a corepressor and binds with the repressor as a complex to the operator, thereby preventing the bacteria from making its own tryptophan, which would be energetically wasteful.

> ## Key Concept
>
> Much as we want to be able to turn genes on when it is necessary, we would also like to be able to turn these genes off when necessary. Repressible systems allow us to do this.

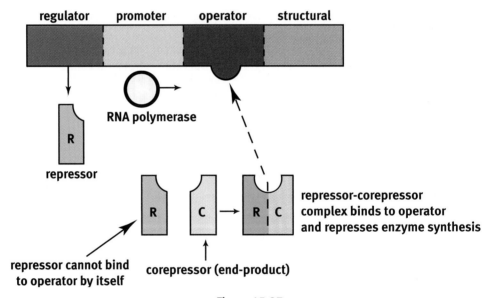

Figure 15.27

Conclusion

Molecular genetics is the field of science that underlies the Mendelian genetics that we learned in Chapter 14. Mendelian genetics allows us to predict that a flower would be tall and purple, and molecular genetics helps us figure out how those traits are coded for. Additionally, we should make the connection that, in order for genetic traits to be passed on in any organism, the genome must be replicated. This chapter has shown us how that can be done in eukaryotes, bacteria, and viruses. DNA's structure is critical to this process because it provides the genome with stability to last over the lifetime of the organism. Shorter-lived messages make use of RNA. In order to make these shorter-lived messages into proteins, we need our trusty genetic code, which serves as a translator between the language of nitrogenous bases and amino acids. Without transcription and translation, DNA can do little more than store the genome. It is the transformation of the genetic code into proteins that allows cells to go about their business. We have examined mutations, which can result in changes to the amino acid sequence and ultimately the structure and function of proteins. These changes in the DNA are the molecular basis by which evolution occurs. The next, and final, chapter will review the key concepts of evolution.

CONCEPTS TO REMEMBER

☐ DNA is deoxyribonucleic acid. It is a double-stranded, antiparallel double helix that exhibits base pairing between complementary nitrogenous bases. Its purpose is to store the genome.

☐ RNA is ribonucleic acid. It substitutes ribose for deoxyribose and uracil for thymine. It is usually single-stranded and exists in the forms of mRNA, tRNA, rRNA, and hnRNA.

☐ Replication of the genome requires enzymes to separate the strands (helicase) and insert the appropriate complmentary bases (DNA polymerase) in a $5' \rightarrow 3'$ manner.

☐ Generation of a eukaryotic mRNA from an hnRNA requires addition of a 5'-guanosyl cap and poly-A tail. Introns must also be spliced out.

☐ The genetic code is degenerate. Multiple codons may code for the same amino acid. This is one of the mechanisms by which silent mutations occur.

☐ Translation consists of three phases: initiation, elongation, and termination. The initiation and termination steps have specific codons to signify them.

☐ Post-translational modifications may include addition of covalent moieties (e.g., methylation, carboxylation, glycosylation). In addition, large peptides may be cleaved before they are active.

☐ Viral genomes are more diverse than the genomes of cellular organisms. They may be single- or double-stranded; they may also be made of DNA or RNA.

☐ Bacteria may use transduction, conjugation, and transformation to increase genetic diversity.

☐ Bacteria use inducible and repressible systems to control gene expression at the transcriptional level.

Practice Questions

1. In the DNA of a fruit fly (*Drosophila melanogaster*), 20% of the bases are cytosines. What percent are adenines?

   A. 20%
   B. 30%
   C. 40%
   D. 60%

2. In a single strand of a nucleic acid, nucleotides are linked by

   A. hydrogen bonds.
   B. phosphodiester bonds.
   C. ionic bonds.
   D. van der Waals forces.

3. What role does peptidyl transferase play in protein synthesis?

   A. It transports the initiator aminoacyl–tRNA complex.
   B. It helps the ribosome to advance three nucleotides along the mRNA in the 5' to 3' direction.
   C. It holds the protein in its tertiary structure.
   D. It catalyzes the formation of a peptide bond.

4. Which stage of protein synthesis does NOT require energy?

   A. Initiation
   B. Elongation
   C. Termination
   D. All of the above require energy.

5. Topoisomerases are enzymes involved in

   A. DNA replication.
   B. DNA transcription.
   C. RNA processing.
   D. RNA translation.

6. You have just sequenced a piece of DNA that reads:

   5'—TCTTTGAGACATCC—3'

   What would be the base sequence in the mRNA transcribed from this DNA?

   A. 5'-AGAAACUCUGUAGG-3'
   B. 5'-GGAUGUCUCAAAGA-3'
   C. 5'-AGAAACTCTGTAGG-3'
   D. 5'-GGATGTCTCAAAGA-3'

7. Which of the following statements regarding differences between DNA and RNA is FALSE?

   A. DNA is double-stranded, whereas RNA is single-stranded.
   B. DNA uses the nitrogenous base thymine; RNA has uracil.
   C. The sugar in DNA is deoxyribose; the sugar in RNA is ribose.
   D. DNA strands replicate in a 5' to 3' direction, whereas RNA is synthesized in a 3' to 5' direction.

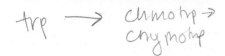

trp → chmotrp →
chymotrp

8. When trypsin converts chymotrypsinogen to chymotrypsin, some molecules of chymotrypsin bind to a repressor, which in turn binds to the operator and prevents further transcription of trypsin. To which gene regulation system is this process most similar?

   A. Transduction
   B. *lac* operon
   C. *trp* operon
   D. Lysogenic cycle

9. Which of the following DNA sequences would have the highest melting temperature?

   A. CGCAACCATGCG 8   MOST G's and C's
   B. CGCAATAATACA 4
   C. CGTAATAATACA 3
   D. CATAACAAATCA 3

10. Chemical analysis of some viral DNA has given the following results: 20 percent of the bases are adenines, 35% are thymines, 15% are cytosines, and 30% are guanines. What must be true of this DNA?

   A. It is in the process of being transcribed into mRNA.   A 20%
   B. It is mitochondrial DNA.   T 35%
   C. It is single-stranded.   C 15%
   D. It is in the S stage of the cell life cycle.   G 30%

11. Herpes is a virus that enters the human body and remains dormant in the nervous system until it produces an outbreak, without any particular reason. Which of the following statements correctly describes herpes?

   A. While it remains dormant in the nervous system, the virus is in its lysogenic cycle.
   B. During an outbreak, the virus is in the lytic cycle.
   C. Herpes integrates itself into the DNA of the cell.
   D. All of the above are true statements.

12. What does a polycistronic mRNA mean?

   A. It contains a large number of cytosine bases.
   B. It is translated to a protein that contains many cysteine amino acids.
   C. It codes for more than one polypeptide.
   D. It is translated to a protein involved in polycystic fibrosis.

13. Resistance to antibiotics is a well-recognized medical problem. What mechanisms account for a bacterium's ability to increase its genetic variability, and thus adapt itself to different antibiotics?

   A. Binary fission
   B. Conjugation
   C. Transduction
   D. Both B and C are true.

Small Group Questions

1. Many point mutations do not have an effect on the gene product. What are two possible explanations for this observation?

2. Why does DNA molecule with a high G-C content have a higher boiling point?

3. Why might a virus prefer to enter a lysogenic versus a lytic cycle?

Explanations to Practice Questions

1. B

If 20% of the bases are cytosines, 20% of the bases must also be guanines because they base pair. The remaining 60% $(100 - 20 - 20 = 60)$ of bases are adenines and thymines. Again, because of complementary base pairing, 30% must be adenines and 30% thymines. (B) is the correct answer.

2. B

Nucleotides bond together to form polynucleotides. The 3′ hydroxyl group of one nucleotide's sugar joins the 5′ hydroxyl group of the adjacent nucleotide's sugar by a phosphodiester bond. (B) is therefore the correct answer.

3. D

Peptidyl transferase is an enzyme that catalyzes the formation of a peptide bond between the amino acid attached to the tRNA in the A site and the one attached to the tRNA in the P site. (D) is therefore the correct answer.

4. D

All three stages of protein synthesis (initiation, elongation, and termination) require a large amount of energy, making (D) the correct answer.

5. A

Topoisomerases, such as DNA gyrase, are involved in DNA replication. DNA gyrase is a type of topoisomerase that enhances the action of helicase enzymes by the introduction of negative supercoils into the DNA molecule. These negative supercoils facilitate DNA replication by keeping the strands separated and untangled.

6. B

In order to answer this question correctly, we must remember that mRNA will be antiparallel to DNA. Our answer should be 5′ to 3′ mRNA, with the 5′ end complementary to DNA's 3′ end. Thus, the desired mRNA strand will be 5′-GGAUGUCUCAAAGA-3′, which matches with (B).

7. D

Since we are looking for the false statement, we have to read every choice and eliminate those that are true. Let's quickly review the main differences between DNA and RNA. DNA is double-stranded, with a deoxyribose sugar and the nitrogenous bases A, T, C, and G. RNA, on the other hand, is usually single-stranded, with a ribose sugar and the bases A, U, C, and G. (A), (B), and (C) all state correct differences between DNA and RNA. (D) is incorrect because both DNA replication and RNA synthesis proceed in a 5′ to 3′ direction. (D) is therefore the correct answer.

8. C

The question stem is basically telling us that the end product of an enzyme-catalyzed reaction binds to a repressor, which in turn binds to the operator to prevent further transcription of the enzyme. This is a repressible system of gene regulation similar to *trp* operon, in which transcription is the norm as long as there is no co-repressor present. The co-repressor (in this case, chymotrypsin) binds to the repressor, forming a complex that binds to the operator and prevents transcription. (C) is therefore the correct answer.

9. A

The melting temperature of DNA is the temperature at which a DNA double helix separates into two single strands. To do this, the hydrogen bonds linking the base pairs must be broken. Cytosine binds to guanine by three hydrogen bonds, whereas adenine binds to thymine with two hydrogen bonds. The amount of heat needed to disrupt the bonding is proportional to the number of bonds. Thus, the more C and G present in a DNA segment, the higher the melting point. Therefore, (A) will have the highest melting temperature, and (D) would have the lowest. (A) is therefore the correct answer.

10.   C

The main conclusion we can draw from the information given in the question stem is that the percentages of C and G are not equal, and the percentages of A and T are also not equal. The only explanation for this is that the DNA is single stranded, as (C) indicates.

11.   D

Viruses can exist in either the lytic or lysogenic cycle; they may even switch between them throughout their lifetime. During the lytic cycle, the virus's DNA takes control of the host cell's genetic machinery, manufacturing numerous progeny. In the end, the host cell bursts (lyses) and releases new virions, each capable of infecting other cells. In the lysogenic cycle, viral DNA is integrated into the host cell's genome, but can remain dormant for days or years. Either spontaneously or as a result of environmental circumstances, the provirus can reemerge and enter a lytic cycle. Thus, all of the answer choices correctly describe the herpes virus, making (D) the correct answer.

12.   C

The term *polycistronic* refers to prokaryotic mRNA and its ability to code for more than one polypeptide (usually a group of related proteins). (C) is therefore the correct answer.

13.   D

Bacterial cells reproduce by binary fission, an asexual process in which the progeny is identical to the parent. However, several mechanisms exist to allow for genetic variance within a population: transformation, conjugation, and transduction. Transformation is the process by which a foreign chromosome fragment is incorporated into the bacterial chromosome via recombination, creating new inheritable genetic combinations. Conjugation can be described as a sexual mating in bacteria; it is the transfer of genetic material between two bacteria that are temporarily joined. Transduction occurs when fragments of the bacterial chromosome accidentally become packaged into viral progeny produced during a viral infection. (D) is therefore the correct answer.

Evolution

We've done it! We have made it to the final chapter in our Biology Review Notes. Our final topic, evolution, is quite fitting. **Evolution** is the process of adaptation and change leading to genetic diversity and new life forms. It may be accomplished by **natural selection**, **mutation**, **genetic drift**, and **genetic shift**. Certainly over the course of reading these few hundred pages, you have evolved as a critical thinker and test taker. You have become an expert in the MCAT Biological Sciences and have emerged a new species of test taker that is meaner, leaner, and all the more ready to go out and earn a 15 on the Biological Sciences section of the MCAT. Before you can do that, though, you need to finish this chapter! It will cover different hypotheses that have been suggested to explain evolution, as well as empirical observations to support them. Evolution is a theory; it is only as good as the evidence behind it. Let's examine that evidence.

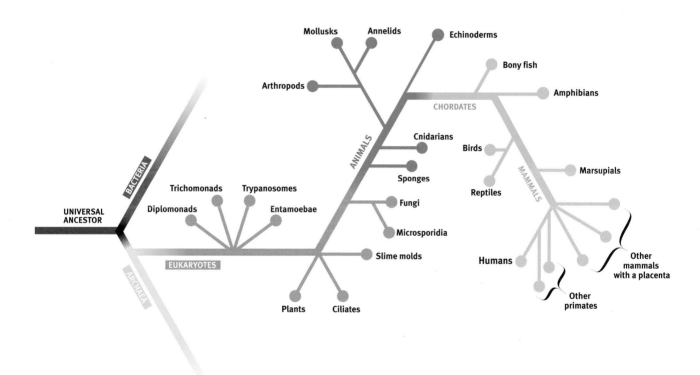

Figure 16.1

Theories of Evolution ★★★★☆

The development of evolutionary thought has a relatively short history; the first theories suggesting that new species may arise from older ones were proposed in the 19th century. Significant "evolution" of these evolutionary theories has occurred since then. We will examine four of the major contributions to the field.

LAMARCK'S INHERITANCE OF ACQUIRED CHARACTERISTICS THEORY

One of the earliest (and eventually disproven) theories of evolution was that of Jean Baptiste Lamarck. He proposed that the concept of **use and disuse** was behind the generation of newer species from older ones. Organs that were used extensively would develop, whereas those that were not used would atrophy. This would suggest, for example, that the diminutive size of the human appendix is due to its relative disuse by our evolutionary forebears. These changes were termed **acquired characteristics** by Lamarck and were proposed to underlie the emergence of new, more complex species. Lamarck is best remembered for having the first organized approach to evolution. We now know that his theory was incorrect, because traits are inherited, not acquired. This makes for an interesting concept in MCAT terms, as we must recognize that Lamarck's ideas, although testable, are spurious.

DARWIN'S NATURAL SELECTION THEORY

Darwin published *On the Origin of Species*, his masterwork, in 1859. In it, he detailed a mechanism for evolution that had several main tenets.

1. Organisms produce offspring, few of which survive to reproductive maturity.
2. Chance variations within individuals in a population may be **inheritable**. If these variations give an organism a slight survival advantage, they are termed **favorable**.
3. Individuals with a greater preponderance of these favorable variations are more likely to survive to reproductive age and produce offspring; the overall result will be an increase in these traits in future generations. This process is known as **natural selection**. Over long periods of time, aggregations of these favorable traits will result in the separation of organisms into distinct species. **Fitness** is defined as the reproductive success of an individual. Reproductive success is directly related to the relative genetic contribution of an individual to the next generation.

Darwin's theory was ultimately proven to be correct in many ways, though not completely. Carrying our appendix example forward, Darwin would suggest that having a small appendix is somehow favorable, leading to the current anatomical state of affairs. The elucidation of the larger field of genetics in the 20th century led to refinements and the currently accepted theory known as **Neo-Darwinism** or the **modern synthesis**.

NEODARWINISM (THE MODERN SYNTHESIS)

Once scientists proved that genes ultimately changed due to mutation or recombination (Chapter 14), Darwin's theory was updated to the current form. When mutation or recombination results in a change that is favorable to the organism's survival, that change is more likely to pass on to the next generation; the opposite is also true. This

Key Concept

If we see any hint of the buzz phrases *use and disuse* or *inheritance of acquired characteristics* on Test Day, think Lamarck. And don't forget—Lamarck was wrong!

Key Concept

Evolution is not equivalent to natural selection. The MCAT likes to test your ability to understand that natural selection is simply a *mechanism* for evolution. Natural selection is equivalent to *survival of the fittest*.

Key Concept

Natural Selection:

- Chance variations occur as a result of mutation and recombination.
- If the variation is "selected for" by the environment, that individual will be more "fit" and more likely to survive to reproductive age.
- Survival of the fittest leads to an increase of those favorable genes in the gene pool.

process is termed **differential reproduction**. After time, those traits passed on by the more successful organisms will become pervasive in the **gene pool**. The gene pool is the sum total of all genes from all individuals in the population at a given time. Because it is the gene pool that changes over time, we must be careful to say that populations, not individuals or species, evolve.

PUNCTUATED EQUILIBRIUM

One final theory to consider was proposed as a result of research into the fossil record. Upon examination, it was discovered that little evolution within a lineage of related forms would occur for long periods of time, followed by a massive burst. Niles Eldredge and Stephen Jay Gould proposed the theory of punctuated equilibrium to explain this in 1972. In contrast to Darwin's theory, punctuated equilibrium suggests that changes in species occur in rapid bursts rather than evenly over time. An example with which we might be familiar is that of the dinosaurs. When examining rock layers, there are many dinosaur fossils present until the Cretaceous–Tertiary Boundary, about 65 million years ago. After this, there are none but there is a relative flourishing of mammalian species. Dinosaurs did not disappear gradually from the face of the Earth; rather, there was a massive catastrophic event that fundamentally altered the course of their evolution.

Evidence of Evolution ★★★☆☆

As our sidebar pointed out, evolution is a theory that explains the origins of species. The theory of evolution functions in the same way that the theory of gravity functions to explain the behavior of mass: a scientific hypothesis supported by evidence and observation. The evidence that underlies it comes from a wide variety of scientific disciplines, including **paleontology**, **biogeography**, **comparative anatomy**, **comparative embryology**, and **molecular biology**.

PALEONTOLOGY

You may remember paleontology from when you learned about dinosaurs in middle school. Certainly, it is a wider field than that, encompassing the study of the complete fossil record. Using radioactive dating that employs some of the same principles we saw with autoradiography in Chapter 1, scientists are able to determine a fossil age. By relating the ages of different fossils to their anatomies and relative abundances, paleontologists can determine the chronological succession of species in the fossil record.

BIOGEOGRAPHY

Evolution is an interesting phenomenon because it does not occur equally in all places around the globe. Darwin made many of his observations in the Galapagos Islands, which contain a number of unique flora and fauna. On one island, he found that the species present were more similar to those on the mainland than the organisms found on the other islands. He hypothesized that these animals and plants must have migrated to the island and then evolved in isolation from one another, thereby leading to species **divergence**.

COMPARATIVE ANATOMY

By comparing similar structures between species, it is possible to determine the degree of evolutionary similarity between them. **Homologous structures** are similar in structure and share a common evolutionary origin even if they don't have a similar appearance, shape, or form. If we were to look at a bat, we initially might think that its wings are different from our arms. However, both are forearm structures that are common among mammals. So, too, are whales' flippers, which evolved from the homologous structural precursor in the common ancestor of mammals.

Analogous structures serve a common purpose but evolved separately in each species. Whereas we know that most birds and insects are capable of flight, their wings are analogous, not homologous. The species in each group that was capable of flight benefited (by way of natural selection) from this ability and developed unique mechanisms to achieve flight over time. Bird wings and bee wings serve a similar purpose but are not related in origin through evolutionary development from a common ancestor.

Finally, **vestigial structures** may be present in organisms. These are remnants of organs that have lost their ancestral function. Humans have a coccyx, commonly referred to as the tailbone. Animals with tails, use them for balance. Humans walk upright, and the structure has been lost. The appendix (Figure 16.2) is sometimes debated, but is often considered vestigial because its presence is not necessary for life. When inflamed, it is removed in a routine procedure known as an appendectomy.

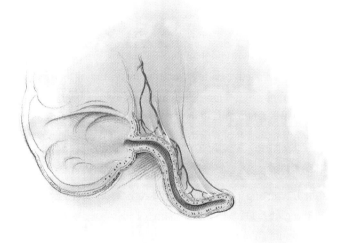

Figure 16.2

COMPARATIVE EMBRYOLOGY

We used model organisms such as sea urchins, in Chapter 5, understand human embryology. We were really doing comparative embryology at that point. By analyzing similarities between the embryos of different species, we can get a greater insight into evolutionary patterns. For example, the coccyx that we mentioned in the last paragraph as vestigial is actually present as a tail for about four weeks during human embryogenesis. Another example would be gills, which are present in all chordates (a group that includes fish, birds, and humans) during embryogenesis.

MOLECULAR BIOLOGY

As we saw in Chapter 14, DNA is capable of undergoing changes by mutation. By comparing the DNA sequence between different species, scientists can predict the degree of similarity between two organisms. For example, the chimpanzee shares over 95% of its genome with humans, whereas the mouse shares only about 85%. As species become more taxonomically distant, the amount of shared genome will decrease. One way of indirectly comparing DNA sequences is by comparing protein structures. The figure below shows how differences in protein structure indicated when new species originated.

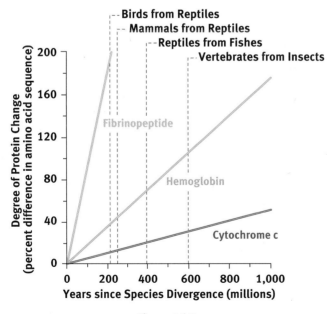

PROTEIN EVOLUTION REFLECTS SPECIES DIVERGENCE

Figure 16.3

Genetic Basis of Evolution

If evolution works by selecting those variations that are more favorable, we must have a method to generate those differences at the level of the genome. This can be accomplished through mutations, random base changes in the DNA sequence, and recombination, novel genetic combinations that result from sexual reproduction and crossing over.

HARDY-WEINBERG EQUILIBRIUM

How often an allele appears in a population is known as the **gene frequency**. For example, in your college biology course, the number of people with alleles for type A blood, divided by the total number of blood type alleles in the class, would be the gene frequency for type A blood in this group of people. Evolution results from changes in these gene frequencies in reproducing populations over time. When the gene frequencies of a population are not changing, the gene pool is stable and, no evolution is occurring. Five criteria must be met for this to be true.

1. The population is very large.
2. There are no mutations that affect the gene pool.
3. Mating between individuals in the population is random.
4. There is no net migration of individuals into or out of the population.
5. The genes in the population are all equally successful at reproducing.

Provided all these conditions are met, we can state that the population is in **Hardy-Weinberg equilibrium**, and use a pair of equations to predict the allelic and phenotypic frequencies.

Let us define a gene as having only two possible alleles, T and t. Further, we will say that p is the frequency of the dominant allele T, and q is the frequency of the recessive allele t. There are only two possible choices at the gene locus, so $p + q = 1$, because the combined frequency of the alleles must total 100%. We can square both sides of the equation to get $(p + q)^2 = 1^2$. Expanding the binomial on the left, we derive a second equation

$$p^2 + 2pq + q^2 = 1$$

Where p^2 = frequency of TT (dominant homozygotes)

$2pq$ = frequency of Tt (heterozygotes)

q^2 = frequency of tt (recessive homozygotes)

Key Concept

All you need to know to solve any MCAT Hardy-Weinberg problem is the value of p (or p^2) or q (or q^2). From there, you can calculate everything else using $p + q = 1$ and $p^2 + 2pq + q^2 = 1$.

We should be aware that each equation provides us with different information. The first tells us about the frequency of *alleles* in the population, whereas the second provides information about the frequency of a *phenotype* in the population. Both are useful pieces of information. We should also be aware that there will always be two times as many alleles in the population as there are individuals; this is because each person has two alleles. For example, if we have 100 people in the sample, there would be 200 alleles.

These equations can be used to show that if microevolution is not occurring in a population (guaranteed by the previous conditions), the gene frequencies will remain constant from generation to generation. We will show this in the example below.

Let's say that we have a population in which the frequency for the gene for tallness, T, is 0.80. This means that q is 0.20 by subtraction. Setting up our F_1 cross below for two heterozygotes, we can see the results of such a mating.

	$p = 0.80$	$q = 0.20$
$p = 0.80$	$p^2 = 0.64$ TT = 64%	$pq = 0.16$ Tt = 16%
$q = 0.20$	$pq = 0.16$ Tt = 16%	$q^2 = 0.04$ tt = 4%

We see that we get 64% homozygous tall, 32% heterozygous tall, and 4% homozygous short. These are the phenotypic frequencies. To calculate the gene frequencies, we need to look at the next table.

$$64\% \text{ TT} = 64\% \text{ T allele} + 0\% \text{ t allele}$$
$$32\% \text{ Tt} = 16\% \text{ T allele} + 16\% \text{ t allele}$$
$$4\% \text{ tt} = 0\% \text{ T allele} + 4\% \text{ t allele}$$
$$\text{Gene frequencies} = 80\% \text{ T allele} + 20\% \text{ t allele}$$

Notice that the gene frequencies are unchanged compared to the parent generation. T is still 0.80 and t is still 0.20. Species in Hardy-Weinberg equilibrium will exhibit this property.

MICROEVOLUTION

In all populations, eventually one or more of the tenets will be violated. After all, mutations in the human genome are introduced about once every 10 million base pairs during DNA replication. This alone would be enough to upset Hardy-Weinberg equilibrium, which is more a theoretical model than an assessment of real-world situations. There are five agents of microevolutionary change that we need to define briefly.

Natural Selection

Genotypes with favorable variations are selected through natural selection, and the frequency of favorable genes increases within the gene pool. If a bird has a mutation that causes its wings to be more efficient, it will have more energy to contribute instead to reproduction. Thus, it will produce more offspring and this trait will be selected for.

Mutation

Gene mutations change allelle frequencies in a population, shifting gene equilibria.

Assortive Mating

If mates are not randomly chosen, but rather, selected according to criteria such as phenotype and proximity, the relative genotype ratios will be affected, and will depart from the predictions of the Hardy-Weinberg equilibrium. On the average, allele frequencies in the gene pool remain unchanged. An example of this can be seen with Tay-Sachs disease, which is a recessive lysosomal storage disorder. The frequency of carriers in the general population is 1 in 300, meaning a random mating would only result in a 1 in 360,000 chance of having a child afflicted with the disease ($1/300 \times 1/300 \times \frac{1}{4}$). Remember that we have to multiply by $\frac{1}{4}$ because two heterozygotes only have a one-in-four chance of having an affected child. In the Ashkenazi Jewish population, the carrier rate is much higher, 1 in 30. If these individuals select mating partners within their ethnic group, they have a 1 in 3,600 chance of having an affected child. The chances are 100-fold greater owing to assortive mating.

Genetic Drift

Genetic drift refers to changes in the composition of the gene pool due to chance. Genetic drift tends to be more pronounced in small populations, where it is sometimes called the founder effect. This can happen when a small population of a species finds itself in reproductive isolation from other populations, as a result of natural barriers or catastrophic events.

Gene Flow

Migration of individuals between populations will result in a loss or gain of genes, and thus change the composition of a population's gene pool.

Modes of Natural Selection ★★★☆☆

Whereas the previous section discussed several mechanisms for microevolution, which deals with changes in a population over a short period of time (tens to hundreds of years), natural selection is the only method capable of generating stable evolutionary changes over long periods of time (thousands to millions of years).

 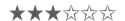

It may occur as **stabilizing selection**, **directional selection**, or **disruptive selection** (see Figure 16.4).

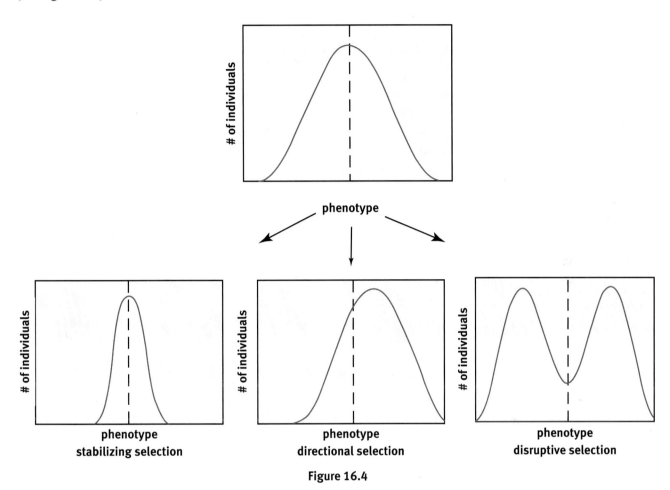

Figure 16.4

STABILIZING SELECTION

Stabilizing selections work to keep phenotypes within a specific range by eliminating extremes. For instance, human birth weight is maintained within a narrow band by stabilizing selection. Fetuses that weigh too little may not be healthy enough to survive, and fetuses that weigh too much can experience trauma during delivery through the relatively narrow birth canal. In addition, the larger the fetus, the more resources it requires from the mother. For all of these reasons, it is advantageous to keep birth weights within a narrow range.

DIRECTIONAL SELECTION

Adaptive pressure leads to the emergence and dominance of an initially extreme phenotype. If we have a heterogeneous plate of bacteria, very few may have resistance to antibiotics. If we then treat the plate with ampicillin (a type of antibiotic), only those colonies that exhibit resistance will survive. A new standard phenotype emerges as a result of differential survivorship. Natural selection is the history of differential survivorship over time. The emergence of mosquitoes resistant to DDT, a type of pesticide, is attributed to directional selection.

DISRUPTIVE SELECTION

In disruptive selection, both extreme phenotypes are selected over the norm. When Darwin studied finches on the Galapagos islands, he noted that although there were many species, they arguably all had a common ancestor. However, when he compared beak sizes, they were all either large or small. No animals exhibited the intermediate phenotype of medium-size beaks. Darwin hypothesized that the sizes of seeds, the food of the finches, on the island led to this effect. Seeds were either quite large or fairly small, requiring a large or small beak, respectively. Thus, if the original ancestor had a medium-size beak, over time, the animals with slightly larger or smaller beaks would be selected for.

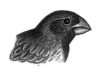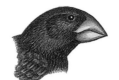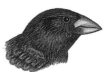

Figure 16.5

Altruistic Behavior ★★☆☆☆

Darwin's theory is not without exceptions. It has been observed in several species, including many insect species such as bees and ants, that certain individuals will endure sacrifices to benefit others. These social insects have large castes of workers that are sterile but work for the benefit of the whole colony, including the sexually reproducing insects. Such selfless behavior is termed **altruistic**.

Some attempted to explain this phenomenon by proposing group selection, suggesting that there was a gene that led certain individuals within the population not to reproduce. Can we see the flaw in this theory? How would the gene that coded for decreased or no reproduction be passed on? It couldn't; if its whole purpose was to prevent reproduction, it would be exterminated from the gene pool immediately, because it would have no way to be passed to future generations.

A related theory to group selection is **kin selection**, which suggests that organisms will behave altruistically if they are closely related to successfully reproducing organisms. This would explain our social insect example above, because the workers are related to the fertile queen of the colony. This theory is consistent with

MCAT Expertise

Like all theories, evolution also has detractors and problems. These challenges may seem to make the answers less clear on Test Day because they open up gray areas, but remember that the MCAT is written in a one-right, three-wrong format. If an answer isn't completely *right*, it is completely *wrong*. Keep your basic facts in mind for Test Day success.

neo-Darwinism. **Inclusive fitness** refers to the number of alleles that an individual passes on to the next generation, even if only indirectly through altruistic behavior.

Speciation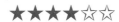

Speciation is defined as the emergence of new species, a group of individuals who can interbreed freely with each other, but not with members of other species. If we took two groups of the same species and separated them geographically for a long period of time, different evolutionary pressures would lead to different adaptive selections. If enough time passed, the changes would be sufficient to lead to **reproductive isolation**. We would now consider the two groups separate species. Reproductive isolation may occur either prezygotically or postzygotically. Prezygotic mechanisms prevent formation of the zygote completely; postzygotic mechanisms allow for gamete fusion, but yield either inviable or sterile offspring. Mules are an example of postzygotic reproductive isolation. Although a horse and donkey can produce a viable mule, the mule will be sterile and thus unable to contribute to a self-perpetuating mule lineage.

PREZYGOTIC ISOLATING MECHANISMS

Temporal Isolation
Two species may breed during different seasons or times of the day, thus preventing interbreeding.

Ecological Isolation
Two species living in the same territory but in different habitats. They rarely meet, and therefore, rarely mate.

Behavioral Isolation
Members of two species are not sexually attracted to each other because of differences in such things as pheromones (chemical signals) and courtship displays.

Reproductive Isolation
The genitalia of two species are incompatible, so interbreeding cannot occur.

Gametic Isolation
Intercourse can occur, but fertilization cannot.

POSTZYGOTIC ISOLATING MECHANISMS

Hybrid Inviability
Genetic incompatibilities between two species abort hybrid zygote development, even if fertilization does occur.

Hybrid Sterility

Hybrid offspring are sterile, and thus incapable of producing functional gametes.

Hybrid Breakdown

First-generation hybrids are viable and fertile, but second-generation hybrid offspring are inviable and/or infertile. The potential for hybrid breakdown exists whenever closely related but reproductively isolated species are introduced to each other, and occurs more in plants than in animals.

Adaptive Radiation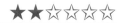

When a single ancestral species gives rise to a number of different species, **adaptive radiation** has occurred. Each species diverges to the point that it is able to occupy a unique ecological **niche**. Going back to the finches we mentioned previously, they exhibit adaptive radiation because the single ancestor led to 13 distinct species, each of which has a specific environmental role that is not filled by another species. What would be the benefit of such rapid evolution? It decreases competition for limited resources.

Patterns of Evolution

When we look at similarities between two species, we must be careful to determine whether those similarities are due to sharing a common ancestor or sharing a common environment with the same evolutionary pressures. When analyzing species this way, three patterns of evolution emerge: **convergent evolution**, **divergent evolution**, and **parallel evolution** (see Figure 16.6).

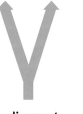 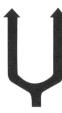 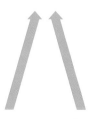

divergent evolution   parallel evolution   convergent evolution

Figure 16.6

CONVERGENT EVOLUTION

Convergent evolution refers to the independent development of similar characteristics in two or more lineages not sharing a recent common ancestor. For example, fish and dolphins have come to resemble one another physically, although they belong to different classes of vertebrates. They evolved certain similar features in adapting to the conditions of aquatic life.

DIVERGENT EVOLUTION

Divergent evolution refers to the independent development of dissimilar characteristics in two or more lineages sharing common ancestry. For example, seals and cats are both mammals belonging to the order Carnivora, yet differ markedly in general appearance. These two species live in very different environments, and adapted to different selection pressures while evolving.

PARALLEL EVOLUTION

Parallel evolution refers to the process whereby related species evolve in similar ways for a long period of time in response to analogous environmental selection pressures.

Origin of Life

Although we have discussed some very simple organisms, we have not suggested how life began. The earliest evidence of life appears in stromatolites, the trace evidence of photosynthetic bacteria, which have been dated to about 3.5 billion years ago. These organisms were primitive prokaryotes. In the 1920s, Oparin and Haldane proposed a mechanism for the origin of life, which was tested in the 1950s by Stanley Miller.

FORMATION OF ORGANIC MOLECULES

The Original Origin-of-Life Experiment

In the early 1950s Stanley L. Miller, working in the laboratory of Harold C. Urey at the University of Chicago, did the first experiment designed to clarify the chemical reactions that occurred on the primitive earth (*right*). In the flask at the bottom, he created an "ocean" of water, which he heated, forcing water vapor to circulate (*arrows*) through the apparatus. The flask at the top contained an "atmosphere" consisting of methane (CH_4), ammonia (NH_3), hydrogen (H_2) and the circulating water vapor. Next he exposed the gases to a continuous electrical discharge ("lightning"), causing the gases to interact. Water-soluble products of those reactions then passed through a condenser and dissolved in the mock ocean. The

experiment yielded many amino acids and enabled Miller to explain how they had formed. For instance, glycine appeared after reactions in the atmosphere produced simple compounds—formaldehyde and hydrogen cyanide—that participated in the set of reactions shown below. Years after this experiment, a meteorite that struck near Murchison, Australia, was shown to contain a number of the same amino acids that Miller identified (*table*) and in roughly the same relative amounts (*dots*); those found in proteins are highlighted in blue. Such coincidences lent credence to the idea that Miller's protocol approximated the chemistry of the prebiotic earth. More recent findings have cast some doubt on that conclusion.

HOW GLYCINE FORMED

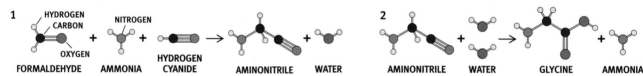

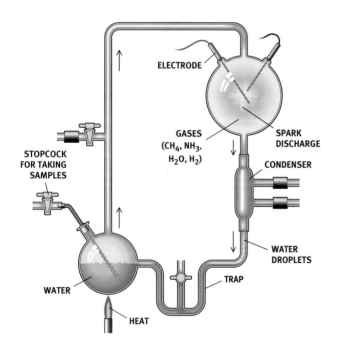

AMINO ACID	MURCHISON METEORITE	DISCHARGE EXPERIMENT
GLYCINE	• • • •	• • • •
ALANINE	• • • •	• • • •
α-AMINO-*N*-BUTYRIC ACID	• • •	• • • •
α-AMINOISOBUTYRIC ACID	• • • •	• •
VALINE	• • •	• •
NORVALINE	• • •	• • •
ISOVALINE	• •	• •
PROLINE	• • •	•
PIPECOLIC ACID	•	‹
ASPARTIC ACID	• • •	• • •
GLUTAMIC ACID	• • •	• •
β-ALANINE	• •	• •
β-AMINO-*N*-BUTYRIC ACID	•	•
β-AMINOISOBUTYRIC ACID	•	•
γ-AMINOBUTYRIC ACID	•	• •
SARCOSINE	• •	• • •
N-ETHYLGLYCINE	• •	• • •
N-METHYLALANINE	• •	• •

Figure 16.7

Oparin and Haldane suggested that the conditions of early Earth favored the creation of organic molecules such as simple amino acids. The very early planet contained high amounts of carbon, hydrogen, and nitrogen, along with lesser amounts of oxygen. The mixture of these atoms in the seas has been termed **primordial soup**. With massive energy input from many sources including the sun, lightning, radioactive decay, and volcanic activity, it was hypothesized that bonds formed between these atoms. Miller carried out an experiment in which he mixed these gases and exposed them to an electrical discharge. At the end of a week, many simple amino acids were found in the reaction apparatus. Further experimentation led to creation of all 20 amino acids, lipids, and all five of the nitrogenous bases of DNA and RNA.

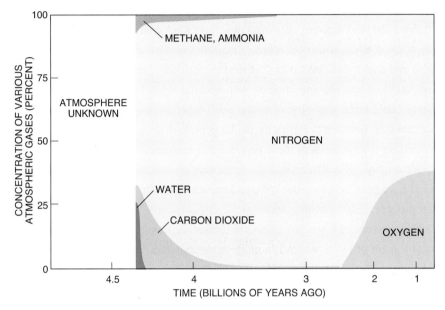

ATMOSPHERIC COMPOSITION, shown by the relative concentration of various gases, has been greatly influenced by life on the earth. The early atmosphere had fairly high concentrations of water and carbon dioxide and, some experts believe, methane, ammonia and nitrogen. After the emergence of living organisms, the oxygen that is so vital to our survival became more plentiful. Today carbon dioxide, methane and water exist only in trace amounts in the atmosphere.

Figure 16.8

FORMATION OF PROTOBIONTS

In laboratory experiments, abiotically produced polymers in an aqueous solution were found to spontaneously assemble into tiny proteinaceous droplets called microspheres. These microspheres had a selectively permeable membrane that separated them from their surroundings and maintained an independent internal environment. Colloidal droplets called coacervates had been formed in Oparin's laboratory from a solution of polypeptides, nucleic acids, and polysaccharides. They are capable of carrying out enzymatic activity within their membrane if enzymes and substrate are present. Although microspheres and coacervates have some properties characteristic of life, they are not living cells. The collection of organic polymers that are believed to have been the primitive ancestors of living cells are called *protobionts*.

FORMATION OF GENETIC MATERIAL

These hypothetical protobionts had the ability to grow in size and divide, but did not have a way of transmitting information to the next generation. The evolution of genetic material is difficult to map out, but it is believed that short strands of RNA were the first molecules capable of self-replication, and storing and transmitting information from one generation to the next. Experiments in the laboratory have shown that free bases can align with their complementary bases on a short RNA sequence and bind together, creating a new short RNA chain. Natural selection probably favored RNA sequences whose three-dimensional conformations were more stable and could replicate faster. The next evolutionary step may have involved the association of specific amino acids with specific RNA bases. Thus, an RNA sequence could bring a number of amino acids together in a particular sequence and facilitate their bonding to form a particular peptide. Natural selection may also have selected for the synthesis of those peptides that enhanced the replication and/or the further activity of the RNA. Once this hereditary mechanism developed, protobionts would have been able to grow, split, and transmit important genetic information to their progeny. Self-replicating molecules eventually evolved to code for many of the molecules needed by primitive cells. Evolutionary trends then led to the eventual establishment of DNA, which is a more stable molecule than RNA, as the primary warehouse of genetic information.

Conclusion

Our final chapter in the review of biology for the MCAT has been a journey through the relatively short history of the development of the theory of evolution. We have reviewed one of the earliest theories, Lamarck's "use and disuse", Darwin's theory of natural selection, and the modern neo-Darwinian theory founded on the understanding of molecular genetics. We noted the vast body of evidence supporting evolution, including findings in paleontology, biogeography, comparative anatomy, comparative embryology, and molecular biology. The genetic basis of evolution explains both macro- and microevolutionary development, which can result in speciation and subspeciation, respectively. Within the realm of microevolution, the MCAT will expect you to be able to analyze allelic frequencies in genetically stable populations using the Hardy-Weinberg equations. We reviewed the key concepts of natural selection and patterns of macroevolution. Finally, we discussed an important theory on the origin of life and the development of organic molecules that became the basis for RNA and DNA.

Although our time together has been brief, we would like to congratulate you on a job well done completing these review notes. The MCAT is an exam that requires you to be an expert on a great deal of content. It is our sincere hope that these pages have illuminated you. As you continue your studies approaching Test Day, return to these chapters when you are feeling a little unsure of a topic; let them be your constant guide to the highest yield material for the MCAT. We hope that we have accomplished our goal of reviewing the biology content clearly and concisely. Furthermore, we hope that we have been able to assure you of your ability to perform well on the MCAT. Your success on the exam is based on the hard work you invest now. You can be sure that your time and effort will pay off in points on Test Day. Finally, we hope that we have been able to help you enjoy the learning process. We know and understand that this is not an easy test for which to prepare. We know that it is not always fun. We know that it can be frustrating, stressful, and anxiety provoking. But we also know that the art and science of medicine is your passion. Biology—and physics and chemistry—is the foundation upon which your future medical practice is built. What could be more fun and more rewarding than the opportunity to prove yourself intellectually capable of success in your passionate pursuit of excellence in the medical sciences? We wish you all the best on your MCAT and in your future career as a physician!

CONCEPTS TO REMEMBER

- ☐ Evolution is the process of adaptation and change leading to genetic diversity and new life forms.

- ☐ Lamarck wrongly suggested that evolution occurred by increased or decreased use of a structure.

- ☐ Darwin's theory of natural selection in its modern synthesis is capable of explaining much of the evolutionary record. Natural selection states that those organisms with more favorable traits will have greater reproductive success, thereby leading to those traits being expressed to a greater degree in the next generation.

- ☐ Punctuated equilibrium is an alternative theory of evolution stating that evolution occurs in rapid bursts rather than gradually over time.

- ☐ Hardy-Weinberg equilibrium can be used to predict phenotypic and allelic frequencies in a nonevolving population.

- ☐ Whereas microevolution may occur by many mechanisms, long-term evolutionary changes may be carried out only by natural selection. Natural selection may be classified as stabilizing, directional, or disruptive selection based on the new species deviation from the original normative standard.

- ☐ Altruistic behavior benefits one individual at the direct reproductive expense of another.

- ☐ Evolution may be described as convergent, divergent, or parallel.

- ☐ Experimental evidence from Stanley Miller demonstrates that the primordial environment of the earth was sufficient to create the organic molecules necessary for life.

- ☐ RNA is thought to be the first molecule capable of passing genetic information on to the next generation.

Practice Questions

1. Which of the following statements is INCORRECT regarding inheritance of traits?

   A. A mutation due to excessive amounts of ultraviolet light in a female occurs in an unfertilized egg; this will affect the child who is born from that egg.
   B. The muscular strength gained by a weightlifter during his lifetime is inherited by his children.
   C. A green-feathered bird that survived all of the predators in the forest will pass on the green feather genes to its offspring.
   D. A flower with tasty nectar that is eaten by a butterfly is more likely to pass on its delicious genes through the pollen spread by the butterfly than one that is not tasty and falls on the ground.

2. Which of the following statements is FALSE based on Darwin's theory of evolution?

   A. Natural selection is the driving force of evolution.
   B. Favorable genetic variations become more and more common in individuals throughout their lives.
   C. Natural selection drives organisms to live in groups and ultimately become distinct species.
   D. Fitness is measured in terms of reproductive success.

3. Which of the following is NOT a necessary condition for the Hardy-Weinberg equilibrium?

   A. Large population size
   B. No mutations
   C. Mating partners are monogamous
   D. There is no net migration into or out of the population

4. As the climate got colder during the Ice Age, a particular species of mammal evolved a thicker layer of fur. This is an example of what kind of selection?

   A. Stabilizing selection
   B. Directional selection
   C. Disruptive selection
   D. Speciation

5. At what point are two populations descending from the same ancestral stock considered separate species?

   A. When they can no longer produce viable, fertile offspring
   B. When they look significantly different from each other
   C. When they can interbreed successfully and produce offspring
   D. When their habitats are separated by a significantly large distance so that they cannot meet

6. In a nonevolving population, there are two alleles, R and r, which code for the same trait. The frequency of R is 30%. What are the frequencies of all the possible genotypes?

   A. 49% RR, 42% Rr, 9% rr
   B. 30% RR, 21% Rr, 70% rr
   C. 0.09% RR, 0.42% Rr, 0.49% rr
   D. 9% RR, 42% Rr, 49% rr

7. As the ocean became saltier, whales and fish independently evolved mechanisms to maintain the concentration of salt in their bodies; this can be explained by

   A. divergent evolution.

   B. parallel evolution.

   C. convergent evolution.

   D. analogous evolution.

8. In a particular Hardy-Weinberg population, there are only two eye colors: brown and blue. 36% of the population has blue eyes, the recessive trait. What percentage of the population is heterozygous for brown eyes?

   A. 24%

   B. 48%

   C. 60%

   D. 64%

9. In a certain population, 64% of individuals are homozygous for curly hair (CC). The gene for curly hair is dominant to the gene for straight hair, c. What percentage of the population has curly hair?

   A. 4%

   B. 32%

   C. 64%

   D. 96%

10. Which of the following was NOT a belief of Darwin's?

   A. Evolution of species occurs gradually and evenly over time.

   B. There is a struggle for survival among organisms.

   C. Genetic mutation and recombination are the driving forces of evolution.

   D. Those individuals with fitter variants will survive and reproduce.

11. The proposed primordial soup was composed of organic precursor molecules formed by interactions between all the following gases EXCEPT

   A. oxygen and hydrogen.

   B. helium.

   C. nitrogen.

   D. carbon.

12. Microspheres can be characterized by all of the following statements EXCEPT

   A. they are composed of tiny, abiotically produced proteinaceous droplets.

   B. they are also known as colloidal droplets called coacervates.

   C. they have a selectively permeable membrane.

   D. they have an internal chemical environment distinct from that of their surroundings.

Small Group Questions

1. Why is it incorrect to regard evolution as progressive (i.e., proceeding from lowest or simplest to highest or most complex)?

2. Adaptive radiation results when an ancestral species gives rise to many descendants, which are adapted to different parts of the environment. How would scenarios for adaptive radiation differ if speciation occurred allopatrically (different ranges) versus sympatrically (overlapping ranges)?

3. Typically, r-selected species produce many offspring, each of which has a relatively low probability of surviving to adulthood. On the other hand, k-selected species invest more heavily in fewer offspring, each of which has a relatively high probability of surviving to adulthood. In the scientific literature, r-selected species are occasionally referred to as "opportunistic," whereas k-selected species are described as in "equilibrium." Using natural selction, explain the advantage of each.

4. Can Hardy-Weinberg equilibrium be achieved in nature? Why or why not?

Explanations to Practice Questions

1. B

In order to find the correct answer, we have to read each choice in part and eliminate the ones that fit with the modern-day theories of inheritance. Basically, any statement that will argue that acquired characteristics are passed on to the offspring will be incorrect. Based on this, we can tell right away that (B) is incorrect because the muscular strength is an acquired characteristic and thus cannot be transmitted on to the offspring. Lamarck argued that a giraffe that stretches its neck to reach for high trees will produce offspring with longer necks, but modern evolutionary theories proved this argument to be incorrect. (B) therefore is the correct answer.

2. B

Darwin's theory of natural selection, in a nutshell, argues that chance variations in our genes occur thanks to mutation and recombination, and that if the variation helps the individual survive to reproductive age and produce many offspring, the variation of the fit individual will be transmitted to the next generation. The survival of the fittest leads to an increase of those favorable genes in the gene pool. Basically, Darwin strongly believed that, as (A) states, natural selection is the driving force of evolution and that the fitness of an individual is measured in terms of reproductive success, as (D) indicates. Through natural selection, organisms become separated in groups, depending on how adapted they are to a particular environment, and these groups eventually separate to the point of becoming distinct species. Thus, based on Darwin's theory, (B) is the false statement. The theory of natural selection applies to a population of organisms, not to a particular individual. As such, favorable genetic variations become more and more common from generation to generation, not during the lifetime of an individual. In fact, the chance mutations an individual organism accumulates over its lifespan are more likely to be harmful than helpful. (B) is therefore the correct answer.

3. C

The Hardy-Weinberg equilibrium exists in certain ideal conditions which, when satisfied, allow one to calculate the gene frequencies within a population. The Hardy-Weinberg equation can be applied only under these five conditions: 1) the population is very large; 2) there are no mutations that affect the gene pool; 3) mating between individuals in the population is random; 4) there is no net migration of individuals into or out of the population; 5) the genes in the population are all equally successful at reproduction. Thus, from the given choices, only (C) is incorrect. Monogamy is not a necessary condition for the Hardy-Weinberg equilibrium to be applied, making (C) the correct answer.

4. B

The situation described in the question stem is an example of directional selection. In directional selection, the phenotypic norm of a particular species shifts toward an extreme to adapt to a selective pressure, such as an increasingly colder environment. Only those individuals with a thicker layer of fur were able to survive during the Ice Age, thus shifting the phenotypic norm. (B) is the correct answer.

5. A

Two populations are considered separate species when they can no longer interbreed and produce viable, fertile offspring. (A) is therefore the correct answer.

6. D

Let's use the information provided by the question stem to set up our equations.

We are told that the frequency of R equals 30%, and as such, $p = 0.30$. The frequency of the recessive gene $r = 100\% - 30\% = 70\%$; thus, $q = 0.70$. The frequency of the genotypes, according to the Hardy-Weinberg equilibrium, is $p^2 + 2pq + q^2 = 1$, where $p^2 = $ RR, $2pq = $ Rr, and $q^2 = $ rr. We can now calculate the frequencies of all the possible genotypes:

$$p^2 = (0.3)^2 = 0.09 = 9\% \text{ RR}$$
$$2pq = 2(0.3)(0.7) = 0.42 = 42\% \text{ Rr}$$
$$q^2 = (0.7)^2 = 0.49 = 49\% \text{ rr}$$

Choice (D) matches our results and is therefore the correct answer.

7. C

When two or more lineages not sharing a recent common ancestor independently developed similar characteristics, a convergent evolution is said to have taken place. Whales and fish do not share a recent common ancestor; whales are mammals, but fish are not. Since they both independently developed a similar mechanism to maintain the concentration of salt in their bodies, convergent evolution must have occurred. (C) is therefore the correct answer.

8. B

Using the information given to use in the question stem, we can determine that the percentage of the population with blue eyes (genotype = bb) = 36%= $q^2 = 0.36$; therefore, $q = 0.6$. Since this is a Hardy-Weinberg population, we can assume that $p + q = 1$, so $p = 1 - 0.6 = 4$. The frequency of heterozygous brown eyes is therefore $2pq = 2(0.4)(0.6) = 0.48$. So, 48% of the population is heterozygous for brown eyes, making (B) the correct answer.

9. D

We can assume that this is a Hardy-Weinberg population since we are not told otherwise. Let us denote P, the frequency of the dominant allele (C), and q the frequency of the recessive allele (c). The CC frequency is 64%, which means that $p^2 = 0.64$, or $p = 0.80$. Since $p + q = 1$, $q = 1 - 0.80 = 0.20$. The problem asks for the percentage of the population with curly hair; this includes both homozygous and heterozygotes (CC and Cc). The genotype frequencies can be found using the equation $p^2 + 2pq + q^2$.

$$CC = p^2 = (0.8)^2 = 0.64 = 64\% \text{ homozygous curly}$$
$$Cc = 2pq = 2(0.8)(0.2) = 0.32 = 32\% \text{ heterozygous curly}$$
$$Cc = q^2 = (0.20)^2 = 0.04 = 4\% \text{ straight hair}$$

Therefore, the percentage of the population with curly hair is 64% + 32% = 96%, making (D) the correct answer.

10. C

Darwin's main argument was that natural selection is the driving force of evolution. He argued that chance variations occur thanks to mutations and recombination. If the variation is selected for by the environment, that individual will be more fit and more likely to survive to reproductive age. Survival of the fittest leads to an increase of those favorable genes in the gene pool. Based on this, (C) is the correct answer, because it does not match Darwin's beliefs regarding evolution.

11. B

According to Oparin and Haldane, the conditions during the early years of Earth's existence favored the abiotic synthesis of organic molecules. Carbon, hydrogen, nitrogen, and small amounts of oxygen present in the atmosphere and seas bonded together in various ways and accumulated, forming a primordial soup. Thus, out of the answer choices, the molecule that did not participate in the formation of the precursor molecules was helium, (B).

12. B

In laboratory experiments, abiotically produced polymers in an aqueous solution can spontaneously assemble into tiny proteinaceous droplets called microspheres. These microspheres have selectively permeable membranes and their internal chemical environment is distinct from that of their surroundings. Colloidal droplets are called coacervates. Thus, from the given choices, the one that does not describe microspheres is (B), the correct answer.

High-Yield Problem Solving Guide for Biology

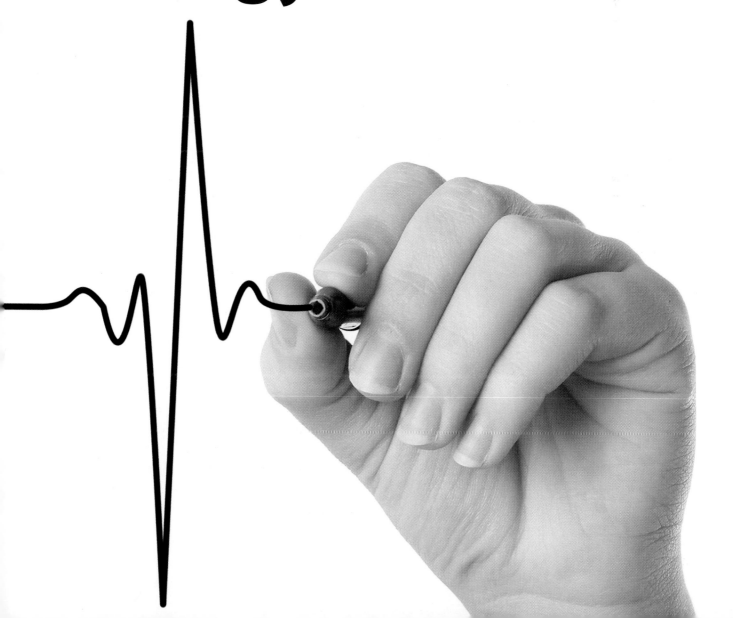

High-Yield MCAT Review

This is a special **High-Yield Questions spread**. These questions tackle the most frequently tested topics found on the MCAT. For each type of problem, you will be provided with a stepwise technique for solving the question and key directional points on how to solve for the MCAT specifically.

At the end of each topic you will find a "Takeaways" box, which gives a concise summary of the problem-solving approach; and a "Things to watch out for" box, which points out any caveats to the approach discussed above that usually lead to wrong answer choices. Finally, there is a "Similar Questions" box at the end so you can test your ability to apply the stepwise technique to analogous questions.

We're confident that this guide can help you achieve your goals of MCAT success and admission into medical school!

Good luck!

Key Concepts

Chapter 5

Fetal circulation

Fetal structures

Fetal Circulation

Fetal lungs are supplied with only enough blood to nourish the lung tissue itself because fetal lungs do not function prior to birth. Obstruction of which fetal structure would cause an increase in blood supply to fetal lungs?

1) Identify the unique structures involved in fetal circulation.

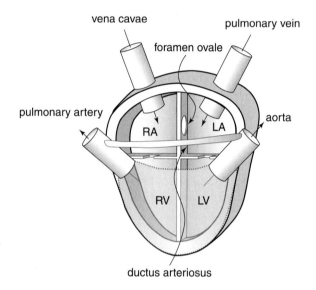

Fetal circulation differs from adult circulation in several important ways. The major difference is that in fetal circulation, blood is oxygenated in the placenta because, as the question states, fetal lungs are nonfunctional before birth. The fetal circulatory route contains three shunts that divert blood flow away from the developing fetal liver and lungs. The umbilical vein carries oxygenated blood from the placenta to the fetus. The blood bypasses the fetal liver by way of a shunt called the ductus venosus, before converging with the inferior vena cava. The inferior and superior vena cavae return deoxygenated blood to the right atrium. Because the oxygenated blood from the umbilical vein mixes with the deoxygenated blood of the vena cavae, the blood entering the right atrium is only partially oxygenated. Most of this blood bypasses the pulmonary circulation and enters the left atrium directly from the right atrium by way of the foramen ovale, a shunt that diverts blood away from the right ventricle and pulmonary artery. The remaining blood in the right atrium empties into the right ventricle and is pumped to the lungs via the pulmonary artery. Most of this blood is shunted directly from the pulmonary artery to the aorta via the ductus arteriosus, diverting even more blood away from the fetal lungs.

2) Examine the normal flow of blood to fetal lungs.

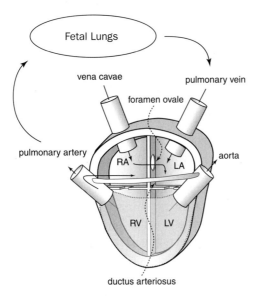

Takeaways

Understand the differences in fetal circulation and adult circulation and be able to apply that knowledge to situations in which the normal flow of blood is altered.

In the fetus, the pulmonary arteries carry oxygenated blood to the lungs, though this blood is by no means saturated with oxygen. The blood that is delivered to the lungs is further deoxygenated there because the blood unloads its oxygen to the fetal lungs, which need it for proper development. Remember, gas exchange does not occur in the fetal lungs—it occurs in the placenta. The deoxygenated blood then returns to the left atrium via pulmonary veins. Despite the fact that this blood mixes with the partially oxygenated blood that crossed over from the right atrium (via the foramen ovale) before being pumped into the systemic circulation by the left ventricle, the blood delivered via the aorta has an even lower partial pressure of oxygen than the blood that was delivered to the lungs. Deoxygenated blood is returned to the placenta via the umbilical arteries.

Things to Watch Out For

Remember that the umbilical vein in the fetus carries oxygenated blood.

3) Determine which structure is most critical in bypassing fetal lungs.
The ductus arteriosus and foramen ovale shunt blood from the pulmonary arteries to the systemic circulation, bypassing the lungs. Obstruction of either structure would cause an increase in blood supply to the fetal lungs because all of the blood pumped into the pulmonary arteries by the right ventricle would then have to flow through the lungs—there would be no place else for it to go.

Remember: There are three important shunts that divert blood flow in the fetus: the ductus venosus, the foramen ovale, and the ductus arteriosus.

Similar Questions

1) What symptoms might a baby have if the ductus arteriosus fails to close at birth?

2) What symptoms might a baby have if the foramen ovale fails to close at birth?

3) At birth, there is a reversal in the pressure gradient between the atria. What is responsible for this reversal?

Digestive System

In the gastric phase of digestion, food in the stomach, particularly the presence of amino acids and peptides, causes G cells to secrete gastrin, which in turn stimulates parietal cells. Gastrin secretion is normally inhibited once acidic chyme, with a pH less than 3, reaches the duodenum. What physiological condition would be the result of a gastrin-secreting tumor?

1) Determine the role of gastrin in the stomach.

According to the question stem, gastrin stimulates parietal cells when food is present in the stomach. Parietal cells secrete HCl, and therefore gastrin is a physiological agonist of HCl secretion. Once the chyme reaches a certain acidity (pH < 3) and moves into the small intestine, gastrin secretion is inhibited and therefore HCl secretion is decreased.

2) Determine the role of HCl in the stomach.

In the stomach, HCl is necessary for the proper function of pepsin because the proper pH for pepsin is between 1 and 3.

3) Examine what occurs when acidic chyme reaches the small intestine.

Once the chyme moves into the small intestine, the pH needs to be increased in order to reach the optimal pH (≈ 8) for pancreatic proteases and lipases. Therefore, gastrin release is inhibited and the pancreas is stimulated to secrete bicarbonate in order to neutralize the acid. The pancreas also releases hydrolytic enzymes such as amylase, trypsinogen, chymotrypsinogen, and pancreatic lipases.

4) Examine the effect of a gastrin-secreting tumor.

A gastrin-secreting tumor will secrete gastrin at all times and will not be inhibited by normal feedback mechanisms such as the presence of chyme in the small intestine. This gastrin will continually stimulate parietal cells to produce HCl. This excess of acid will move with the chyme into the small intestine. Normal amounts of bicarbonate will be released; however, this is not enough to neutralize such an excess of HCl.

5) Determine the effects of an acidic environment in the small intestine.

Pancreatic juices require a less acidic environment than do stomach enzymes. If the environment in the small intestine is too acidic, then pancreatic secretions will be unable to function normally. While proteins and carbohydrates are partially digested before they reach the small intestine, fats do not begin digestion until they reach the duodenum. If pancreatic lipases are unable to function due to an excessively acidic environment, they will not be able to digest lipids. This hypersecretion of gastrin will lower the pH of the duodenum so that pancreatic lipases are inactivated. This will result in the malabsorption of lipids, also known as steatorrhea.

Remember: *The pH levels of the stomach and the small intestine affect the ability of enzymes to function properly.*

Similar Questions

1) A patient with a peptic ulcer takes a large overdose of antacid. This would affect the activity of what enzyme?

2) Pancreatic ductal cells secrete bicarbonate, which is moved into the intestinal lumen. What would be the physiological results if these ductal cells were destroyed by an autoimmune disorder?

3) Pancreatitis is a disease that prevents the pancreas from being able to produce adequate amounts of lipase enzymes. What will be the physiological results of this disease?

Key Concepts

Chapter 1

Hypertonic solution

Hypotonic solution

Sodium potassium pump

Takeaways

Questions that involve osmosis are usually combined with other biology topics (particularly kidney function) to create a multistep solution. The key is to have a solid understanding of what hypertonic and hypotonic mean, and how the terms can be used interchangeably to describe the same state.

Things to Watch Out For

Some students presume that the scenario presented will eventually return to equilibrium and may actually predict that ATP consumption will decrease and then increase. However, the question stem does not speak of a return to equilibrium. Be wary of trying to read too much into the question.

Osmosis

The sodium potassium pump is an ATPase that pumps 3 Na^+ out of the cell and 2 K^+ into the cell for each ATP hydrolyzed. Cells can use the pump to help maintain cell volume. What would most likely happen to the rate of ATP consumption if a cell were moved to a hypertonic environment?

1) Determine the relationship between two solutions to predict the flow of water.

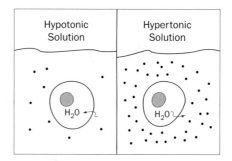

A hypertonic environment means that the environment is more concentrated than the cell is. Note that you can similarly express this condition by stating that the cell is hypotonic to the environment. A hypotonic solution is one that is less concentrated than the solution to which it is being compared.

The cell is being moved into a hypertonic environment, which means that the environment is more concentrated with solutes than the interior of the cell. Thus, we can predict that water will flow out of the cell.

2) Given the flow of water, determine how the biological function in the question will be affected.

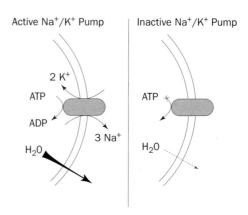

Water will flow out of the cell, thus decreasing cell volume. To counter this effect, ATP consumption will decrease to maintain cell volume.

The sodium potassium pump moves in two potassium ions as it moves out three sodium ions. The net effect is to decrease cell solute concentration as the cell loses one ion per each pump. The pump is dependent upon ATP consumption; therefore, relative to its current rate of ATP consumption, an increase in consumption will decrease cell volume whereas a decrease in consumption will increase cell volume.

Similar Questions

1) Antidiuretic hormone (ADH) directly increases the ability of the blood to reabsorb water from the nephron. If an individual's blood becomes hypotonic with respect to the filtrate, would ADH secretion increase or decrease?

2) The reabsorption of water from the filtrate increases as the concentration of the interstitial fluid increases. Using the terms "hypertonic" and "hypo-osmotic," describe the relationship between the interstitial fluid and the filtrate as well as the relationship between the filtrate and the interstitial fluid.

3) Alcohol and caffeine block the activity of ADH, a hormone that increases the ability of the blood to reabsorb water from the filtrate. An individual drinks a large coffee in the morning, and when he goes to the restroom finds that his urine is nearly colorless. Was the urine produced hypotonic, isotonic, or hypertonic to the blood?

Respiratory System

The volume of the lungs that does not participate in gas exchange is considered physiological dead space. There are two types of dead space that are seen at rest: anatomical and alveolar. Anatomical dead space is in the conducting areas, such as the mouth and trachea, where oxygen enters the respiratory system but does not contact alveoli. Alveolar dead space is the area in the alveoli that does contact air but lacks sufficient circulation to participate in gas exchange. How can physiological dead space be reduced?

1) Examine each type of dead space separately.
Anatomical dead space refers to the air that remains in the mouth and trachea with every breath. Because the size and length of the mouth and trachea are set and relatively unchangeable, it is unlikely that physiological dead space can be decreased through the anatomical dead space.

Alveolar dead space involves alveoli that contact air but do not participate in gas exchange. Because the alveoli are normal, they are capable of participating in gas exchange under the right conditions; therefore, alveolar dead space can be reduced.

---

2) Review the method of gas exchange at the tissues and in the lungs.

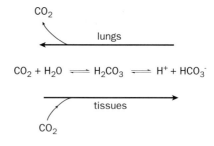

In the normal lung, O_2 will diffuse from alveolar air into the pulmonary capillary. When the partial pressures of O_2 in alveolar air and capillary blood equilibrate, the diffusion stops. Normally this occurs before the blood in the pulmonary capillary passes out of the lungs and is considered perfusion-limited gas exchange. This O_2 is bound to hemoglobin and is taken and released to the tissues. CO_2 is produced by the tissues and diffuses into capillary blood, where it is carried to the lungs as HCO_3^-. At the lungs, the reaction is reversed and CO_2 is exhaled.

---

3) Determine why some alveoli do not participate in gas exchange.

There is not sufficient blood flow through the capillaries of these "dead space" alveoli to induce them to participate in gas exchange. There must be blood flow in order for gas exchange to occur.

---

4) Determine how to increase blood flow through the lungs.

If pulmonary blood flow were increased, then more alveoli would be perfused with blood and would therefore participate in gas exchange. Increasing pulmonary blood flow would require increasing the output of the right ventricle. Cardiac output increases during exercise because there is an increased heart rate and increased venous return due to skeletal muscle activity. Therefore, exercise would increase the amount of pulmonary blood flow. This increased flow of blood through the lungs would recruit more alveoli for gas exchange and therefore reduce alveolar and physiological dead space.

Remember: Gas exchange occurs between alveolar air and the pulmonary capillaries. In order to increase the number of alveoli being used for gas exchange, the amount of pulmonary blood available for gas exchange must also be increased.

Similar Questions

1) What is the result if blood flow to the left lung is completely blocked by a pulmonary embolism?

2) If an area of the lung is not ventilated due to an obstruction, what is the partial pressure of oxygen (Po_2) of the pulmonary capillary in that area?

3) At what point will the diffusion of air from the alveoli to the capillary stop?

Circulation

Increased O_2 consumption in the left ventricle coupled with left ventricular hypertrophy and a heart murmur is most likely the result of what condition, and what symptoms would be seen in a patient with this condition?

1) Examine the reasons for increased O_2 consumption in the heart.

O_2 consumption in the heart increases when there is increased afterload (or increased aortic pressure), increased heart rate, increased contractility, and/or increased size of the heart.

2) Examine the reasons for left ventricular hypertrophy.

Left ventricular hypertrophy is the abnormal enlargement of the muscle of the left ventricle. This thickening occurs when the left ventricle has to work harder to generate enough force to overcome greater pressure as it is pumping (greater afterload).

3) Review the flow of blood through the heart.

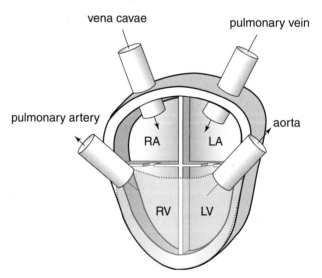

Takeaways

It's important to be able to integrate knowledge from different areas, in this case O_2 consumption, blood flow, and the pathway of the heart, when examining a question.

Blood travels into the right atrium through the vena cava. It moves through the tricuspid valve into the right ventricle and is then passed into the pulmonary artery, which carries it to the lungs. After leaving the lungs, blood travels through the pulmonary vein to the left atrium, then through the mitral valve into the left ventricle. The left ventricle pumps blood through the aortic valve into the aorta.

4) Determine the cause of the heart murmur.

Heart murmurs result from turbulent blood flow through the heart, particularly through the valves. Deformities of a valve will cause blood flow through the valve to become turbulent and create a heart murmur.

5) Determine the cause of the left ventricular hypertrophy and the increased O_2 consumption.

The left ventricle thickens and uses more oxygen because it cannot easily pump the blood through the aortic valve into the aorta. Stenosis is a condition in which the leaves of a heart valve adhere to each other, decreasing the volume of blood flow through the valve. Therefore, a stenotic aortic valve would make pumping blood through the aortic valve more difficult and lead to increased O_2 consumption and left ventricular hypertrophy.

6) Determine the effects of decreased blood flow due to aortic stenosis.

If less blood can be pumped from the left ventricle into the aorta, the ability to supply the body with blood will be reduced. This can cause blood to back up into the lungs and cause shortness of breath, especially with activity, as well as chest pain. Also, because less blood will be going out to the body, weakness can result; further, because less blood will be going to the brain, fainting is also a symptom of aortic stenosis.

Remember: *Knowing the pathway that blood takes through the heart is essential!*

Similar Questions

1) Where would a patient diagnosed with stenosis of the mitral valve experience the greatest increase in blood pressure?

2) If a tracer substance were injected into a patient's superior vena cava, which structure would it reach last before leaving the heart?

3) The decrease in the number of pulmonary capillaries due to the loss of functional lung tissue will most likely result in a pressure overload. Where will this overload occur?

Normal Oxygen Dissociation Curve

How does the oxygen dissociation curve of arterial blood differ from the curve for venous blood, and what accounts for this difference?

1) Review the normal oxygen dissociation curve.

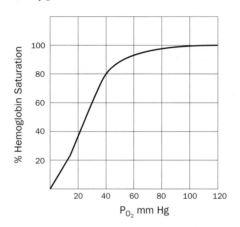

The oxygen dissociation curve shows the percent saturation of hemoglobin as a function of the partial pressure of O_2 (P_{O_2}). At $P_{O_2} = 100$ mm Hg, hemoglobin saturation is 100%, which means that four oxygen molecules are bound to the hemoglobin. At $P_{O_2} = 40$ mm Hg, hemoglobin is 80% saturated and at $P_{O_2} = 25$ mm Hg, hemoglobin is 50% saturated with oxygen molecules. The cooperative binding of O_2, meaning the binding of the first O_2 molecule, facilitates the binding of the next and results in a sigmoidal, or S-shaped, curve.

2) Examine how arterial blood differs from venous blood.

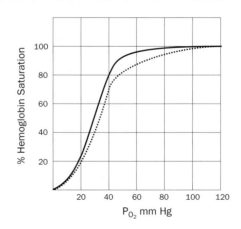

After blood passes through the lungs and into the arteries, the hemoglobin is 100% saturated with oxygen. The tissues of the body produce CO_2 as waste. The increase in CO_2 at the tissues decreases the pH of the tissues. Increases in CO_2 or decreases in pH decrease the affinity of hemoglobin for oxygen and cause the curve to shift slightly to the right, increasing the P_{O_2} and facilitating the unloading of O_2 at the tissues. The tissues keep P_{O_2} low by consuming O_2 for aerobic metabolism, so that the O_2 diffusion gradient is maintained. In arterial blood, the hemoglobin saturation at 40 mm Hg is 80%, but in venous blood the Hb saturation at 40 mm Hg is 75%. Therefore, about 5% more oxygen is released. This right shift of the curve is known as the Bohr effect. An increase in temperature also causes a right shift.

At the lungs, alveolar gas has a P_{O_2} of 100 mm Hg. O_2 diffuses from the alveolar air into the capillaries. O_2 is bound very tightly to hemoglobin because at a P_{O_2} of 100 mm Hg, hemoglobin has a very high affinity for O_2. This maintains the partial pressure gradients and facilitates the diffusion of oxygen into the blood.

Similar Questions

1) How is the P_{50} of venous blood different from that of arterial blood?

2) How will the fetal oxygen dissociation curve differ from that of an adult?

3) How will arterial P_{O_2} be affected by living at a high altitude?

Key Concepts

Chapter 9

Oxygen dissociation curve

Carbon monoxide

Hemoglobin

Left shift

Abnormal Oxygen Dissociation Curve

Carbon monoxide (CO) binding to hemoglobin occurs in competition with oxygen (O_2) to hemoglobin binding; hemoglobin's affinity for CO is over 200 times its affinity for O_2. However, the binding of CO at one site increases the affinity for O_2 at the remaining sites. Draw the oxygen dissociation curve for CO poisoning, measuring hemoglobin oxygen content (in units of mL O_2/dL) on the vertical axis.

1) Visualize the normal oxygen dissociation curve.

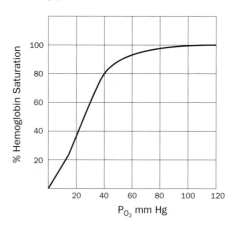

The oxygen dissociation curve shows the percent saturation of hemoglobin as a function of the partial pressure of O_2 (P_{O_2}). At P_{O_2} = 100 mm Hg, hemoglobin saturation is 100%, which means that four oxygen molecules are bound to the hemoglobin. At P_{O_2} = 40 mm Hg, hemoglobin is 80% saturated and at P_{O_2} = 25 mm Hg, hemoglobin is 50% saturated with oxygen molecules. The cooperative binding of O_2, meaning the binding of the first O_2 molecule, facilitates the binding of the next and results in a sigmoidal, or S-shaped, curve.

Takeaways

Be familiar with the concepts of P_{O_2} and P_{CO_2}, what factors change their values, and how they are represented graphically.

2) Examine the effect that CO binding has on O_2 binding.

The question stem states that CO competes with O_2 when binding hemoglobin. Because hemoglobin affinity is 200 times greater for CO than for O_2, hemoglobin will preferentially bind CO first on a hemoglobin molecule. This will decrease the amount of O_2 that can bind to hemoglobin and therefore decrease the amount of O_2 that is in the blood.

3) Determine the effect that CO binding will have on the oxygen dissociation curve.

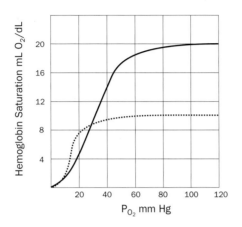

The question stem also states that the binding of CO increases hemoglobin affinity for O_2 at the remaining sites. Any physiological factor (i.e., decreased Pco_2, increased pH, or decreased temperature) that increases the affinity of hemoglobin for oxygen has the effect of shifting the curve to the left. Any physiological factor (i.e., increased Pco_2, decreased pH, or increased temperature) that decreases the affinity of hemoglobin for oxygen has the effect of shifting the curve to the right. The right shift is known as the Bohr effect. However, in this case the affinity of hemoglobin for oxygen is increased and there will be a left shift in the oxygen dissociation curve. It is this left shift that makes CO poisoning so deadly; with CO bound to hemoglobin, the O_2 molecules are bound so tightly that they cannot be off-loaded at the tissues and thus asphyxia occurs.

Remember: *The oxygen dissociation curve can be shifted to the left or to the right based on physiological conditions.*

Similar Questions

1) How will exercise affect the oxygen dissociation curve?

2) What type of physical reaction would high Pco_2 cause?

3) What would the oxygen dissociation curve look like in a patient with metabolic alkalosis?

Lymphatic System

Approximately 20 L/day of fluid filters across capillaries. Reabsorption across capillaries is approximately 16 L/day, and therefore the excess fluid must be returned to circulation by the lymphatic system. Lymphatic vessels are attached to the underlying connective tissue by fine filaments. What purpose do these filaments serve?

1) Examine the structure of lymph vessels.

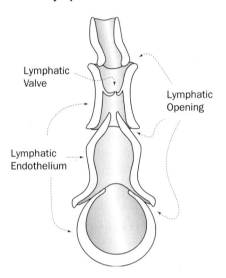

Lymphatic Valve

Lymphatic Opening

Lymphatic Endothelium

Lymphatic vessels have very thin walls that do not contain the smooth muscle that is found in arteries. Lymph vessels contain valves that ensure the unidirectional flow of lymph through the vessels. Filtrate from blood vessels, including cells and protein that have moved into the interstitial fluid compartment, is picked up by the lymphatic vessels. Lymphatic vessels called lacteals absorb fats from the gastrointestinal tract. The filtrate is moved through the system of lymphatic vessels, passing through lymph nodes where foreign particles are destroyed and removed. It rejoins blood circulation at the thoracic duct and superior vena cava.

2) Determine how interstitial fluid moves through lymph vessels.

Because lymphatic vessels do not have smooth muscle in their walls, they must rely on outside forces to move the lymph fluid through the vessels. The movement of skeletal muscles around the lymphatic vessels aids in moving lymph along, and their one-way valves prevent backflow of this fluid.

3) Determine how interstitial fluid enters lymphatic vessels.

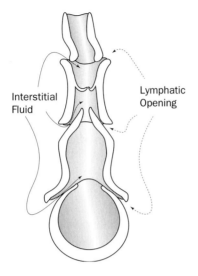

Interstitial Fluid

Lymphatic Opening

Capillaries have tight junctions between their endothelial cells. These tight junctions prevent unregulated passage of solutes in and out of the capillary lumen. Lymphatic vessels do not possess these tight junctions but rather have openings through which the interstitial fluid, complete with cells and proteins, can pass into the vessel. Because the lymph vessels are attached by fine filaments to their underlying connective tissue, skeletal muscle contraction will pull on these filaments and distort the lymphatic vessel. This distortion causes spaces to open between the endothelial cells of the vessel and allows the interstitial fluid to enter.

Remember: Lymphatic vessels differ from blood vessels in that they lack smooth muscle around the vessel and lack tight junctions between endothelial cells.

Key Concepts

Chapter 11

Plasma osmolarity

Filtrate osmolarity

ADH

Aldosterone

Water reabsorption

Kidney Function

A student discovers that drinking diet caffeinated soda results in a significant increase in urine volume and frequency. What are the physiological factors driving this phenomenon?

1) Identify the relevant kidney function affected: filtration, secretion, and/or reabsorption.

Excessive urine output means that there is a failure to reabsorb water from the nephron. Thus, the problem is at the reabsorption level.

Renal failure relating to filtration usually results in irregular plasma osmolarity (i.e., the urea concentration is too high or the albumin concentration is too low). Secretion plays a critical role in maintaining blood pH, K^+ concentration in blood, and nitrogenous waste concentration in the filtrate. Reabsorption also affects filtrate concentration as essential substances such as glucose, salts, and blood are returned to the blood.

2) Identify the role of plasma osmolarity and ADH.

Caffeine (as well as alcohol) inhibits ADH activity, thus decreasing water reabsorption activity from the collecting duct. Presuming the solution is isotonic to the blood, no change in plasma osmolarity is expected.

ADH works directly on the collecting duct by increasing its permeability to water; thus, a decrease in ADH levels will lead to a decrease in water reabsorption. ADH secretion is triggered by a sustained increase in plasma osmolarity. Note that if the solution is hypertonic to the blood plasma, osmolarity increases momentarily, but water from the interstitial fluid will move in to stem the increase (notice that the end result leads to an increase in arterial pressure).

Takeaways

Questions related to the nephron appear in varying contexts. The key is to isolate the relevant component of the kidney function being tested and then to tease apart which particular step(s) above (i.e., filtrate osmolarity) are being affected.

3) Identify the role of blood pressure, renin, and aldosterone.

Ingestion of a large volume of soda increases arterial pressure, leading to a decrease in renin and aldosterone and therefore a decrease in water reabsorption.

Recall that aldosterone increases sodium reabsorption, and because water follows sodium on its way out of the tubules of the nephron, it also increases water reabsorption. Keep in mind that aldosterone is regulated by renin, which is secreted when blood pressure is low.

4) Identify the role of filtrate osmolarity.

An abnormally high filtrate osmolarity will decrease the osmotic gradient between the tubule and the interstitial fluid, causing a drop in water reabsorption levels.

Diet sodas substitute sugar with Nutrasweet®, but unlike glucose the Nutrasweet® cannot be reabsorbed back into the blood from the nephron—hence the high filtrate osmolarity. Even if you did not know that Nutrasweet® cannot be reabsorbed from the nephron, it is imperative to recognize the role that filtrate osmolarity can play in water reabsorption. Recall that with diabetes mellitus a similar mechanism is at play: due to the high glucose concentration, not all of the sugar is reabsorbed from the nephron, leading to an abnormally high filtrate concentration, less water reabsorption, and ultimately the excretion of urine with glucose.

Similar Questions

1) A patient has been found to have insufficient levels of ADH. What symptoms would be prevalent?

2) Diabetics who fail to take insulin experience dehydration. What are the physiological factors driving this phenomenon?

3) A patient with renal failure has nephrons that lack the ability to actively secrete or reabsorb any substances. What type of actions can the kidney still perform?

Things to Watch Out For

The function of the kidney is to produce urine hypertonic to the blood, but in the situation described above the urine produced is likely to be hypotonic to the blood. Alcohol consumption produces similar physiological effects. However, frequent urination does not always mean that the urine is hypotonic to the blood. Patients who excrete protein in their urine (filtration failure) have low levels of blood osmolarity, and thus there is a low level of water reabsorption. Therefore, the urine produced will still be hypertonic to the blood.

Key Concepts

Chapter 11

Starling Forces

Capillary filtration

Plasma proteins

Glomerular capillaries

Takeaways

As blood flows through a capillary, fluid that is lost at the arterial end is reabsorbed at the venule end when normal blood proteins are present. Changes in Starling forces alter the conditions where capillaries are present. An increase in capillary hydrostatic pressure or an increase in interstitial oncotic pressure will lead to capillary filtration. An increase in capillary oncotic pressure or interstitial hydrostatic pressure will oppose capillary filtration.

Things to Watch Out For

Remember that proteins act as a solute, and water will flow to the areas of higher solute concentration.

Starling Forces

A patient with kidney disease has extensive damage to the glomerular capillaries. These capillaries have become permeable to plasma proteins. What other symptoms will this patient have as a result of this kidney damage?

1) Determine the effect of glomerular capillaries that are permeable to proteins.
Glomerular capillaries do not normally allow the passage of plasma proteins or red blood cells. If the capillaries are damaged so that plasma proteins enter the renal tubule, these proteins will be lost because they cannot be reabsorbed along the tubule.

2) Examine the forces at work on capillaries.
The relationship of the different forces at work in the capillaries is explained by Starling forces as follows. Capillary hydrostatic pressure (P_c) is blood pressure, and it is the major force in capillary filtration. Osmotic pressure is the major force that keeps fluid from leaving the capillaries and is considered the oncotic pressure (π_c) of the plasma proteins. The interstitial fluid also has hydrostatic pressure (P_i), which opposes filtration out of the capillary. The proteins of the interstitial fluid exert oncotic pressure (π_i) and tend to favor filtration out of the capillary. To recap in simpler terms, the blood pressure in the capillary tries to force fluid out the capillary, whereas the pressure of the fluid in the interstitial space tries to hold the fluid in the capillary. The proteins in the interstitial space try to "suck" fluid out of the capillary, whereas the proteins in the blood try to hold the fluid in the capillary.

When blood enters the arterial end of a capillary, the P_c pressure acts to force fluids to leave the capillary and enter the interstitial space. This loss of fluid along the capillary increases the concentration of the solute, or proteins, in the blood. This increase in oncotic pressure "pulls" fluid back into the capillary at the venous end. Any fluid that is not returned to the capillary is generally picked up by the lymphatic system.

3) Determine the effect when proteins are lost from the blood.

The loss of plasma proteins will cause a drop in oncotic pressure in the blood. As a result, water that leaves the arteriole end of the capillary will not be reabsorbed at the venule end. Fluid in large quantities cannot be picked up by the lymphatic system, so this fluid will remain in the interstitial space and back up in the extremities, a condition known as edema. The failure of fluid to be reabsorbed from the interstitial space also leads to a large drop in blood volume and therefore blood pressure.

Similar Questions

1) What factors increase the loss of fluid to the interstitial space at the arterial end of a capillary?

2) What physiological conditions can increase capillary oncotic pressure?

3) What symptoms will patients with inadequate lymphatic function have?

Key Concepts

Chapter 12

Menstrual cycle

FSH

LH

Estrogen

Progesterone

Positive/negative feedback

Takeaways

It is important to have a good understanding of the normal way that systems such as the menstrual cycle function. Using that knowledge, different variables, such as disease or dysfunction, can be applied to the system and the results of that dysfunction can be found in a methodical way.

Menstrual Cycle

During the follicular phase of the menstrual cycle, a dominant follicle is produced that secretes estrogen. If this follicle produces normal amounts of estrogen during the early days of its maturity but declines in estrogen production by day 10 of the menstrual cycle, what would be the result?

1) Visualize the menstrual cycle, focusing on the follicular phase.

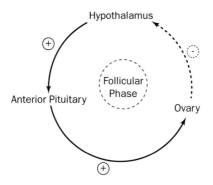

In the follicular phase, the hypothalamus secretes GnRH, which acts on the anterior pituitary to promote the release of FSH. FSH acts on the ovary and promotes the development of several ovarian follicles. The mature follicle begins secreting estrogen.

2) Determine the normal role of estrogen up until day 10.

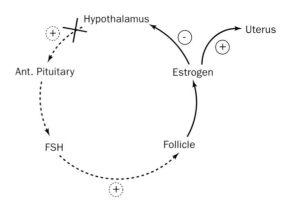

Estrogen has both positive and negative feedback effects in the menstrual cycle. Early in the follicular phase, the estrogen acts on the uterus, causing vascularization of the uterine wall. It also acts in a negative feedback loop to inhibit the release of FSH from the anterior pituitary in order to prevent the development of multiple eggs. Because the question stem states that early levels of estrogen are normal, vascularization of the uterus and inhibition of FSH will both occur normally.

Things to Watch Out For

Estrogen has both negative and positive feedback effects on FSH and LH at different times in the menstrual cycle. Remember that estrogen levels fall dramatically after the LH surge but rise again during the luteal phase. During this phase, however, both estrogen and progesterone are now produced by the corpus luteum, and both have a negative feedback effect.

3) Determine the normal role of estrogen after day 10.

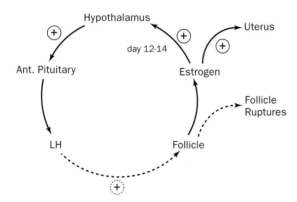

The question also states that estrogen levels decline after day 10. Now focus on the role of estrogen after day 10. Estrogen levels increase rapidly around day 12 of the cycle, and this burst of estrogen has a positive feedback effect on the secretion of FSH and LH. This results in the LH surge. The LH surge is responsible for ovulation, or the release of an egg.

Similar Questions

1) At what point in the follicular phase is FSH inhibited?

2) What are the actions of estrogen in the follicular phase of the menstrual cycle?

3) How can ovulation during the menstrual cycle be prevented?

4) Examine the consequence a decrease in estrogen after day 10.

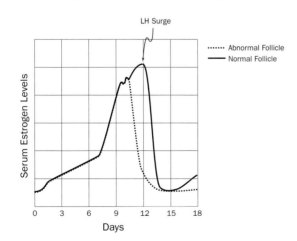

Therefore, if estrogen levels decrease after day 10 rather than increase as they normally should, then there will be no ovulation.

Key Concepts

Chapter 13

Action potentials

Depolarization

Refractory periods

Action Potential

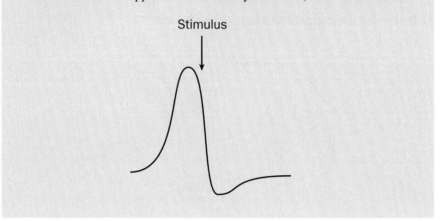

A nerve action potential is depicted below. If, during the action potential, a stimulus were to be applied as indicated by the arrow, what would result?

1) Visualize the graph of the action potential.

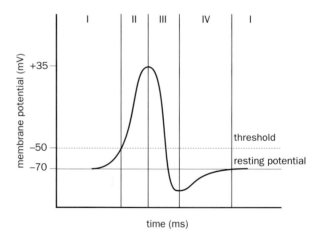

Takeaways

It is important to understand each stage of the action potential, including which gates are open or closed and which ions are flowing.

Region I—The cell is at rest and all gates are closed.

Region II—Depolarization: sodium gates are open and sodium flows into the cell, moving the membrane towards the sodium equilibrium potential.

Region III—Repolarization: sodium gates close and potassium gates open, moving the cell closer to the potassium equilibrium potential.

Region IV—Hyperpolarization: all gates are closed and the cell is ready to undergo another action potential, but the distance to the threshold is farther so it is harder to stimulate the cell. This is known as the relative refractory period.

2) Review the characteristics of the action potential.

Action potentials propagate by the spread of currents to adjacent membranes; they are considered "all or nothing" because once threshold is reached, an action potential will continue. During an action potential (regions II and III) no other action potential can be elicited, no matter how large the stimulus. This is known as the absolute refractory period.

3) Evaluate the region in which the new stimulus is being applied.

The new stimulus being applied to the action potential occurs during repolarization. This is also during the absolute refractory period, a time during which no new action potentials can be elicited. Therefore, the new stimulus will not produce a new action potential.

Remember: Action potentials are all or nothing. Once one begins it will continue, and a new action potential cannot be stimulated until after the absolute refractory period.

Similar Questions

1) At what point in the action potential is sodium closest to its electrochemical equilibrium?

2) What forces can increase the speed of an action potential?

3) How can an action potential be inhibited?

Classical Genetics—Probability & Penetrance

Dystonia is a syndrome of involuntary spasms and sustained contractions of the muscles. One form of the disease is childhood dystonia, in which dystonia begins in the leg or foot and eventually spreads to involve the entire body. If one parent has this type of dystonia, while the other parent has no alleles for the disease, a child of those parents has a 50% chance of having the genotype for the disease. Given that the gene's penetrance is 40%, if a man with the disease (his mother was homozygous recessive) and a woman with no alleles for the disease have two children, what is the probability that both children will be healthy?

1) Identify the inheritance pattern.

No generation is skipped, and gender does not matter; thus, dystonia is an autosomal, dominant trait.

Whether it is presented in a pedigree diagram or indirectly given in the question stem, the inheritance pattern should be identified quickly. In the question stem above, we are told that if just one parent has the disease, there is at least a 50% chance she will pass it on to a child; thus, the trait must be dominant. The probabilities cited in the question stem are independent of the gender of the parent or the child; thus, sex-linked inheritance is ruled out.

Takeaways

After identifying the pattern of inheritance for the gene and the genotypes of the parental generation, set up the Punnet square to aid in the calculations of the probability questions posed. Unless otherwise stated, it is safe to assume that the penetrance of a gene in a given question is 100%.

2) Identify the relevant genotypes to set up the Punnet square.

Because the man is afflicted with the disease, and we have determined that the disease is autosomal dominant, he must be homozygous (DD) for the trait or heterozygous (Dd). Because his mother was homozygous recessive (dd), he must be heterozygous for the disease, as he received one recessive allele from his mother. The woman has no alleles for the disease and thus must be homozygous recessive (dd).

	D	d
d	Dd	dd
d	Dd	dd

The relevant genotypes may vary depending on the question. In this question, the relevant genotypes are those of the parents because we are interested in the probability of conceiving a healthy child.

3) Use the Punnet square to calculate the probability for each event.

The probability that the couple will bear two healthy children is $(80\%)^2 = 64\%$.

There is a 50% chance that a child will be homozygous recessive (healthy) and a 50% chance that the child will inherit the genotype for the disease. However, because penetrance is only 40%, there is only a 20% ($50\% \times 40\%$) chance of the child actually expressing the disease. Therefore, there is an 80% chance that the child will be healthy.

Recall that penetrance is the dependence of an organism's phenotype on the genotype. One hundred percent penetrance signifies no environmental effects, whereas 0% penetrance signifies no genetic influence of a particular gene on a physical trait. Here, we have 40% penetrance, which means that only 40 percent of the heterozygotes will actually suffer from childhood dystonia.

Remember: To find the probabilities of both events occurring, multiply the probabilities of each event.

Things to Watch Out For

Beware of tricky probability questions. One typical trap was on your diagnostic: a disease is expressed in individuals who are homozygous recessive for the gene. Given parents who are both heterozygotes, what is the probability that a healthy child will be homozygous dominant? The Punnet square indicates 25%, but the trick is that we know the child is healthy; thus, there are only three possible outcomes—not four. Therefore, the probability is $\frac{1}{3}$ instead of $\frac{1}{4}$.

Similar Questions

1) The phenotype of an individual is known, but her genotype is not. Given a pedigree, could you determine the probability that she is homozygous dominant for this trait?

2) If normal parents have a colorblind son, what is the probability that he inherited the gene for colorblindness from his mother? What is the probability that he inherited the gene from his father?

3) A woman with blood genotype B marries a man with blood genotype A. What is the chance that their first child will have blood type B? What is the chance that their first and second children will have blood type B?

DNA Transcription

An RNA strand with the sequence 5′-GACTGAUCAGACTA-3′ was erroneously created when a mutant RNA polymerase substituted a thymine for the second cysteine when it encountered a GG in the reading frame of the DNA. What is the antisense strand of the DNA from which this RNA was transcribed? (Assume that "GA" is not in the antisense strand.)

Takeaways

When solving any transcription problems, follow these rules:

- G pairs with C and T pairs with A.
- In RNA, T is replaced with U.
- The sense strand of the DNA = the transcribed hnRNA with U replacing T.
- The antisense strand and the sense strand are complements of each other.

Things to Watch Out For

Note that the sequence described above is for problems that ask for DNA sequence from RNA sequence. In problems that ask for RNA sequence from DNA sequence, perform step 3 first, followed by step 2 and then step 1.

Be careful to maintain the correct polarity in every step of the problem. The newly synthesized strand is built in the 5′ to 3′ direction, and the reading frame is read in the 3′ to 5′ direction.

1) Determine the correct primary structure of RNA.
We can substitute CC for CT in the fragment in order to produce the correct sequence of RNA:

$\quad$ 5′-GACCGAUCAGACCA-3′.

In this case, when C precedes T, we know that it is due to the mutant polymerase. The first G in the DNA sequence GG will correctly have been transcribed as C, but the second G will have been incorrectly transcribed as T, yielding CT instead of CC.

2) Determine the sense strand.
We can simply replace the uracils with thymines to get the following sense strand:

$\quad$ 5′-GACCGATCAGACCA-3′.

Transcription always proceeds in the 5′ to 3′ direction starting at the 3′ end of the anti-sense strand. The RNA corresponds to the sense strand (minus any introns that were spliced out—in this problem we will assume there were no introns).

We are working backwards, going from RNA to DNA. The RNA produced represents the sense strand with the thymines replaced by uracil.

3) Determine the antisense strand.
$\quad$ 5′-GACCGATCAGACCA-3′ → sense strand
$\quad$ 3′-CTGGCTAGTCTGGT-5′ → anti-sense strand

The antisense strand of DNA is the complement of the sense strand of DNA. We can determine the sense strand by remembering that G pairs with C, that T pairs with A, and that the antisense strand is antiparallel to the sense strand (meaning that the 3′ end of the sense strand will line up with the 5′ end of the antisense strand and vice versa).

Similar Questions

1) What is the base sequence of the mRNA produced from the following sense strand of DNA: 3'-TAGGGTACGTACCTA-5'?

2) What are the possible primary structures of mRNA produced from the antisense strand 3'-GAATACCAGTAGTATTTGCCGATGACTAGTTAGCCGTTAGC-5' after splicing by a splisosome that makes blunt end cuts between GG in the sequence 5'-CGGC-3'?

Key Concepts

Chapter 14

Semiconservative replication

DNA

Takeaways

DNA replication is semiconservative. The newly synthesized strand of DNA will be identical to the old complementary strand, provided that there are no mutations.

DNA Replication

The following molecule of DNA is replicated using two cycles of PCR in the presence of N^{15} labeled guanine. What percentage of the DNA strands will contain the labeled guanine in both strands (sense and antisense strands)?

5'- CATACTGATCATCTAGCGTATGCGT-3'
3'- GTATGACTAGTAGATCGCATACGCA-5'

1) Determine what happens after the first round of replication.
DNA replication is semiconservative, which means that for every strand of original DNA, one new strand of DNA is synthesized as its new complement.

Our templates for this first round of replication are:

5' – CATACTGATCATCTAGCGTATGCGT – 3'
3' – GTATGACTAGTAGATCGCATACGCA – 5'

Neither of these original strands contains the labeled guanine. So the first round of replication gives us:

5' – CATACTGATCATCTAGCGTATGCGT – 3'
3' – GTATGACTAGTAGATCGCATACGCA – 5'∗

and

5' – CATACTGATCATCTAGCGTATGCGT – 3'∗
3' – GTATGACTAGTAGATCGCATACGCA – 5'

where the ∗ marks strands containing the labeled guanine.

The original strand with the 5' to 3' polarity at the site of replication will be the lagging strand because nucleotides can only be added in the 5' to 3' direction. Primase lays down a new primer to which DNA polymerase can bind in intervals of about 500 nucleotides, so that its new complementary strand can be created in short fragments called Okazaki fragments. The primer for these Okazaki fragments is RNA and is replaced with DNA before ligase joins the short fragments together. This process eliminates the need to create the replicate strand in the 3' to 5' direction.

2) Determine what happens after the second round of replication.
Our templates for the second round of replication are:

5' – CATACTGATCATCTAGCGTATGCGT – 3'
3' – GTATGACTAGTAGATCGCATACGCA – 5'∗

and

5′ – CATACTGATCATCTAGCGTATGCGT – 3′
3′ – GTATGACTAGTAGATCGCATACGCA – 5′*

So this second round of replication gives us:

5′ – CATACTGATCATCTAGCGTATGCGT – 3′
3′ – GTATGACTAGTAGATCGCATACGCA – 5′*

and

5′ – CATACTGATCATCTAGCGTATGCGT – 3′*
3′ – GTATGACTAGTAGATCGCATACGCA – 5′*

and

5′ – CATACTGATCATCTAGCGTATGCGT – 3′*
3′ – GTATGACTAGTAGATCGCATACGCA – 5′*

and

5′ – CATACTGATCATCTAGCGTATGCGT – 3′*
3′ – GTATGACTAGTAGATCGCATACGCA – 5′

with the asterisks again indicating strands containing labeled guanine.

In the second round of replication, the new strands from the first round of replication are used as templates to create newer strands.

---

3) Determine the percentage of DNA molecules that only have "new" strands.
50% of the double stranded DNA molecules will have both strands with the labeled N^{15} guanine.

After two rounds of replication, the middle two double-stranded DNA molecules have both strands labeled with the N^{15} guanine, whereas the outer two double strands of DNA still maintain one original strand.

Similar Questions

1) What is the product after 5′-ACGAGCTATGCTACTATATG-3′ goes through two rounds of replication?

2) A molecule of DNA is replicated using three cycles of PCR in the presence of N^{15} labeled nuclei acids. What percentage of the newly formed DNA will contain an unlabeled strand?

Key Concepts

Chapter 16

Hardy-Weinberg

$p^2 + 2pq + q^2 = 1$

Gene frequency

Takeaways

Remember the Hardy-Weinberg equation for geneotypes: $p^2 + 2pq + q^2 = 1$. Note that p^2 is the homozygous dominant genotype (GG), $2pq$ is the heterozygous genotype (Gg), and q^2 is the homozygous recessive genotype (Gg).

Be sure to understand what category each percent or frequency falls under. For phenotype frequencies, consider either dominant or recessive. For genotype frequencies, consider either homozygous dominant, heterozygous, or homozygous recessive. For allele frequencies, consider dominant or recessive.

Hardy-Weinberg

The gene for gigantism is known to be on a recessive allele. The dominant allele for the same gene codes for a normal phenotype. In North Carolina, 9 people out of a sample of 10,000 were found to have gigantism phenotypes, whereas the rest had normal phenotypes. Assuming Hardy-Weinberg equilibrium, calculate the frequency of the recessive and dominant alleles as well as the number of heterozygotes in the population.

1) **Solve for the frequency of the recessive allele.**
   gigantism = homozgygous recessive = gg = q^2
   q^2 = 9/10,000 = 0.0009
   q = 0.03
   Recessive allele frequency = 3%

Refer back to the Hardy-Weinberg equation:

$$p^2 + 2pq + q^2 = 1$$

Because gigantism will only emerge with a recessive genotype, it will be represented as gg. From the Hardy-Weinberg equation, the recessive genotype is depicted as q^2. By taking the square root of q^2 we get the frequency of the recessive gigantism allele or 0.03.

2) **Solve for the frequency of the dominant allele.**
   $p + q = 1$
   $p = 1 - q$
   $1 - 0.03 = 0.97$
   Dominant allele frequency = 97%

The frequency of the dominant allele plus the recessive allele equals 1. To solve for the frequency of the dominant allele, you subtract the recessive allele frequency from 1.

3) Solve for the heterozygous population.

$2pq$ = frequency of heterozygotes

Gg = 2 (0.97) × (0.03)

Gg = 0.058 or 6%

0.058 × 10,000 = 580 people

To find the heterozygous population, we need to use the heterozygous portion of the Hardy-Weinberg equation. Plugging in $2pq$ gives us the frequency of the heterozygous genotype.

Things to Watch Out For

There are five circumstances in which the Hardy-Weinberg law may fail to apply. These five are: mutation, gene migration, genetic drift, nonrandom mating, and natural selection.

Similar Questions

1) Suppose a similar survey was done in New York. However, this time they found 90 people with gigantism out of a survey of 200,000 people. Calculate the same parameters with the new survey.

2) An allele x occurs with a frequency of 0.8 in a wolf pack population. Give the frequencies of the genotypes XX, Xx, and xx.

3) If the homozygous recessive frequency of a certain allele is 16%, determine the percentage of phonetically normal individuals.

Art Credits for Biology

Figure 1.1—Image credited to Bryan Christie Design. From Working Knowledge: Lab Tests by Mark Fischetti. Copyright © 2002 by Scientific American, Inc. All rights reserved.

Figure 1.3a—Image credited to Eye of Science/Photo Researchers, Inc. From The Challenge of Antibiotic Resistance by Stuart B. Levy. Copyright © 1998 by Scientific American, Inc. All rights reserved.

Figure 1.3b—Image credited to E. Gray/Photo Researchers, Inc. From The Challenge of Antibiotic Resistance by Stuart B. Levy. Copyright © 1998 by Scientific American, Inc. All rights reserved.

Figure 1.4—Image credited to Jeff Johnson Hybrid Medical Animation/Photo Researchers, Inc. From The Once and Future Nanomachine by George M. Whitesides. Copyright © 2001 by Scientific American, Inc. All rights reserved.

Figure 1.7—Image created by Jeff Johnson Hybrid Medical Animation/Photo Researchers, Inc. From Sweet Medicines by Thomas Maeder. Copyright © 2002 by Scientific American, Inc. All rights reserved.

Figure 1.8. Image credited to Jeff Johnson Hybrid Medical Animation/Photo Researchers, Inc. From The Once and Future Nanomachine by George M. Whitesides. Copyright © 2001 by Scientific American, Inc. All rights reserved.

Figure 1.9—Image credited to Tomo Narashima. From Budding Vesicles in Living Cells by James E. Rothman and Lelio Orci. Copyright © 1996 by Scientific American, Inc. All rights reserved.

Figure 1.10—Image credited to Dana Burns Pizer and Tomo Narashima. From Caloric Restriction and Aging by Richard Weindruch. Copyright © 1996 by Scientific American, Inc. All rights reserved.

Figure 1.11—Image credited to Christoph Blumrich. From Uprooting the Tree of Life by W. Ford Doolittle. Copyright © 2000 by Scientific American, Inc. All rights reserved.

Figure 1.12 (Cell surface illustration)—Image credited to Ryota Matsuura, Robert Ezzell, and Donald E. Ingber. From The Architecture of Life by Donald E. Ingber. Copyright © 1998 by Scientific American, Inc. All rights reserved.

Figure 1.12 (MF, MT, IF illustrations)—Images credited to Laurie Grace. From The Architecture of Life by Donald E. Ingber. Copyright © 1998 by Scientific American, Inc. All rights reserved.

Figure 1.12 (MF and MT photographs)—Images credited to Donald E. Ingber. From The Architecture of Life by Donald E. Ingber. Copyright © 1998 by Scientific American, Inc. All rights reserved.

Figure 1.12 (IF photograph)—Image credited to Robert D. Goldman, Northwestern University Medical School. From The Architecture of Life by Donald E. Ingber. Copyright © 1998 by Scientific American, Inc. All rights reserved.

Figure 1.16—Image credited to Daniela Naomi Molnar. From Are Aliens Among Us? by Paul Davies. Copyright © 2007 by Scientific American, Inc. All rights reserved.

Figure 2.2—Image credited to Michael Goodman. From Drugs by Design by Charles E. Bugg, William M. Carson and John A. Montgomery. Copyright © 1993 by Scientific American, Inc. All rights reserved.

Figure 3.7—Image credited to Dana Burns Pizer and Tomo Narashima. From Caloric Restriction and Aging by Richard Weindruch. Copyright © 1996 by Scientific American, Inc. All rights reserved.

Figure 3.8—Image credited to Tomo Narashima. From The 1997 Nobel Prizes in Science, The Mechanism of Life by Staff Editor. Copyright © 1998 by Scientific American, Inc. All rights reserved.

Figure 4.1—Image credited to Dimitry Schidlovsky. From How Cancer Arises by Robert A. Weinberg. Copyright © 1996 by Scientific American, Inc. All rights reserved.

Figure 4.4. Image credited to Dimitry Schidlovsky. From The Centrosome by David M. Glover, Cayetano Gonzalez and Jordan W. Raff. Copyright © 1993 by Scientific American, Inc. All rights reserved.

Sidebar Page 80—Image credited to Lucy Reading—Ikkanda. From The Real Life of Pseudogenes by Mark Gerstein and Deyou Zheng. Copyright © 2006 by Scientific American, Inc. All rights reserved.

Figure 4.10—Image credited to Tomo Narashima. From Future Contraceptives by Nancy J. Alexander. Copyright © 1995 by Scientific American, Inc. All rights reserved.

Figure 4.12.—Image credited to Tomo Narashima. From Mother Nature's Menders by Mike May. Copyright © 2000 by Scientific American, Inc. All rights reserved.

Chapter 5 Cover—Image credited to Bradley R. Smith. From Visualizing Human Embryos by Bradley R. Smith. Copyright © 1999 by Scientific American, Inc. All rights reserved.

Figure 5.1—Image credited to Gamma Presse. From Blastomere Blowup by Charles Q. Choi. Copyright © 2006 by Scientific American, Inc. All rights reserved.

Figure 5.2—Image credited to Jason Burns/Phototake. From Embryonic Stem Cells for Medicine by Roger A. Pederson. Copyright © 1999 by Scientific American, Inc. All rights reserved.

Figure 5.5—Image credited to Andrew Swift. From The Stem Cell Challenge by Robert Lanza and Nadia Rosenthal. Copyright © 2004 by Scientific American, Inc. All rights reserved.

Chapter 6 Cover—Image credited to Aaron Goodman. From Regrowing Human Limbs by Ken Muneoka, Manjong Han, and David M. Gardiner. Copyright © 2008 by Scientific American, Inc. All rights reserved.

Figure 6.1—Image credited to John Gurche. From Food for Thought by William Leonard. Copyright © 2002 by Scientific American, Inc. All rights reserved.

Figure 7.3—Image credited to Biomedial Imaging Unit/Southhampton General Hospital/Photo Researchers, Inc. From Bugs and Drugs by Gunjan Sinha. Copyright © 2005 by Scientific American, Inc. All rights reserved.

Figure 7.4—Image credited to Jeff Johnson Hybrid Medical Animation/Photo Researchers, Inc. From Atherosclerosis: The New View by Peter Libby. Copyright © 2002 by Scientific American, Inc. All rights reserved.

Chapter 9 Cover—Image credited to Jeff Johnson Hybrid Medical Animation. From Atherosclerosis: The New View by Peter Libby. Copyright © 2002 by Scientific American, Inc. All rights reserved.

Figure 9.20—Image credited to Roberto Osti. From Surgical Treatments of Cardiac Arrhythmias by Alden H. Harken. Copyright © 1993 by Scientific American, Inc. All rights reserved.

Sidebar Page 192—Image credited to Roberto Osti. From Surgical Treatments of Cardiac Arrhythmias by Alden H. Harken. Copyright © 1993 by Scientific American, Inc. All rights reserved.

Figure 9.6 (illustration and chart). Image credited to Johnny Johnson; Source: Biology, by Neil Campbell. From The Search for Blood Substitutes by Mary L. Nucci and Abraham Abuchowski. Copyright © 1998 by Scientific American, Inc. All rights reserved.

Figure 9.6 (erythrocytes)—Images credited to Dr. Dennis Kunkel/Phototake. From The Search for Blood Substitutes by Mary L. Nucci and Abraham Abuchowski. Copyright © 1998 by Scientific American, Inc. All rights reserved.

Glossary

Abductor A muscle that moves a limb away from the center of a body.

Absorption The process by which substances are taken up into, or across, tissues (e.g., from the intestinal lumen into the blood).

Acetylcholine A neurotransmitter found throughout the nervous system (e.g., somatic motor neurons, preganglionic parasympathetic and sympathetic nerves, and postganglionic parasympathetic nerves). It is metabolized by acetylcholinesterase.

Acrosome The large vesicle at the head of a sperm cell containing enzymes that degrade the ovum cell membrane to allow fertilization.

Actin A protein found in the cytoskeleton and muscle cells; it is the principal constituent of the thin filament.

Action potential An abrupt change in the membrane potential of a nerve or muscle caused by changes in membrane ionic permeability. Results in conduction of an impulse in nerves or contraction in muscles.

Active immunity An immune response (antibody production or cellular immunity) acquired in response to exposure to an antigen.

Active site Substrate-binding region of an enzyme.

Active transport The use of energy to move a substance across a membrane against a concentration gradient.

Adaptation The development of characteristics that enable an organism to survive and reproduce in its habitat.

Adaptive radiation The evolutionary process by which one species gives rise to several species, each specialized for different environments.

Adductor A muscle that moves a limb toward the center of a body.

Adenine A purine base present in DNA and RNA; it forms hydrogen bonds with thymine and uracil.

Adenosine triphosphate A nucleotide molecule consisting of adenine, ribose, and three phosphate moieties. The outer two phosphates are bound by high-energy bonds. ATP plays a central role in energy exchange in biological systems. (Adenosine diphosphate [ADP] contains two phosphate groups and one high-energy bond.)

Adipose Referring to fatty tissue, fat-storing tissue, or fat within cells.

Adrenaline (Epinephrine) A hormone synthesized by the adrenal medulla; it stimulates the fight-or-flight response. It is also a neurotransmitter in the sympathetic nervous system.

Adrenocorticotropic hormone (ACTH) A hormone secreted by the anterior pituitary that stimulates hormone production in the adrenal cortex.

Aerobic A biological process that occurs in the presence of molecular oxygen (O_2); organisms that cannot live without molecular oxygen.

Afferent (sensory) neurons A neuron that picks up impulses from sensory receptors and transmits them toward the central nervous system.

Allantois One of four embryonic membranes, it contains the growing embryo's waste products.

Allele Alternative forms of the same gene coding for a particular trait. Alleles segregate during meiosis.

Alveolus Basic functional unit of the lung; a tiny sac specialized for passive gas exchange between the lungs and the blood.

Amino acids The building blocks of proteins, each containing an amino group, a carboxylic acid group, and a side chain (or R group) attached to the alpha carbon.

Amnion The innermost fluid-filled embryonic membrane; it forms a protective sac surrounding the embryos of birds, reptiles, and mammals.

Amylase An enzyme found in saliva and pancreatic juices that hydrolyzes starch to maltose. Also known as ptyalin, diastase, or amylopsin.

Anabolism The process by which complex molecules (macromolecules) are synthesized from simple ones.

Anaerobic A biological process that can occur without oxygen; organisms that can live without molecular oxygen.

Analogous structures Structures that are similar in function but of different evolutionary origins (e.g., whale flippers and fish fins).

Anaphase The stage of mitosis or meiosis characterized by the migration of chromatids or homologous chromosomes to opposite poles of the dividing cell.

Androgen Any male sex hormone (e.g., testosterone and dihydrotestosterone).

Anterior Front of an organism.

Antibiotic Substance that kills or inhibits the growth of bacteria or fungi (usually by disrupting cell wall assembly or by binding to ribosomes, thus inhibiting protein synthesis).

Antibody (Immunoglobulin) Immune or protective protein evoked by the presence of foreign substances (antigens) in the body. Each antibody binds to a specific antigen in an immune response.

Anticodon The three nucleotide sequence on tRNA that is complimentary to the mRNA codon.

Antidiuretic hormone (ADH, vasopressin) A hormone synthesized by the hypothalamus; it inhibits urine excretion by increasing water reabsorption in the kidneys.

Archenteron The central cavity in the gastrula stage of embryological development; it is lined by endoderm and ultimately gives rise to the adult digestive tract.

Asexual reproduction Any reproductive process that does not involve the fusion of gametes (i.e., budding).

Atrioventricular node (AV node) A small mass of nodal tissue that serves as an electrical bridge between the atria and the ventricles; located in the lower portion of the wall that separates the atria.

Autosome Any chromosome other than the sex chromosomes.

Axon The long fiber of a neuron; it conducts impulses away from the cell body toward the synapse.

Bacillus Rod-shaped bacterium.

Bacteriophage A virus that invades bacteria and sometimes uses bacterial RNA and ribosomes to self-replicate. (See *transduction*.)

Bile A solution of salts, pigments, and cholesterol produced by the liver and stored in the gall bladder; it emulsifies large fat droplets when secreted into the small intestine via the bile duct.

Binary fission A type of asexual reproduction characteristic of prokaryotes in which there is equal nuclear and cytoplasmic division.

Blastocoel The fluid-filled central cavity of the blastula.

Blastopore Opening of the archenteron to the external environment in the gastrula stage of embryonic development.

Blastula The early embryonic stage during which the embryo is a hollow fluid-filled sphere of undifferentiated cells.

Bowman's capsule The cuplike structure of the nephron; it collects the glomerular filtrate and channels it into the proximal convoluted tubule.

Budding A type of asexual reproduction in which the offspring starts out as an outgrowth of the parent that subsequently splits off to exist as an independent organism.

Bundle of His Part of the conducting system of the heart; it carries impulses from the AV node to the ventricles.

Calcitonin A polypeptide hormone secreted by the thyroid; it causes the deposition of calcium and phosphate in bones and thus lowers their concentrations in the blood.

cAMP (See *cyclic adenosine monophosphate.*)

Cartilage A firm, elastic, translucent connective tissue produced by cells called chondrocytes.

Catabolism The chemical breakdown of complex substances (macromolecules) to yield simpler substances and energy.

Catalyst A substance that speeds up a chemical reaction by lowering the activation energy without being altered or consumed during the reaction.

Cecum A cavity open at one end, such as the blind pouch (diverticulum) at the junction of the large and small intestines.

Central nervous system (CNS) The brain and spinal cord.

Centriole A small organelle in the cytoplasm of animal cells; it organizes the spindle apparatus during mitosis or meiosis.

Centromere The area of a chromosome at which sister chromatids are joined; it is also the point of attachment to the spindle fiber during mitosis and meiosis.

Cerebellum The section of the mammalian hindbrain that controls muscle coordination and equilibrium.

Cerebral cortex The outer layer of the forebrain, consisting of gray matter; it is the site of higher cognitive functions in humans. Neurons of the cerebral cortex initiate voluntary muscle action and constitute the final reception area for sensory impulses.

Chiasmata Site at which crossing over occurs between homologous chromosomes during meiosis.

Chondrocyte A differentiated cartilage cell that synthesizes cartilage matrix.

Chromatid Each of the two chromosomal strands formed by DNA replication in the S phase of the cell cycle, held together by the centromere.

Chromosome A filamentous body found within the nucleus of a cell, composed of DNA and proteins (histone and nonhistone) and containing the cell's genetic information.

Circadian rhythm A behavioral pattern based on a 24-hour cycle.

Citric acid cycle (See *Krebs cycle.*)

Cleavage A series of mitotic divisions of the zygote immediately following fertilization, resulting in progressively smaller cells with increased nucleus-to-cytoplasm ratios.

Cocci Spherically shaped bacteria.

Cochlea The coiled tube that comprises the auditory sensory organ of the inner ear.

Codominance (Incomplete dominance) A genetic effect in which the phenotype of a heterozygote is a reflection of both alleles at a particular locus.

Codon A three-base sequence on an mRNA strand; it codes for a specific tRNA anticodon, and thus for a specific amino acid.

Coenocytic Cells consisting of many nuclei housed within the same cytoplasm (i.e., skeletal muscle tissue).

Coenzyme An organic cofactor required for enzyme activity.

Cofactor Nonprotein molecules required by many enzymes for activity.

Colon The large intestine.

Conjugation The temporary joining of two organisms via a tube called a pilus, through which genetic material is exchanged. A form of sexual reproduction used by bacteria, fungi, algae, and protozoans.

Connective tissue Animal tissue composed of cells lying in an extracellular proteinaceous network, which supports, connects, and/or surrounds the organs and structures of the body.

Convergent evolution The process by which unrelated organisms living in a similar environment develop analogous structures.

Cornea The thin transparent layer that covers the front of the eye.

Corpus callosum A thick bundle of nerve fibers that connects the two cerebral hemispheres.

Corpus luteum The remnant of the ovarian follicle, which after ovulation continues to secrete progesterone; its degeneration leads to menstruation. Maintains uterine lining during pregnancy.

Cortex The external layer found in many organs of the body, including the brain, adrenal glands, and kidney.

Crossing over The exchange of genetic material between homologous chromosomes during meiosis.

Cyclic adenosine monophosphate (cAMP) An intracellular participant in one of the mechanisms of hormonal action. Synthesized from ATP by adenylate cyclase. It is also referred to as a "second messenger."

Cytochromes Iron-containing proteins that function in the electron transport chain in mitochondria, and in photophosphorylation in chloroplasts.

Cytokinesis The division and distribution of parent cell cytoplasm to the two daughter cells during mitotic and meiotic cell division.

Cytoplasm The fluid and solutes within a cell membrane, external to the nucleus and cellular organelles.

Cytosine A pyrimidine base found in nucleic acids; it hydrogen bonds with guanine.

Deletion A type of genetic mutation in which one of the bases in the DNA template is deleted during replication.

Dendrite The portion of a neuron that receives stimuli and conveys them toward the cell body.

Deoxyribose The five-carbon cyclic (pentose) sugar found in DNA.

Dermis The layer of skin cells under the epidermis. Contains sweat glands, hair follicles, fat, and blood vessels.

Diastole The period of relaxation of cardiac muscle during which the atrioventricular valves open and the ventricles fill with blood.

Diencephalon Posterior forebrain containing the thalamus and hypothalamus.

Differentiation The process by which unspecialized cells become specialized. Involves selective transcription of the genome.

Diffusion The flow of molecules from a region of high concentration to a region of low concentration as dictated by the laws of thermodynamics.

Digestion The breakdown of macromolecular nutrient material via mechanical and chemical means to simple molecular building blocks; this facilitates absorption.

Diploid (2N) Having two chromosomes of each type per cell.

Disaccharide A sugar composed of two monosaccharide units.

Divergent evolution A process of change whereby organisms with a common ancestor evolve dissimilar structures (e.g., dolphin flippers and human arms).

DNA (Deoxyribonucleic acid) Nucleic acid composed of monomers consisting of the five-carbon sugar deoxyribose, a phosphate group, and a nitrogenous base (adenine, cytosine, guanine, or thymine); contains the cell's genetic information.

Dominant Refers to an allele in a diploid cell whose phenotypic effect is the same in both homozygotes and heterozygotes.

Dorsal Situated towards the back of an organism.

Duodenum First segment of the small intestine; the contents of the stomach and the pancreatic and bile ducts empty into it. Site of digestion and some absorption.

Ectoderm Outermost embryonic germ layer; it gives rise to the skin and nervous system.

Effector An organ, muscle, or gland used by an organism to respond to a stimulus.

Efferent (motor) neuron A neuron that transmits nervous impulses from the spinal cord to an effector.

Electron transport chain The chain of cytochromes in mitochondria that transfers electrons from NADH to oxygen with the release of energy, which is then used to synthesize ATP via oxidative phosphorylation.

Embryo The early developmental stage of an organism. In humans it refers to the first two months after fertilization.

Endocrine Refers to ductless glands that produce or secrete hormones.

Endoderm Innermost embryonic germ layer; it later gives rise to the linings of the alimentary canal and of the digestive and respiratory organs.

Endoplasmic reticulum Membrane-bound channels in the cytoplasm that transport proteins and lipids to various parts of the cell.

Endotherms (Homeotherms) Organisms that maintain a constant internal temperature.

Enzyme A protein that catalyzes a biochemical reaction.

Epidermis The outermost layer of the skin.

Epididymis The coiled tube in which sperm gains motility and is stored after its production in the testes.

Epiglottis The small flap of cartilage covering the glottis during swallowing.

Epinephrine (See *adrenalin.*)

Epithelium The cellular layer that covers internal and external surfaces.

Erythrocyte Red blood cell; a biconcave disk-shaped cell that contains hemoglobin and has no nucleus.

Esophagus Portion of the alimentary canal connecting the pharynx and the stomach.

Estrogen Female sex hormone that stimulates the development of secondary sexual characteristics and is secreted by the ovarian follicle.

Estrous cycle The regular changes in the behavior and physiology of a female mammal throughout her fertile life.

Eukaryote A unicellular or multicellular organism composed of cells that contain a membrane-bound nucleus and other membrane-bound organelles.

Evolution The changes in the gene pool from one generation to the next caused by mutation, nonrandom mating, natural selection, and genetic drift.

Excretion The release of metabolic wastes by an organism.

Exocrine glands Glands that release their secretions into ducts (e.g., the liver, sweat glands).

Extensor A muscle used in the straightening of a limb.

F_1 generation The first generation of offspring from a cross-fertilization of individuals.

F_2 generation The offspring from the cross-fertilization of individuals from the F_1 generation.

Facultative anaerobes Prokaryotes that can exist with or without oxygen.

Fallopian tube (See *oviduct.*)

Feedback inhibition The process by which the concentration of a product or intermediate in a metabolic pathway inhibits the pathway that led to its formation.

Fermentation Catabolism of macromolecules in the absence of oxygen.

Fertilization Fusion of the nuclei of two gametes.

Fetus A developing organism that has passed the early developmental stages. In humans, the term refers to an embryo from the third month of pregnancy until birth.

Fibrin The insoluble protein that forms the bulk of a blood clot.

Fight-or-flight response An organism's reaction to danger, which includes increased heartbeat, pupil dilation, increased respiration, constriction of the peripheral blood vessels, and reduced digestive activity. It is stimulated by adrenalin release and by innervation of the sympathetic nervous system.

Filtration In the nephron, the process by which blood plasma is forced (under high pressure) out of the glomerulus into Bowman's capsule. Also, a process used to separate and purify aqueous solutions.

Fixation The process of preparing tissues for microscopic examination.

Flagellum A microscopic, whiplike filament that functions in locomotion of sperm cells and some unicellular organisms, and is composed of microtubules.

Flexor A muscle used in the bending of a limb.

Follicle The set of cells surrounding a developing or mature ovum. Secretes nutrients and estrogen, and atrophies into the corpus luteum after ovulation.

Follicle stimulating hormone (FSH) The anterior pituitary hormone that stimulates the maturation of ovarian follicles and spermatogenesis.

Fovea An area in the center of the retina containing the greatest concentration of cones, and therefore the area of sharpest vision.

Gamete Sperm or ovum; a cell that has half the number of chromosomes of a somatic cell (haploid) and can fuse with another gamete to form a zygote.

Ganglion A mass of neuron cell bodies; ganglia integrate and coordinate impulses.

Gastrin A hormone released by the pyloric mucosa of the stomach when food enters the stomach. Stimulates the secretion of gastric juices.

Gastrula The embryonic stage characterized by the presence of endoderm, ectoderm, the blastocoel, and the archenteron. The early gastrula is two-layered; later a third layer, the mesoderm, develops.

Gene The basic unit of heredity, it is a region on a chromosome that codes for a specific product.

Gene flow The movement of alleles into and out of a population's gene pool.

Gene pool All of the alleles for every gene in every individual in a given population.

Genetic code The system of nucleotide triplets (codons) in DNA and RNA that codes for individual amino acids.

Genetic drift Variations in the gene pool caused by chance.

Genome An organism's complete set of chromosomes.

Genotype The genetic composition of an entire organism, or reference to a particular trait.

Genus A taxon of closely related species.

Glomerulus The network of capillaries encapsulated by Bowman's capsule. Acts as a filter for blood entering the nephron.

Glottis The opening to the trachea.

Glucagon A hormone produced in the alpha cells of the pancreas that increases the concentration of blood glucose.

Glycogen The principal storage form of glucose in animals.

Glycolysis The anaerobic catabolism of glucose to pyruvic acid.

Golgi bodies Organelles that play a role in the packaging and secretion of proteins and other molecules produced intracellularly.

Gonad Ovary or testis; the reproductive organ in which gametes are produced.

Gray matter Any region in the central nervous system that consists largely of neuron cell bodies, dendrites, and synapses.

Guanine A purine base present in DNA and RNA; it forms hydrogen bonds with cytosine.

Haploid (N) Having only one of each type of chromosome per cell.

Hardy-Weinberg law States that gene ratios and allelic frequencies remain constant through the generations in a nonevolving population.

Haversian system The structural unit of compact bone. Consists of a hard, inorganic matrix surrounding a central canal.

Hemoglobin Iron-containing protein found in red blood cells that binds O_2 and transports it throughout the body.

Hepatic Of or pertaining to the liver.

Heterotrophic An organism that requires preformed organic nutrients because it cannot form them from inorganic precursors.

Heterozygous Having two different alleles for a particular trait.

Histone Structural protein found in eukaryotic chromosomes.

Homeostasis Maintenance of a stable internal physiological environment in an organism.

Homologous chromosomes Chromosomes in a diploid cell that carry corresponding genes for the same traits at corresponding loci.

Homologous structures Structures that are similar in function and are of the same evolutionary origin.

Homozygous Having two identical alleles for a given trait.

Hormones Chemical messengers secreted by cells of one part of the body and carried by the bloodstream to cells elsewhere in the body, where they regulate biochemical activity.

Hybrid The resultant offspring of a cross (mating) either between two different gene types or between two different species.

Hydrolysis The breaking apart of a molecule by the addition of water.

Hyperplasia An increase in the number of cells in a tissue or organ.

Hypertonic solution A solution that, when compared to another, has a greater concentration of solute particles and, consequently, a greater osmotic concentration.

Hypertrophy An increase in the size of individual cells within a given site or tissue.

Hyphae Branched filaments of a fungus.

Hypothalamus The region of the vertebrate forebrain that controls the autonomic nervous system, and is the control center for hunger, thirst, body temperature, and other visceral functions. Also secretes factors that stimulate or inhibit pituitary secretions.

Hypotonic solution A solution that, when compared to another, has a lower concentration of solute particles and, consequently, a lower osmotic concentration.

Ileum The terminal portion of the small intestine.

Immune reaction The process by which the body defends itself in response to an antigen; e.g., the production of antibodies.

Immunoglobulin (See *antibody*.)

Incomplete dominance (See *codominance*.)

In situ At the site of (origin).

In vitro In a test tube or in culture.

In vivo In a living organism.

Independent assortment Unlinked genes within a primary germ cell separate randomly during gametogenesis (see *Mendel's second law*).

Induction The initiation of cell differentiation in a developing embryo due to the influence of other cells.

Insulin A hormone produced by the beta cells in the pancreas that lowers blood glucose concentration.

Interneuron A neuron which has its cell body and nerve terminals confined to one specific area.

Interphase The stage between successive nuclear divisions; it is divided into the G_1, S, and G_2 stages. Cell growth and DNA replication occur during interphase.

Inversion A chromosomal mutation in which a section of a chromosome breaks off, flips over, and then reattaches in its original spot.

Invertebrate An animal that does not possess a backbone.

Iris The part of the eye that contracts or dilates to regulate the amount of light passing through the pupil.

Isolation Mechanism that prevents genetic exchange between individuals of different species or populations.

Isotonic A solution that, when compared to another, has the same concentration of solute particles and, consequently, the same osmotic concentration.

Jejunum The middle portion of the small intestine.

Kidney Vertebrate organ that regulates water and salt concentration in the blood and is responsible for urine formation.

Krebs cycle (citric acid cycle, TCA cycle) A metabolic pathway used in cellular respiration, in which acetyl CoA combines with oxaloacetic acid to form citric acid, which then undergoes a series of reactions to yield NADH, FADH, ATP, and CO_2. Occurs in aerobes.

Latent period The short interval between the application of a stimulus to a muscle and the contraction of the muscle.

Leukocyte White blood cell; the four principal types of leukocytes are granulocytes, macrophages, monocytes, and lymphocytes.

Ligament Connective tissue that joins two bones.

Linkage Tendency for certain alleles to be inherited together due to proximity on the same chromosome.

Lipases Enzymes that specifically cleave the bonds of lipids.

Lipids A group of molecules that are insoluble in water but are soluble in a variety of organic solvents: oils, waxes, fats, steroids, glycolipids, phospholipids.

Locus In genetics, an area or region of a chromosome.

Loop of Henle The U-shaped section of a mammalian nephron.

Lumen The opening within a tube or a sac.

Luteinizing hormone (LH) A hormone secreted by the anterior pituitary. In females, it transforms a follicle into a corpus luteum and triggers ovulation. In males, it stimulates testosterone secretion.

Lymph Clear tissue fluid derived from blood plasma and transported through lymph vessels to the lymphatic ducts, which empty into the circulatory system.

Lymphocyte A type of white blood cell involved in an organism's immune response.

Lysogenic cycle (lysogeny) Bacteriophage infection involving the integration of viral DNA into the bacterial genome without disrupting or destroying the host. The virus may subsequently reemerge and enter a lytic cycle.

Lysosome A membrane-bound organelle that stores hydrolytic enzymes.

Lytic cycle Bacteriophage infection involving the destruction (lysis) of the host bacterium.

Macrophage A phagocytic white blood cell.

Marsupial A mammal with a ventral pouch in which its young develop after birth.

Medulla The internal section of an organ (e.g., the adrenal glands and the kidney); the medulla oblongata of the mammalian hindbrain (see below).

Medulla oblongata The part of the brainstem closest to the spinal cord. It controls functions such as breathing and heartbeat.

Meiosis A process of cell division in which two successive nuclear divisions produce four haploid gametes from one diploid germ cell.

Mendel's first law Alleles segregate during meiosis.

Mendel's second law Alleles of unlinked genes independently assort during meiosis.

Meninges The three membranes that envelop the brain and spinal cord: the dura mater, arachnoid, and pia mater.

Menstruation The shedding of the uterine lining that occurs every four weeks in a nonpregnant, sexually mature human female.

Mesoderm The middle embryonic germ layer; it later gives rise to the muscular, skeletal, urogenital, and circulatory systems.

Messenger RNA (mRNA) This class of RNA is the product of the transcription process and acts as a template for the synthesis of polypeptides (translation).

Metabolism The sum of all biochemical reactions that occur in an organism.

Metamorphosis Transformation of an immature animal into an adult; change in the form of an organ or structure.

Metaphase The stage of mitosis or meiosis during which single chromosomes or tetrads line up on the central axis of the dividing cell and become attached to spindle fibers.

Metencephalon The anterior portion of the hindbrain of vertebrates; it includes the cerebellum and the pons.

Microtubule A small hollow tube composed of two types of protein subunits, serving numerous functions in the cell (e.g., microtubules comprise the internal structures of cilia and flagella).

Mitochondria Membrane-bound cellular organelles in which the reactions of aerobic respiration and ATP synthesis occur.

Mitosis Cellular division that results in the formation of two daughter cells that are genetically identical to each other and to the parent cell.

Monocyte A white blood cell that transforms into a macrophage in the presence of foreign invaders.

Monosaccharide A sugar consisting of one monomer; e.g., glucose, fructose, or galactose.

Morphogenesis The development of structure and form in an organism.

Morula The solid ball of cells that results from the early stages of cleavage in an embryo.

Motor neuron (See *efferent neuron.*)

Mucosa The type of epithelial tissue that lines moist body cavities; a mucous membrane.

Mutagen An agent, either chemical or physical, that can cause mutations.

Mutation An inheritable change in the genetic composition of an organism.

Mycelium A collection of filamentous hyphae which makes up a fungus.

Myelin The white, lipid-containing material surrounding the axons of many neurons in the central and peripheral nervous systems.

Myoglobin Heme-containing protein that binds molecular oxygen in muscle cells.

Myosin A protein found in muscle cells that functions in muscle contraction. Myosin fibers are also called thick filaments

NAD (Nicotinamide adenine dinucleotide) A coenzyme that functions in cell respiration.

NADH The reduced form of NAD.

NADP$^+$/NADPH (Nicotinamide adenine dinucleotide phosphate). An electron acceptor/donator system that functions, primarily, in biosynthetic processes.

Natural selection An ongoing evolutionary process resulting in changes in gene frequencies. It leads to the differential development of different phenotypes in a population.

Negative feedback (See *feedback inhibition.*)

Nephron The functional unit of the vertebrate kidney.

Nerve A bundle of nerve fibers.

Nerve impulse The self-propagating change in electric potential across the axon membrane.

Neural tube Embryonic hollow tube that subsequently gives rise to the central nervous system.

Neuron A cell that conducts electrical impulses; the functional unit of the nervous system.

Neurotransmitter A chemical agent released into the synaptic cleft by the synaptic bouton of a neuron. Binds to receptor sites on postsynaptic neurons or effector membranes to alter activity.

Niche The role of a given organism within the environment, including its interactions with other organisms and with the physical environment.

Nitrogen fixation Incorporation of atmospheric nitrogen into inorganic nitrogen compounds. Performed by bacteria.

Nodes of Ranvier Points on a myelinated axon that are not covered by myelin.

Nondisjunction Failure of homologous chromosomes to separate during meiosis.

Noradrenaline *See norepinephrine.*

Norepinephrine A hormone secreted by the adrenal medulla that stimulates the fight-or-flight response. It is also a neurotransmitter.

Notochord A supportive rod running just ventral to the neural tube in lower chordates and in vertebrate embryos.

Nuclear membrane Double membrane enveloping the nucleus, interrupted periodically by pores; found in eukaryotic cells only.

Nucleic acid Polymer of nucleotides; e.g., DNA and RNA.

Nucleoid The region in prokaryotic cells where the chromosome is located.

Nucleolus Dense body visible in a nondividing nucleus. Site of ribosomal RNA synthesis.

Nucleosome Packaging unit of DNA in eukaryotic cells, consisting of DNA and histone proteins complexed together.

Nucleotide An organic molecule composed of three subunits: a five-carbon sugar, a phosphate group, and a purine or a pyrimidine (nitrogenous base). The basic subunits of DNA and RNA.

Nucleus The eukaryotic membrane-bound organelle that contains the cell's chromosomes.

Oocyte An undifferentiated cell that undergoes meiosis to produce an egg cell (ovum).

Oogenesis Gametogenesis in the ovary, leading to the formation of mature ova.

Operator A site on DNA that interacts with a repressor protein, regulating transcription of an operon.

Operon A segment of DNA consisting of a promoter, operator, and structural genes. The structural genes code for products of a specific biochemical pathway; their transcription is regulated by a repressor protein.

Organ A body part composed of a group of tissues that form a functional and structural unit.

Organelle Any specialized cytoplasmic structure.

Osmosis The diffusion of water across a semipermeable membrane from a region of low solute concentration to a region of high solute concentration.

Ovary The female egg-producing gonad.

Oviduct (Fallopian tube) The tube leading from the outer extremity of the ovary to the uterus; generally, the site of fertilization.

Ovulation The release of the mature ovum from the ovarian follicle.

Ovum The female gamete; egg cell.

Oxidation The loss of electrons or hydrogen from an atom, ion, or molecule; the addition of oxygen to an atom, ion, or molecule.

Oxidative phosphorylation The synthesis of ATP using the energy released from the reactions of the electron transport chain.

Oxygen debt The amount of oxygen needed to reconvert lactic acid to pyruvate following strenuous exercise of muscle tissue.

Pancreas A gland that secretes digestive enzymes into the duodenum via a duct, and synthesizes and secretes the hormones insulin, glucagon, and somatostatin. It is located between the stomach and the duodenum.

Parasympathetic The subdivision of the autonomic nervous system involved in restor-nervous systeming homeostasis; it is antagonistic to the sympathetic nervous system.

Parathyroids Two pairs of glands located on the thyroid that secrete hormones that regulate calcium and phosphorous metabolism.

Parthenogenesis A form of asexual reproduction yielding progeny without fertilization of the ovum by spermatozoa.

Passive immunity Immunity conferred by the transfer or injection of previously formed antibodies.

Passive transport The movement of a substance across a membrane without the expenditure of energy.

Patella The bone of the kneecap.

Pathogen A disease-causing agent.

Pepsin A stomach enzyme that cleaves peptide bonds of proteins.

Peptide bond The bond between two amino acids that results from a condensation reaction between the carboxyl end of one amino acid and the amino end of the other.

Peripheral nervous system Includes all neurons outside the central nervous system including sensory and motor neurons; it is subdivided into somatic and autonomic nervous systems.

Peristalsis Rhythmic waves of muscular contraction that move a substance through a tube (e.g., food through the digestive tract).

Peritoneum Membrane lining of the abdomen and pelvis that also covers the visceral organs.

Permeable Allowing solutes to pass through; a term usually applied to biological membranes.

Phagocytosis A type of endocytosis in which large particles are engulfed by a cell.

Phenotype The physical manifestation of an organism's genotype.

Phylogeny The evolutionary history of related organisms.

Physiology The study of the life processes of plants or animals.

Pinocytosis A type of endocytosis in which small particles or liquid are engulfed by a cell.

Pituitary The bilobed endocrine gland that lies just below the hypothalamus; because many of its hormones regulate other endocrine glands, it is known as the master gland.

Placenta The structure formed by the wall of the uterus and the chorion of the embryo, containing a network of capillaries through which exchange between maternal and fetal circulation occurs.

Plasma The fluid component of blood containing dissolved solutes, minus the red blood cells.

Plasma cells Derived from B lymphocytes; have the ability to produce and secrete antibodies.

Platelets Small, enucleated disk-shaped blood cells that play an important role in blood clotting.

Polar body A small nonfunctional haploid cell created during oogenesis.

Polypeptide A polymer composed of many amino acids linked together by peptide bonds.

Polyploid A cell or an organism that has more than two alleles per trait.

Polyribosome A group of ribosomes attached to a strand of mRNA, simultaneously translating it.

Population A group of organisms of the same species living together in a given location.

Portal system A circuit of blood in which there are two capillary beds in tandem connected by an artery or vein.

Posterior Pertaining to the rear, or tail end.

Potential An electrical difference or gradient between two points or structures (e.g., across axon membranes).

Progesterone A hormone secreted by the corpus luteum and the placenta; it prepares the uterine wall for implantation and maintains the thickened wall during pregnancy.

Prokaryote Cell lacking a nuclear membrane and membrane-bound organelles, such as a bacterium.

Promoter A specific site on the DNA strand to which RNA polymerase attaches to initiate operon transcription.

Prophase The stage of mitosis or meiosis during which the DNA strands condense to form visible chromosomes; during prophase I of meiosis, homologous chromosomes align.

Prostate A gland in the mammalian male that secretes alkaline seminal fluid.

Prosthetic group A nonpolypeptide unit tightly bound to an enzyme that is essential for that enzyme's activity.

Proteins Complex organic polymers of amino acids linked together by peptide bonds.

Proximal Closer to some point of reference; that point usually being the midline of the body (e.g., the elbow is proximal to the hand).

Purines Double-ringed nitrogenous bases such as adenine and guanine.

Purkinje fibers The terminal fibers of the heart's conducting system; located in the walls of ventricles.

Pyloric sphincter The valve that regulates the flow of chyme from the stomach into the small intestine.

Pyrimidines Single-ringed nitrogenous bases such as cytosine, thymine, and uracil.

Recessive An allele that does not express its phenotype in the presence of a dominant allele.

Recombination New gene combinations achieved by sexual reproduction or crossing over in eukaryotes, and by transformation, transduction, or conjugation in prokaryotes.

Reduction The process whereby an atom, ion, or molecule gains electrons or hydrogens; the loss of oxygen from an atom, ion, or molecule.

Reflex An involuntary nervous pathway consisting of sensory neurons, interneurons, motor neurons, and effectors; it occurs in response to a specific stimulus.

Refractory period The period of time following an action potential, during which the neuron is incapable of depolarization.

Regeneration A type of asexual reproduction in which an organism replaces lost body parts.

Releasing hormones Proteins synthesized and secreted by the hypothalamus that stimulate the pituitary to synthesize and release its hormones.

Renal Of or pertaining to the kidneys.

Repressor In an operon, the protein that prevents attachment of RNA polymerase to the promoter by binding to the operator. It is coded for by the regulator.

Respiration (1) Cellular respiration: the series of oxygen-requiring biochemical reactions that lead to ATP synthesis.

(2) External respiration: the inhalation and exhalation of gases and their exchange at a respiratory surface.

Resting potential The electrical potential of a neuron at rest; approximately 70mV across the axon membrane.

Retina The innermost tissue layer of the eye; the sensory cells (rods and cones) are located there.

Retrovirus An RNA virus which contains the enzyme reverse transcriptase, which transcribes RNA into DNA.

Rh factor An antigen on a red blood cell whose presence or absence is indicated by a + or – respectively, in blood type notation.

Ribosome Organelle composed of RNA and protein; it translates mRNA during polypeptide synthesis.

RNA (Ribonucleic acid) Nucleic acid composed of monomers consisting of the five-carbon sugar ribose, a phosphate group, and a nitrogenous base (adenine, guanine, cytosine, or uracil); functions in protein synthesis.

Sarcolemma Muscle cell membrane capable of propagating action potentials.

Sarcomere The functional contractile unit of striated muscle.

Sarcoplasmic reticulum The endoplasmic reticulum of a muscle cell; it envelops myofibrils.

Selection pressure A force, resulting from natural selection parameters, that causes changes within the gene pool of a population.

Semen Fluid released during ejaculation consisting of sperm cells suspended in seminal fluid.

Seminal vesicle A gland found in mammalian males that produces seminal fluid.

Sensory neuron (See *afferent neuron.*)

Sex-linked gene A gene located only on a sex chromosome; such genes exhibit different inheritance patterns in males and females.

Sinoatrial node (SA node, pacemaker) A group of cells on the surface of the right atrium of the heart; it initiates and controls cardiac muscle contraction.

Somatic cells Autosomal cells; all cells in the body except germ cells and gametes.

Species A taxonomic classification applied to organisms of common ancestry who possess the ability to produce fertile offspring.

Sperm The mature male gamete, or sex cell.

Spermatogenesis Gametogenesis in the testes, leading to sperm formation.

Sphincter A ring-shaped muscle that closes and opens a tube; e.g., the pyloric sphincter.

Spindle A structure within dividing cells composed of microtubules; it is involved in the separation of chromosomes during mitosis and meiosis.

Spore An asexual reproductive cell that can endure extreme environmental conditions and develop into an adult organism when conditions become favorable.

Stem cells Nondifferentiated, rapidly dividing cells in the marrow of long bones that differentiate into red and white blood cells.

Steroids Four-ringed organic lipid molecules that make up many hormones and vitamins.

Stimulus Any change in an organism's internal or external environment that changes the organism's activity.

Sympathetic nervous system The subdivision of the autonomic nervous system that produces the "fight-or-flight" response.

Synapse The junction between two neurons into which neurotransmitters are released.

Synapsis The paring of homologous chromosomes during prophase I of meiosis.

Syngamy union of gametes.

Systole The period of heart contraction during which the ventricles contract and pump blood into the aorta and pulmonary arteries.

Taxonomy The classification of organisms according to their evolutionary relationships.

TCA cycle (See *Krebs cycle.*)

Telencephalon Anterior portion of the forebrain.

Telophase The final stage of mitosis or meiosis during which the chromosomes uncoil, nuclear membranes reform, and cytokinesis occurs.

Template A molecule that directs the synthesis of another molecule by acting as a model or pattern (e.g., mRNA is the template for protein synthesis).

Tendon A fibrous connective tissue that connects a bone to a muscle.

Testcross A cross between an organism showing a dominant trait and an organism showing a recessive trait, to determine whether the former organism is homozygous or heterozygous for that trait.

Testis The male sperm-producing organ; also secretes testosterone.

Tetanus Sustained muscle contraction that results from continuous stimulation.

Tetrad A pair of homologous chromosomes synapsing during prophase I of meoisis; each chromosome consists of two sister chromatids, thus each tetrad consists of four chromatids.

Thalamus The relay center between the brainstem and the cerebral cortex; located in the posterior part of the forebrain.

Thoracic duct The lymphatic vessel that empties lymph into the bloodstream.

Threshold The lowest magnitude of stimulus strength that will induce a response.

Thrombin An enzyme that participates in blood clotting, it converts fibrinogen into fibrin.

Thymine A pyrimidine present in DNA, but not in RNA; it forms hydrogen bonds with adenine.

Thymus A ductless gland in the upper chest region of vertebrates; it functions in the development of the immune system.

Thyroid A vertebrate endocrine gland located in the neck; it synthesizes thyroxine.

Thyroxine A hormone produced and released by the thyroid that regulates metabolic rate.

Tissue A mass of similar cells and support structures organized into a functional unit.

Tonus A continuous state of muscle contraction.

Trachea The tube that connects the pharynx to the bronchi; the windpipe.

Transcription The synthesis of RNA molecules from a DNA template.

Transduction The transposition of genetic material from one organism to another by a virus.

Transfer RNA (tRNA) RNA molecules that bind to specific amino acids and carry them to ribosome/mRNA complexes during protein synthesis.

Transformation Uptake and incorporation of "naked" DNA by a recipient bacterial cell.

Translation The process by which protein synthesis is directed by an mRNA nucleotide sequence.

Uracil A pyrimidine found in RNA but not DNA; it forms hydrogen bonds with adenine.

Urea A nitrogenous waste product produced in the liver from ammonia and CO_2.

Ureter The duct that carries urine from the kidneys to the bladder.

Urethra The tube that leads from the bladder to the exterior.

Urine Liquid waste resulting from the filtration, reabsorption, and secretion of filtrate in the nephron.

Uterus Organ in the mammalian female reproductive system that is the site of embryonic development.

Vaccine A solution of fractionated, dead, or attenuated live pathogenic material that is introduced into an individual for the purpose of stimulating a primary immune response or "boosting" a previously produced anamnestic state.

Vacuole A membrane-bound organelle in which water soluble nutrients and wastes are stored.

Vagus nerve The tenth cranial nerve; it innervates the pharynx, larynx, heart, lungs, and abdominal viscera. Responsible for maintaining homeostatic activity.

Vas deferens The tube carrying sperm from the testis to the urethra in mammalian males.

Vasopressin (See *antidiuretic hormone.*)

Vena cavae Two large veins, the superior vena cava and the inferior vena cava, that return deoxygenated blood from the periphery to the heart (right atrium).

Ventral Pertaining to the under surface or front surface of an organism.

Ventricles The chambers of the heart that pump blood into pulmonary and systemic circulation.

Vertebrate Member of phylum chordata possessing a backbone composed of vertebrae (member of subphylum vertebrata).

Vestigial Referring to an organ or limb that has no apparent function now but was functional at some time in the organism's evolutionary past.

Villus A small projection from the wall of the small intestine that increases the surface area for digestion and absorption.

Virus A tiny, organism-like particle composed of protein-encased nucleic acid; viruses are obligate parasites.

Vitamin An organic nutrient that an organism cannot produce itself and that is required by the organism in small amounts to aid in proper metabolic functioning; vitamins often function as cofactors for enzymes.

White matter The portion of the central nervous system consisting primarily of myelinated axons.

Wild type A genetics term for the phenotype characteristic of the majority of individuals in a particular species.

X chromosome The female sex chromosome.

Y chromosome The male sex chromosome.

Zygote The diploid (2N) cell that results from the fusion of two haploid (N) gametes.

Zymogen An inactive enzyme precursor that is converted into an active enzyme.

Index